DIVING SCIENCE

Michael B. Strauss, MD
Igor V. Aksenov, MD, PhD

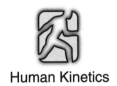

Human Kinetics

Library of Congress Cataloging-in-Publication Data

Strauss, Michael B.
  Diving science / Michael B. Strauss, Igor V. Aksenov.
    p. cm.
  Includes bibliographical references and index.
  ISBN 0-7360-4830-8 (soft cover)
  1. Submarine medicine. 2. Deep diving--Physiological aspects. 3. Underwater physiology. I. Aksenov, Igor V., 1970-II.
Title.
  RC1005.S77 2004
  616.9'8022--dc22

                      2004000181

ISBN-10: 0-7360-4830-8
ISBN-13: 978-0-7360-4830-9

Acquisitions Editor: Michael S. Bahrke, PhD; **Developmental Editor:** D.K. Bihler; **Assistant Editors:** Amanda S. Ewing and Lee Alexander; **Copyeditor:** Joyce Sexton; **Proofreader:** Erin Cler; **Permission Manager:** Dalene Reeder; **Graphic Designer:** Andrew Tietz; **Graphic Artist:** Kathleen Boudreau-Fuoss; **Photo Manager:** Kelly Huff; **Cover Designer:** Keith Blomberg; **Photographer (cover and interior):** Michael B. Strauss; **Art Manager:** Kelly Hendren; **Illustrator:** Sasha Strauss; **Printer:** United Graphics

Human Kinetics books are available at special discounts for bulk purchase. Special editions or book excerpts can also be created to specification. For details, contact the Special Sales Manager at Human Kinetics.

Printed in the United States of America   10 9 8 7 6 5 4 3 2

Human Kinetics
Web site: www.HumanKinetics.com

United States: Human Kinetics
P.O. Box 5076, Champaign, IL 61825-5076
800-747-4457
e-mail: humank@hkusa.com

Canada: Human Kinetics
475 Devonshire Road Unit 100
Windsor, ON N8Y 2L5
800-465-7301 (in Canada only)
e-mail: orders@hkcanada.com

Europe: Human Kinetics
107 Bradford Road, Stanningley
Leeds LS28 6AT, United Kingdom
+44 (0) 113 255 5665
e-mail: hk@hkeurope.com

Australia: Human Kinetics
57A Price Avenue, Lower Mitcham
South Australia 5062
08 8372 0999
e-mail: info@hkaustralia.com

New Zealand: Human Kinetics
Division of Sports Distributors NZ Ltd.
P.O. Box 300 226 Albany
North Shore City, Aukland
0064 9 448 1207
e-mail: blairc@hknewz.com

DIVING SCIENCE

CONTENTS

PREFACE

The underwater environment is a special place, full of mystery and excitement. It is responsible for climate, commerce, ecological habitats, dispersion of pollutants, food, recreation, travel, weather, and more. The biblical statement "Dust thou art, and unto dust shalt thou return" is almost a metaphor for the relationship of the water environment to all life on earth. Life on earth, as well as the embryological development of every individual life form (ontology), has its origin in a water environment. It is no coincidence that the mineral composition of seawater is remarkably similar to that of our blood. Eventually, perhaps over hundreds of thousands of years, everything returns to the sea through the mechanisms of erosion and geological changes. Consequently, the aquatic version of the biblical statement might read "From the sea thou ariseth, and to the sea thou shalt return." Of the 37 phyla of life forms so far identified, 34 (92 percent) can be found in the sea. In contrast, 17 phyla (47 percent) can be found on land. About one-third (39 percent) of the phyla are found on both land and water.

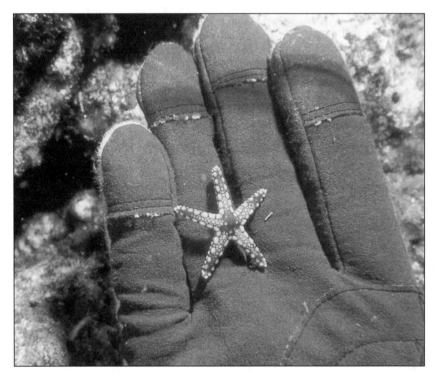

The underwater environment attracts a variety of audiences, from the marine biologist to the seashell collector.

The diver's entrée to the underwater environment is wide-ranging. Through adaptations, acclimatizations, technology, and understanding, the diver can participate in the underwater environment at almost any level of activity. This text is divided into three parts. Each focuses on a different aspect of the underwater environment, but each complements the others. Part I concerns the underwater environment—its challenges, the types of diving with respect to breathing equipment, and the ways in which the diver copes with the inert gas load. Part II explores specific challenges of the underwater environment (e.g., cardiovascular, respiratory, and thermal), the adaptations diving mammals have for meeting these challenges, the counterparts of these adaptations in human divers, and the specific equipment used to meet each challenge. Part III is a synopsis of the medical problems of diving. The synopsis is uniquely organized such that the problems are presented in the order in which they would most likely occur during a dive. This organization makes it easy to focus in on a medical problem of diving without using the table of contents.

Coauthorship can produce a continuity in style and organization that is difficult to achieve with edited texts. The figures and tables in this book contain information that we have used as study aids in over three decades of teaching diving medicine and physiology to a variety of audiences. For many of the subjects we have generated papers and formulated new ideas. We apply physics (gas laws), physiology (how the body works), and anatomy (the structure of the body) to divers and their interaction with the underwater environment. The "Chapter Preview" section in each chapter alerts the reader to the objectives of that chapter. Another feature of out text is the consistent use of case reports and comments for the "Bringing It All Together" sections in the chapters of part III. Text citations have been kept to a minimum and by and large are used only to give credit to scientists who have done the classical research on mammalian adaptations to diving. For readers who seek further information, specially selected recommended readings are listed by chapter at the end of the book.

Our aim is to explain how the diver interacts with the underwater environment in positive as well as undesirable ways, especially for those who wish to know the first-response interventions for medical problems of diving, study the physiological responses to the aquatic environment, teach diving, prepare for missions requiring diving, or simply have the satisfaction of knowing as much about this subject as possible.

ACKNOWLEDGMENTS

In one sense our dive text began 57 years ago with my father, Max B. Strauss. For lack of a better title, he was "Mr. Aquatics" for a small town in western Oregon. Although he was a purported furniture dealer, his true passion was to teach others to love the water. He used any excuse to lock up the furniture store, put a "Gone Swimming" sign on the door, and transport the town kids in his furniture truck to the nearest swimming pool. This evolved to coordinating the county's Red Cross swimming programs and becoming the father of competitive swimming in the county. The "Gone Swimming" sign got a lot of use. From my father I not only gained a great fondness for water-related activities but also learned about managing panic in the water. Many of his admonitions and techniques for the management of panic in the water are as valid today as when he first taught them to me in 1946. This information was the starting point for my papers on diver panic and for the inclusion of this subject in chapter 11.

My second acknowledgment is to the U.S. Navy. Over a 33-year period I received training in and dove with almost every type of equipment discussed in the text. I am especially proud of my 25-year medical association with the Navy Frogmen and SEALS. They reaffirmed my belief that divers can be swimmers as well and were a significant motivating factor for part II of this text concerning the physiological responses to the underwater environment. A third acknowledgment is to retired naval Captain George B. Hart, MD, director emeritus of the department of hyperbaric medicine, Long Beach Memorial Medical Center, Long Beach, California. In 1977, at his invitation and after completion of undersea medicine, orthopedic training, and operational billets in these specialties in the navy, I began working under his auspices as associate director of his department with the mission to define the orthopedic uses of hyperbaric oxygen. Dr. Hart not only helped me to meet this goal, but he encouraged me to maintain my interests in diving. I have collaborated with him in the management of medical problems of diving, and with his support traveled around the world to conduct medical diving seminars and continue my affiliation with the Navy Reserve SEAL teams.

Another person who requires acknowledgment is my Junction City, Oregon, high school classmate, Gary Mortensen. He was the person who rescued me from the episode of breath-holding blackout presented as a case study in chapter 11. Recently, we reminisced at our high school class reunion. Had it not been for Gary's prompt action, the past 45 years could have been very different for me. This experience stimulated my interest in the subject of blackout, resulting in what is now the most complete listing of the no-panic blackout conditions to be found in a diving text.

Finally, I want to acknowledge those who have helped me with the actual production of this text: first, Mike Bahrke, PhD, of Human Kinetics for his invitation (based on his review of one of my dive papers) to submit a proposal to write a dive text. This invitation led to the opportunity to work with many of the Human Kinetics staff, and I sincerely appreciate their constructive criticisms, professionalism, and contributions to the mutual goals of this dive text. Second, for content review, many colleagues helped me, including Marvin Appel, MD; Thomas Asciuto, MD; Andrew Choy, MD; Eknath Deo, MD; Debbie Meeks, Certified PADI instructor; Jon Pegg, MD; Ralph Rozenek, PhD; Ronald Samson, MD; and Donald Winant, MS. Excellent editorial help was received from Zarah Maginot, Julia Ayzenberg, my older son Ari (an electrical engineer), and my younger son Sasha (a brand strategist). The latter I thank especially for his preparation of the illustrations. Finally, my wife, Wendy Groner Strauss, PharmD, deserves special thanks as she was always there to help answer a word or grammar question and to encourage my work on this yearlong project. She substantially contributed to my decision to invite Dr. Aksenov to be the coauthor. With his computer skills, Dr. Askenov made communications between us a "snap." His substantial contributions to part III, the appendixes, and the reference portions of this book made it possible to meet our submission deadlines.

Michael B. Strauss, MD

The writing of this book has been an honor and pleasure for me. Many people have supported me in this endeavor. First of all, I acknowledge my parents, Viktor G. Aksenov and Natalia L. Koustova, who encouraged me to become a physician and attend the St. Petersburg Military Medical Academy. I feel privileged to have received my medical training at one of the oldest and most prestigious medical institutions in Russia. It was there that I was trained as a navy physician and was introduced to diving physiology and medicine. Later, in my capacity as an intensive care physician, I was able to complete postdoctoral studies in diving and hyperbaric medicine at the Academy. More recently, I directed the hyperbaric medicine program at the Saba University School of Medicine and held the position of medical director of the Saba National Marine Park Hyperbaric Facility on the island territory of Saba in the Netherlands Antilles. In this capacity I had extensive experiences in treating medical problems of diving with the able assistance of David Kooistra, park manager, and Janine le Sueur, Hyperbaric Medicine Program Administrator.

For their careful review of selected chapters and their constructive suggestions I give special thanks to Saba University School of Medicine faculty members Angel Kurtev, MD, PhD; Nick Macri, PhD; and Jim Stewart, PhD. Another thanks goes to Ella France, MD, my sister and fellow faculty member at Saba University Medical School. She spent innumerable hours with me discussing issues, shaping ideas, and providing encouragement for this project. Likewise, my wife, Natalya I. Stoyanova, deserves a special acknowledgment for her constant emotional support, patience, understanding, and ability to create a working environment for me while caring for our two sons. Finally, I extend my gratitude to Dr. Michael Strauss, who invited me to coauthor this book. It was a pleasure to work with someone so full of ideas and energy.

Igor Aksenov, MD, PhD

PART I

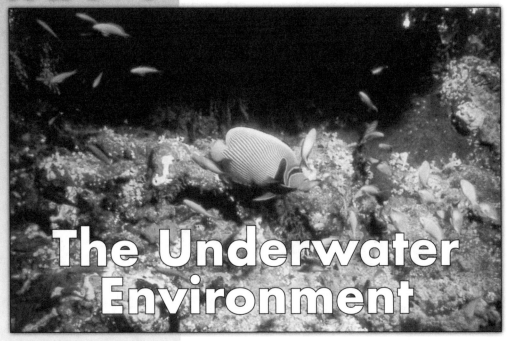

The Underwater Environment

This part of the book focuses on the underwater environment from the perspective of challenges to the diver. One of the fascinations of the underwater environment is that it is so different from our usual terrestrial environment. A diver can literally soar through the underwater environment as a bird flies through a forest. But this freedom from the effects of gravity does not come without costs. The costs are due to the physical properties of water. Water is several hundredfold denser than air and contains about 1/40 the amount of oxygen that air at sea level does. It imposes special considerations relating to the effects of on-gassing of nitrogen or other inert gases to the tissues of the diver's body as the diver descends using a compressed gas supply.

The three chapters in part I address each of these challenges. Chapter 1 covers the physical, physiological, and psychological stresses imposed on the diver underwater. This chapter provides the background for understanding human divers' and diving mammals' adaptations and acclimatizations to the underwater environment as presented in part II. It also provides the basis for understanding what happens when the body's positive feedback responses—used to meet the challenges of the underwater environment—are exceeded, become negative feedback mechanisms, and cause harm to the diver as discussed in part III. Chapter 2 describes the types of diving, dive profiles, and phases of the dive. Chapter 3 deals with the inert gas load. Although this is a complex subject, our aim was to present the material in a manner that would be understandable to our target audiences. This chapter includes a thorough discussion of the advantages and disadvantages of dive tables and the diving computer. Our method of presentation and the thoroughness with which we discuss the subjects in part I are unique to our dive text.

CHALLENGES OF THE UNDERWATER ENVIRONMENT

Chapter Preview

- Principal stresses that the underwater environment imposes on the human diver
- Gas laws and how they help to explain the physical stresses of the underwater environment
- Pressure and how it affects the three pressure-related body compartments
- Physiological stresses of the underwater environment and how they affect the human diver
- Psychological (orientation) stresses of the underwater environment

Both **commercial** (diving for pay) and **sport diving** (diving for enjoyment without consideration for remuneration) expose divers to stresses that are unique to the underwater environment. That is, terrestrial counterparts of the stresses do not exist, or they are ordinarily so minimal that they go unnoticed while a person is on land. **Stress** is a challenge, stimulus, or other signal that initiates a response in an organism. Three main categories of stresses are encountered in the underwater environment: physical, physiological, and psychological (see figure 1.1). In almost all circumstances the diver resolves the stresses of the underwater environment through positive feedback mechanisms.

Stresses themselves are not all undesirable. Most are physiological; that is, they induce responses in the organism that maintain life, protect from injury, or cause the organism to change. These responses are examples of positive feedback. For example, the fundamental physiological stress that initiates breathing is the imperceptible rise in carbon dioxide in the blood that occurs before each breath. Part II of this book deals largely with the physiological stresses of the underwater environment and how they are resolved. When stresses cause harm to the organism, they are labeled pathological. Part III describes the pathological stresses the diver may encounter in the underwater environment, such as the ear squeeze. Underwater, the transition between a physiological stress and a pathological stress is often minimal. Pathological stresses cause negative feedback—responses that are unphysiological and lead to injury.

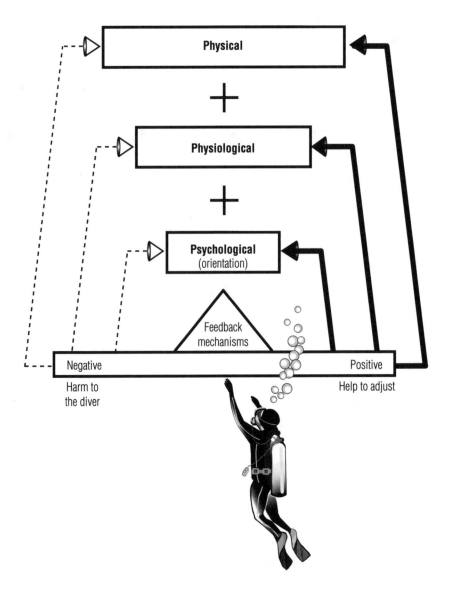

FIGURE
1.1   Stresses in the underwater environment.

Physical Stresses

Physical stresses arise from the physical properties of water. These include the effect of the density of water. Since water is 775 times more dense than air, a few feet of descent in water is equivalent to many hundreds of feet of descent in the atmosphere. Other physical stresses related to the density of water include those from currents and movement through the water. The thermal properties of water are another source of significant physical stress for the diver.

Pressure

The main physical stress of the underwater environment is the effect of hydrostatic (the weight of the water column) pressure. From a mathematical perspective, **pressure** is defined as force per unit area. Two observations cause confusion regarding the concept of pressure. First, multiple units are used to define pressure. Most people are familiar with the designation of pounds per square inch (PSI), used for measuring the amount of air pressure in tires, or millimeters of mercury (mmHg), used for measuring blood pressure. Pressure units like kilopascals and BAR may seem foreign. At least nine different units are used for measuring pressure as enumerated in table 1.1.

Each pressure unit has its own special usage. At least half of the units relate to the underwater environment in one way or another. Fortunately, knowing the equivalent for each unit, based on one-for-one atmosphere of pressure, makes it easy to calculate what a pressure would be in a different unit using simple algebraic principles. Depth is measured in feet of seawater (FSW) (or meters of seawater, MSW). For convenience, unit area is not included among these terms.

For SCUBA (Self-Contained Underwater Breathing Apparatus) diving tanks, PSI is used to designate how full the tanks are, while in mixed-gas diving the tank pressures are measured in BAR. If the diver should be so unfortunate as to develop **decompression sickness** (i.e., a wide spectrum of conditions, from skin itches, to joint pains, to breathing problems, to paralysis, following reductions in ambient pressure), he or she may require treatment in a **recompression chamber** (a vessel that can safely withstand pressurization; it is used to treat diving problems and other medical conditions) where atmospheres absolute (ATA) or feet (meters) of seawater will be used as the pressure unit. Although the use of so many different units to designate pressure may be confusing initially, each particular unit is selected for and determined by convenience and convention, and one unit can be easily converted to another.

> ### *Diving Physics: Pressure Conversion*
>
> *Q:* What would the maximum theoretical height (in feet of seawater) be for blood backing up in a line connected to an artery for someone with a systolic blood pressure of 120mmHg? (Hint: Convert mmHg pressure to feet of seawater.)
>
> *A: 5.2 feet (1.6 meters)*

The second source of confusion associated with pressure is the ubiquitous nature of pressure itself. The surface of the earth is surrounded by the earth's **atmosphere,** the gaseous mass or envelope surrounding the earth and retained by the earth's gravitational field. In essence, at sea level, we live at the bottom of an "ocean of air." This is equivalent to one atmosphere of pressure. As we

TABLE 1.1	Units Used to Designate Pressure*			
Unit (abbreviation)	Equivalent to 1 atmosphere absolute pressure	Usage	Comments	
Atmospheres (ATA) absolute	1.0; the basis for computing equivalents	Hyperbaric oxygen treatments	The weight of the earth's atmosphere at sea level	
Barometer units (BAR)	1.0133	Diving; scientific	The metric equivalent to 1 ATA; used for pressure gauges of rebreather units and for ultrahigh pressure scientific studies	
Centimeters of water (cm H_2O)	1,005.9	Medical	Venous pressure and other fluid-column measurements	
Feet of seawater (FSW)	33.07	Diving	Depth gauge readings	
Inches of mercury (mmHg)	29.82	Weather	Atmospheric pressure	
Kilopascals (kPa)	101.327	Scientific; hyperbaric oxygen treatments	A metric equivalent for BAR; preferred term for reporting studies done at other than 1 ATA (BAR) pressures	
Meters of seawater (MSW)	10.08	Diving	Metric equivalent of FSW	
Millimeters of mercury (mmHg)	760	Medical	Blood pressure	
		Weather	Atmospheric pressure	
Pounds per square inch (PSI)	14.696	Engineering, diving	Pressure, that is, force per unit area	

* For scientific work, absolute pressures, which take into account the pressure of the earth's atmosphere, are used. For convenience (e.g., blood pressure measurements, depth gauges), gauge pressures are set to read zero at the surface. Hence, they automatically subtract the weight of the earth's atmosphere.

rise in altitude, the atmospheric pressure decreases correspondingly. Since the air pressure surrounding us is essentially uniform, that is, equal and undiminished over all parts of our bodies, we normally are unaware of it. This concept corresponds to a corollary of **Pascal's principle.** When fluid such as water or gas surrounds or fills an object, pressure is distributed equally and undiminished to all portions of the object.

Absolute pressure is the total pressure in a system. It takes into account the weight of the earth's atmosphere. Consequently, the absolute pressure at sea level is 1 ATA (atmosphere absolute). Absolute pressure is used for all scientific computations with pressure. **Gauge pressure** refers to the pressure read on the dial of a pressure gauge. Ordinarily, gauge pressure is one atmosphere less than absolute pressure. The depth readings on a diver's depth gauge or **dive computer** (a computer for diving that pairs depths with durations at each depth and then computes safe dive times, ascent rates, and need for decompression stops; the computer may also give information about when it is safe to fly after diving) are gauge pressures. For example, when a diver descends to 33 FSW (10 MSW), the depth gauge will read 33. The 33-FSW depth is actually 2 ATA, that is, one atmosphere of pressure from the earth's atmosphere plus one atmosphere of pressure from the water's pressure (see table 1.2).

The third term associated with pressure is **ambient.** This refers to the pressure around the diver's body and is illustrated in figure 1.2. Thanks to the workings of the regulator, the diver breathes gas at the ambient pressure while underwater. On the earth's surface, at sea level, the ambient pressure is 1 ATA. This is the pressure that surrounds our bodies as well as the pressure of the air we are breathing. If we go up in altitude, the ambient pressure decreases; conversely, as we descend into water, it increases. A difference or differential between the ambient pressure and the pressure within an object, be it in space, in our atmosphere, or underwater, is termed **pressure gradient.** A submarine hull is built to withstand an enormous gradient of pressure between the outside water pressure and its internal atmosphere, which is maintained at about sea level pressure (1 ATA) when it is submerged. Pressure gradients for the human body outside of physiological ranges are harmful and are the source of many pressure-related problems that will be discussed later.

The pressure effects of the underwater environment are due to the density of water. **Density** is the mass of an object as compared to an equal volume of distilled water. Water is approximately 775 times as dense as air. Because of its salt content, seawater is slightly denser than fresh water. This density characteristic of water benefits divers by providing **buoyancy,** the capacity to float in a liquid. If divers are neutrally buoyant, they may hover at any depth, very much like a blimp suspended in air. With few exceptions, submerged divers, as far as water pressure is concerned, will not feel any different when submerged to a shallow depth than when they are submerged to a deep depth. This is because the majority of the human body is like a "bag of water," which can be referred to as the liquid–solid compartment of the body. This compartment transmits pressure, as described by Pascal's principle, equally,

TABLE 1.2 Pressure Changes With Elevations in Altitude Versus Descent Into Water		
Altitudes and depths in feet (meters)	**Pressure (atmospheres)**	**Comments**
68,000 (20,726)	0.055	At this altitude, the pressure is so low that blood "boils" at body temperature.
29,035 (8,850)	0.25	Altitude of Mount Everest (the highest mountain on earth)
18,000 (5,486.4)	0.5	At this altitude, oxygen percentage is 21%, enough to support combustion, but the number of oxygen molecules is reduced by 50% for each lungful of air. Hence, the mountain climber will likely experience shortness of breath.
5,000 (1,524)	0.8	Altitude of Denver, Colorado (the "mile-high city")
6.6 (2)	1.2	Same pressure change differences as ascending in altitude to 5,000 ft
16.5 (5)	1.5	Pressure change equivalent to ascending to an 18,000-ft altitude
33 (10)	2.0	Recommended limit for breathing pure oxygen (2 ATA, 30 min) while underwater
66 (20)	3.0	Maximum depth for pure oxygen breathing in hyperbaric chamber
99 (30)	4.0	SCUBA tank air supply duration about 1/4 what it would be on the surface
130 (40)	5.2	Recommended maximal depth for sport diving
165 (50)	6.0	Maximum depth used in Navy Treatment Table 6A for treating arterial gas embolism
330 (101)	11.0	10% oxygen is sufficient to meet the diver's oxygen needs, but nitrogen partial pressure will likely cause narcosis (sleepiness and confusion)
1,000 (305)	30.5	Breathing mixture with only 0.55% oxygen is sufficient to meet the body's oxygen requirements.

uniformly, and undiminished throughout its contents. There are two other compartments: the air-filled cavities with flexible walls and the air-filled cavities with rigid walls. The three-compartment concept and the effects on pressure for each are summarized in table 1.3.

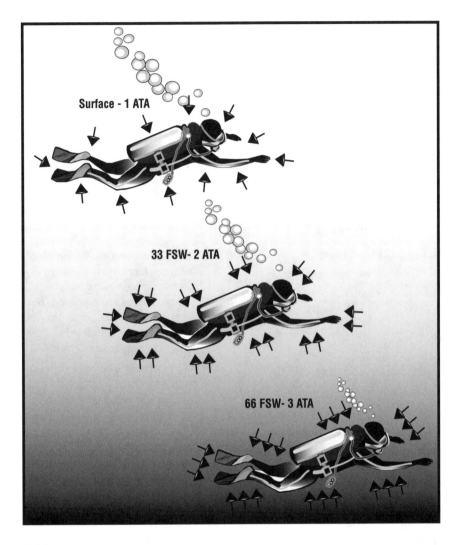

FIGURE 1.2 Pressure changes with descent into water. Except for the air-filled, rigid-walled cavities, the diver is unaware of increases in ambient pressure with descent.

The liquid–solid compartment accounts for over 95 percent of the body mass and includes blood, bones, muscles, solid organs, skin, fat, and so on. These structures transmit pressures equally and undiminished throughout the body mass and thereby avoid pressure gradients (Pascal's principle). Consequently, with respect to this compartment of the body, the diver can descend to any depth without consequences from the effects of pressure since no pressure gradients develop.

The air-filled, flexible-walled compartment consists of air-filled cavities with flexible walls, such as the lungs and the gut. These structures respond

TABLE 1.3	Body Compartment Responses to Pressure Gradients	
Compartment	**Structures**	**Effect with increases in ambient pressure**
Liquid–solid	Blood Bones, joints, teeth Muscles, tendons Solid organs Skin Fat Glands, sex organs Connective tissues Nerves, sensory organs	Transmit pressure equally and undiminished in all directions; consequently, no pressure differentials arise and pressure is tolerated to any depth.
Air-filled flexible wall	Lungs Gut	These compress as the ambient pressure increases, so no pressure differentials develop; in special circumstances the lungs cannot compress beyond a certain point and a pressure differential then arises (see chapters 5 and 13).
Air-filled rigid wall	Middle ear spaces Sinus cavities Face mask airspace Creases in exposure suits	With descent, pressure differentials arise. These must be eliminated by pressure equilibration, or damage to the structures will occur.

to pressure differently than do the liquid–solid structures. As pressure increases, the volumes of the air-filled, flexible-walled structures decrease. **Boyle's Law** describes this effect. As the pressure is increased on a volume of gas, the volume of the gas itself will decrease. The effects of pressure on volume changes of air-filled, flexible-walled compartments are tabulated in table 1.4. With each succeeding increase in atmospheric pressure, there is a proportionately smaller decrease in volume. With ascent, the opposite occurs; the greatest changes in volume occur as the surface is approached. To state Boyle's Law in mathematical terms, the volume of a gas is inversely related to its pressure; that is, $V_1 \times P_1 = V_2 \times P_2$, where the left-hand side of the equation represents the initial volume and pressure and the right side represents the final volume and pressure. The same units for volumes and for pressures must be used consistently in the equation (see table 1.1).

Ordinarily, the air-filled, flexible-walled structures of the body tolerate the effects of pressure well, within the ranges of depths that the sport diver usually encounters. These structures merely decrease in volume as pressure increases, in accordance with Boyle's Law, and no pressure differentials develop. This is analogous to a balloon decreasing in size as it is pulled farther and farther underwater. Consequences of descent in an inanimate

TABLE 1.4	Effects of Pressure on Volume of a Gas With Increasing Ambient Pressure			
Depth in FSW (MSW)	**Atmospheres absolute**	**Volume**	**Percent of original volume**	**Percent decrease in volume from previous pressure**
Surface	1	1	100	Reference point
33 (10)	2	1/2	50	50
66 (20)	3	1/3	33 1/3	17 2/3
99 (30)	4	1/4	25	8 1/3
132 (40)	5	1/5	20	5
165 (50)	6	1/6	16 2/3	3 1/3

With each succeeding increment in pressure, the percent change in volume from the previous pressure becomes proportionally less. This has ramifications for treating decompression sickness, in which bubble reduction is desirable; but the maximum depth for breathing pure oxygen in a chamber is 66 FSW (20 MSW). In addition, with depths deeper than 66 FSW, air or inert gas–oxygen mixtures are needed, adding further nitrogen to the tissues.

air-filled, flexible-walled structure are seen in the buoyancy compensator. If the buoyancy compensator is not equilibrated with descent, the diver will become progressively more negatively buoyant. In rare situations, lung injury occurs in breath-hold diving from lung compression associated with deep breath-hold dives (see chapter 13).

The air-filled, rigid-walled compartment comprises all air-filled, rigid-walled cavities of the body, including the middle ear spaces and the sinus cavities. The air spaces created by face masks, external earplugs, and creases in exposure suits, although equipment related, are examples of air-filled, rigid-walled cavities. With changes in pressure, a gradient develops if the pressures in these cavities are not equalized with the ambient pressure. The liquid–solid supporting structures of these spaces (e.g., the bony wall space of the middle ear and sinuses, solid supporting structures of the face mask, and the creases from the exposure suit) transmit the ambient pressure equally and undiminished (Pascal's principle), while the gas in the cavities tends to remain at the surface pressure.

This pressure differential leads to **barotraumas** (pressure-related injuries) to these structures, termed squeezes (see chapter 13). If one uses the submarine analogy to illustrate the mechanism of squeezes, then a squeeze becomes analogous to a submarine descending beyond its crush depth, the depth at which the pressure hull collapses. When this occurs, seawater fills the submarine. It is no longer a rigid-walled, air-filled structure, but rather converts to a liquid–solid structure. This obliterates the pressure differential between the external environment and the inside of the submarine. The human body, however, has mechanisms of dealing with the pressure differential problems that are different from collapse of the external supporting structures. These are described in the discussion of the clinical aspects of squeezes in chapter 13.

Buoyancy and Viscosity

In addition to the pressure effects of water, which are a consequence of its density, there are other related considerations such as buoyancy and viscosity. Buoyancy is the lifting power of an object in a fluid. Archimedes described the principles of buoyancy over 2,000 years ago, and they are as valid today as they were then. According to **Archimedes' principle,** the buoyancy of an object reflects the ability of an object to sink or float in water and is measured by the weight difference between an object and an equal volume of water. In other words, if the weight of an object is less than the weight of an equal volume of water, it will float; if it is heavier, it will sink, as illustrated in figure 1.3.

Buoyancy is greater in seawater than in fresh water because of the increased density of salt water (64 pounds per square foot vs. 62.4 pounds per square foot for fresh water). The principles of buoyancy have many ramifications for the sport diver. For example, SCUBA divers may be neutrally buoyant at the surface. At depth, however, they may become negatively buoyant due to the compressive effects of water pressure (Boyle's Law) on the partially

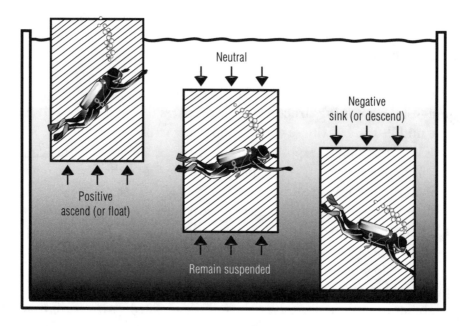

**FIGURE
1.3**   Buoyancy (Archimedes' principle).

air-filled buoyancy compensator and the air cells in the neoprene wet suit. If compensations are not made for this effect, divers may sink or have to swim harder to maintain the desired depth. When one is lifting objects from water with airlift bags, these considerations are crucial. As gas expands in the lifting bag during ascent, buoyancy increases, the rate of ascent may become uncontrolled, and the air in the lifting bag may expand so much that the bag ruptures.

While the density of water provides buoyancy, it also interferes with movement. The reason is the **viscosity** or thickness effect of water. Viscosity causes resistance when moving through water. Diving mammals have adaptations to counteract this effect and improve their propulsive ability in water (see chapter 8). The sport diver, however, must rely on technologies such as fins, hand paddles, and underwater propulsive units to help with mobility in the water.

The viscosity of water poses several other challenges to the diver. These challenges include currents, swells, waves, surges, and turbulence.

- **Current** is the convective flow of one mass of water through another. A current of one knot (one knot = one nautical mile per hour = 6,076 feet per hour) is barely detectable for a powerboat moving through the water. However, a current of this magnitude will cause a diver to make hardly any headway in the water. A rip current is a current caused by a combination of wave action, tides, and bottom contours that moves seawater away from the shoreline.

- **Swells** are upward and downward movements of water generated and propelled by wind.

- **Waves** as swells that approach the shallow water of the shoreline. The kinetic energy of the swell is reflected off the bottom to increase its upward height. The swell eventually breaks over itself as it approaches the shoreline and forms a wave. Because of the density and viscosity of water, crashing waves can impart a tremendous amount of force to divers as they try to pass through the surf zone. The force may be enough to rip off equipment, crash the diver into the ocean floor, cause disorientation, or lead to panic. Past the surf zone, however, swells are barely noticeable. If on the surface, the sport diver may notice gentle upward and downward movement. In the trough of a swell, though, visual references, such as the shoreline or the diving boat, may be blocked by the height of the swell and cause the diver to panic. When a diver is underwater, the effects of swells ordinarily are hardly noticeable.

- **Surge** is the back-and-forth movement of water between waves. Whereas waves tend to prevent divers from passing through the surf zone to deep water, the outbound surge phase tends to carry them out to sea.

- **Turbulence** is a localized current effect that occurs when a current is deflected off another object. In its severest forms, it is an aquatic version of a tornado. In its mildest form, it may merely be a nuisance that interferes with the diver's ability to remain stationary when trying to take an underwater photo. An eddy is a type of turbulent flow in which water flow circles back on itself.

Thermal Properties of Water

Another physical stress associated with water is its thermal properties. This stress presents significant challenges to the sport diver. The specific heat of water is 1,000 times greater than that of air. This means that it takes about 1,000 times more heat energy to warm a given volume of water one degree than to warm an equal volume of air the same amount. In addition, water conducts heat away from an object about 25 times as rapidly as air does. The combination of these two properties of water explains why immersion in cold water is so challenging to the body's heat-conserving mechanisms. Without thermal protection in water, survival can be measured in minutes as compared to hours for survival in air of equal temperature (see chapters 7 and 12).

Technology for mediating cold stresses, which is discussed in part II of this book, has done much to mitigate thermal challenges for the sport diver. Nevertheless, thermal challenges still exist. With descent and increasing pressure, for example, the air cells in the neoprene wet suit compress and lose their effectiveness as insulators. This problem is compounded by the fact that bodies of water typically become colder with increasing depths. In relatively still bodies of water such as lakes, ponds, and quarries, warm and cold masses of water tend to layer. The junction between the layers is termed a **thermocline.** When one is transitioning through a thermocline, change in water temperature is abrupt. In addition, the effect of the decreased insulation properties of the wet suit at increasing depth can quickly lead to chilling and discomfort in the water.

Breathing accounts for about 25 percent of the body's heat loss. This loss of heat is insensible because the diver is not ordinarily aware of heat being lost with exhaled air. Respiratory heat loss occurs almost entirely by convection (moving of masses of warm air) from the body's heat stores. Thermoregulatory mechanisms, such as shunting and vasoconstriction (see chapter 7), do not alter this cause of core heat loss. When air is inhaled, it must be warmed to body temperature and fully saturated with moisture before it reaches the terminal portions of the lungs where gases can be exchanged with the blood. If the air is not warmed and fully saturated, bronchospasms (i.e., constriction of the terminal portions of the airway tree) occur, causing coughing, wheezing, and production of secretions. If the pressure is doubled with diving to a 33-FSW (10-MSW or 2-ATA) depth, the insensible heat loss is twice as great, since each breath will contain twice as many molecules of air as required at sea level (1 ATA). At the 100-FSW (30-MSW or 4-ATA) depth, the requirements are quadrupled because the pressure and the number of molecules of gas to warm are four times as great as on the surface. Insensible respiratory heat loss at a 1,000-foot (305-meter) depth is about 30 times as great as on the surface. Chilling will occur after only a few breaths even when the diver is wearing thermal protection. Chilling not only is a source of discomfort for the sport diver but also has potentially serious medical consequences.

Relationships Between Temperature and Pressure

Charles' Law is the gas law that defines the relationships between temperature and pressure. **Charles' Law** states that in a closed system, the pressure of a gas is directly related to its temperature: $P_1 / T_1 = P_2 / T_2$ (where the left side of the equation equals the initial pressure and temperature and the right side equals the new pressure and temperature). To use Charles' Law, however, Kelvin temperatures are required. Kelvin temperatures are obtained by adding 273 to the Celsius temperature. Fahrenheit (F) temperatures are converted to Celsius (C) temperatures and vice versa with the following formulas:

$$C = (F - 32) \times 5 \div 9$$
$$F = (9 \div 5) \times C + 32$$

From a practical perspective, Charles' Law has few applications to the sport diver. For example, the temperature of the breathing gas changes imperceptibly when pressures increase with descent. The expanding gas from the tank to the regulator has a cooling effect, which more than counteracts the warming effect from breathing the gas under increased ambient pressure. However, one can appreciate the effects of Charles' Law when filling a SCUBA tank rapidly. The temperature of the metal cylinder noticeably increases. When the tank cools, the pressure decreases, and the tank is no longer filled to the maximum allowable pressure. The consequence is a reduction in SCUBA dive time. One can essentially eliminate this problem by filling the SCUBA tank slowly over a 10- to 15-minute period while immersing it in a cool water bath. When Boyle's and Charles' Laws are combined, volumes, pressures, and temperatures can be combined into one formula, the universal gas law, which states that

$$PV = nRT$$

DIVING SCENARIO

APPLICATION OF THE UNIVERSAL GAS LAW

An explosion occurs in a hyperbaric chamber that is at a depth of 100 FSW (30 MSW). If the ambient temperature in the chamber before the explosion was 72 degrees F (22 degrees C), and the pressure gauge on the outside of the chamber shows that the chamber pressure immediately increased to 250 FSW (76.2 MSW), how high did the temperature rise in the chamber? How will this information influence the decision to rescue the victims?

Using the universal gas law, one can determine that the temperature rose to over 670 degrees F (350 degrees C). Any attempt to "rescue" the victims would be futile, and there would be a risk of a fire developing in the chamber facility. The hot gases would act like an enormous blowtorch as they exited the chamber.

where P = pressure, V = volume, n = the number of molecules, R = the universal gas constant, and T = temperature. Since "n" and "R" are constant in a "closed system" such as a SCUBA tank or a hyperbaric chamber, the universal gas law can be expressed as follows:

$$P_1 V_1 / T_1 = P_2 V_2 / T_2$$

Physiological Stresses

Physiological stresses are associated with the normal functions of the body. Physiological stresses associated with diving relate primarily to **ventilation,** that is, the breathing in of oxygen and the exhalation of carbon dioxide. In addition, nitrogen, the **inert gas** that comprises approximately 79 percent of the air we breathe, equilibrates with the nitrogen in our body tissues. Oxygen must be available to all body tissues in order for them to remain alive and carry out their functions. Oxygen is brought into the lungs during the inhalation phase of respiration. In the lungs, it is transferred to the blood and carried to the body's tissues. The human body is not adapted to extract oxygen from water as fish and other species are. The amount of oxygen in seawater is about 1/40 that in air. The ability to breathe fluid with added oxygen when underwater could have many advantages. It would eliminate many of the problems associated with SCUBA diving. However, fluid respiration, as this technique is termed, is in the realm of science fiction at this stage of our knowledge and technology. Two methods mediate the ventilation stresses on a diver while underwater: breath-holding and the supply of an air source to the diver.

Breath-holding meets the ventilation stresses for brief depth excursions. Breath-holding durations are limited, usually one to two minutes for most divers. However, with training these times can improve markedly. Oxygen stores in the lungs, the bloodstream, and some of the other body tissues allow the diver to remain submerged safely for the duration of the breath-hold dive. Although there are many desirable features of breath-hold diving, it has inherent dangers such as blackout during the dive (see chapter 11).

The second method to meet the ventilation stresses underwater is to provide an air supply to the diver. SCUBA diving is one way this may be accomplished. Gas can also be supplied to the diver by air hoses tethered to the surface (i.e., surface-supplied diving). Breathing air under pressure introduces several other ventilation-related challenges. Since air will be breathed at the ambient pressure of the diver, much higher pressures of oxygen and nitrogen—the main constituents of air—will enter the body. Dalton's Law of partial pressures describes how gas pressures change with increases in pressure. According to **Dalton's Law,** the total pressure of gases in a system (e.g., air at sea level) is equal to the sum of the **partial pressures** (the proportion of the total pressure contributed by each gas) of the gases; that is,

$$P_{(Total)} = P_1 + P_2 + \ldots$$

Using this gas law is about as easy as saying 2 = 1 + 1. For example, at sea level the total pressure of 1 ATA equals the sum of the partial pressures of nitrogen (0.79 ATA) and oxygen (0.21 ATA). (For simplification purposes, we have not included argon, carbon dioxide, water vapor, and other gases that are present in miniscule quantities in our atmosphere.)

Oxygen

Oxygen presents unique physiological challenges to the diver. When oxygen supplies are insufficient to meet the body's needs, symptoms such as air hunger, light-headedness, and loss of consciousness occur. However, when oxygen supplies are too great, medical problems arise also. The lungs are amazing filters. They require only a finite number of molecules of oxygen as reflected by the partial pressure of oxygen in the breathing gas. As long as the pressure of oxygen in the inhaled gas remains in the range of 120mmHg (0.158 ATA) to 1,520mmHg (2 ATA), the lungs can extract adequate, safe amounts of oxygen for the body's oxygen requirements. In contrast, combustion is a function of the percentage rather than the partial pressure of oxygen in the breathing medium. If it is less than 18 percent, a flame cannot be kindled. Consequently, for the body's metabolic requirements, there is no depth limitation as long as oxygen is available to the lungs in the range just specified. This means that at a depth of 1,000 FSW (305 MSW, 30 ATA), using an extreme example, only 0.55 percent oxygen (equivalent to 127mmHg, 0.167 ATA) is needed in the breathing gas to meet the body's oxygen requirements. In accordance with Dalton's Law, some other gas or gases must make up the remaining 99.45 percent of the breathing gas. In the air we normally breathe at 1 ATA, nitrogen makes up the difference. At the 1,000-FSW (305-MSW) depth, nitrogen cannot be used because of its narcotic (i.e., sleep producing) properties (see chapter 14).

If the oxygen partial pressure in the breathing gas is too low (less than 120mmHg), the diver will become hypoxic, which is the term for inadequate oxygen availability for the body's needs. The brain is the most sensitive organ in the body with respect to hypoxia, but other tissues are affected also. Initially, they stop functioning—a situation somewhat analogous to suspended animation. The tissues die if adequate oxygen supplies are not restored quickly enough. Different tissues have different tolerances to oxygen deprivation. Damage and death to brain cells occur after only four minutes of oxygen deprivation. Muscle tissues can withstand two hours of oxygen deprivation, while skin, ligaments, tendons, and joint capsules can survive for periods of up to 24 hours. If the oxygen partial pressures are too high, that is, greater than 1,520mmHg (2 ATA), toxicity from breathing oxygen at the increased pressure occurs (see chapter 14). Thus, as shown in figure 1.4, there is a narrow safe range of oxygen partial pressures (oxygen window) for the body.

It is interesting to compare the effects on the body's oxygen requirements of decreased atmospheric pressure associated with mountain climbing, flying,

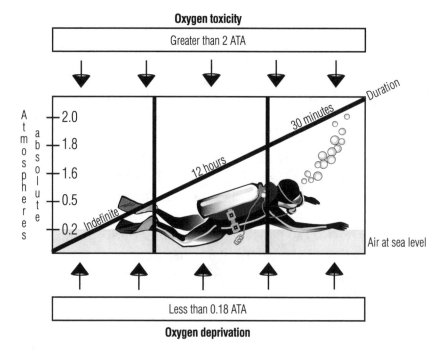

FIGURE 1.4 The physiological range of safe oxygen partial pressures for the human.

and space exploration with the effects of increased atmospheric pressure with diving. With ascents in altitude, there are progressive decreases in ambient pressure. At an 18,000-foot (5,500-meter) altitude, the atmospheric pressure is one-half what it is at sea level. From Dalton's Law (and conversion to mmHg), the one-half atmosphere of pressure equates to an oxygen partial pressure of about 80mmHg. This causes a severe hypoxic stress on the body, which is why supplemental oxygen breathing is used during mountain climbing at high altitudes. However, since the oxygen percentage is greater than 18 percent, a flame can still be kindled. When a person is breathing pure oxygen, again calculated with help from Dalton's Law, the oxygen partial pressure at 18,000 feet (5,500 meters) would be one-half ATA (a little less than 380mmHg), well within the lungs' physiological partial pressure requirements.

In airplanes, the pressures within the cabin are reduced to below one atmosphere of pressure for economic reasons. Typically, commercial aircraft maintain their cabin pressures at about an 8,000-foot (2,450-meter) altitude. Traveling at this altitude places a modest hypoxic stress on the passenger since the oxygen partial pressure for the lungs at this altitude is about 0.15 ATA; this is why pregnant women and patients with heart and lung conditions may be advised not to fly. Changes in oxygen partial pressures have been studied in space capsule flights. For example, a pressure of one-fifth atmosphere of pure oxygen is sufficient to meet the lungs' oxygen partial pressure requirements. Tragically, an explosion occurred in the Apollo 1 space capsule pressurized with pure oxygen. The capsule was pressurized to 1.2 ATA. A spark explosively ignited the combustibles in the cabin. All the astronauts in the cabin were immediately incinerated.

Carbon Dioxide

Carbon dioxide is a waste product of the body's metabolic processes arising from oxygen's interaction with food products and other substances in the body. The production of carbon dioxide is analogous to smoke production from a burning fire. Carbon dioxide diffuses into the bloodstream from the cells' metabolic activity and then is carried via the bloodstream to the lungs. From the lungs, it is exhaled to the outside environment. Although oxygen is necessary for sustaining life, the stimulus to breathe is more responsive to elevated levels of carbon dioxide in the bloodstream than it is to low levels of oxygen. Elevated carbon dioxide levels in the bloodstream cause an irrepressible desire to breathe, whereas the stimulus to breathe from low oxygen levels is not as strong. Ordinarily during SCUBA diving, carbon dioxide accumulation is not a problem since each breath is exhaled through the regulator into the water. However, with special types of diving equipment, carbon dioxide accumulation can be a problem (see chapter 14).

Nitrogen

Another physiological stress that occurs in the body from breathing gas at pressures greater than one atmosphere is that from the inert gas, nitrogen. Nitrogen comprises about 79 percent of the air we breathe. Although the nitrogen gas in air is inert (it ordinarily does not chemically unite with other substances in the body), it does dissolve physically in all tissues in the body. As the partial pressure of nitrogen increases with descent into the water, nitrogen is forced into the body tissues from the air breathed in at the new ambient pressure, as explained by Henry's Law (see figure 1.5). According to **Henry's Law,** in a gas–liquid system, the amount of gas that physically dissolves into the liquid phase is proportional (::) to the pressure of the gas phase: $G_{(PD)}$ :: P (where $G_{(PD)}$ is the gas physically dissolved in the liquid phase and P the pressure in the system). Although the "piston analogy" illustrates Henry's Law, other factors, such as attraction of the liquid for the gas (solubility coefficient), temperature, and metabolism of gas, may modify how much gas physically enters the liquid phase.

Increasing partial pressures of nitrogen affect the sport diver in three ways as summarized in figure 1.6: tissue saturation, narcosis, and density effects. Saturation occurs when the tissue reaches equilibrium with the inert gas. At sea level, all the tissues in the body are fully saturated with nitrogen at approximately 0.79 ATA pressure. With descent to 33 FSW (10 MSW), which is equivalent to 2 ATA, the partial pressure of nitrogen doubles. Some tissues, such as the lungs and blood, equilibrate very rapidly with the inert gas at the new ambient pressure; however, tissues such as ligaments and joint capsules do so very slowly. Eventually all tissues equilibrate with the inert gas at the new ambient pressure if the diver stays at the new pressure long enough. During ascent and decreasing ambient pressure, there is a pressure gradient for the inert gas to leave the tissues and be carried by the bloodstream to the lungs, where it is exchanged with the outside air. If the pressure

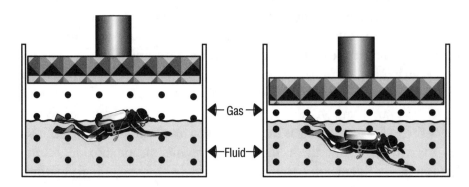

FIGURE 1.5   Piston analogy to explain Henry's Law. Dots represent molecules of gas.

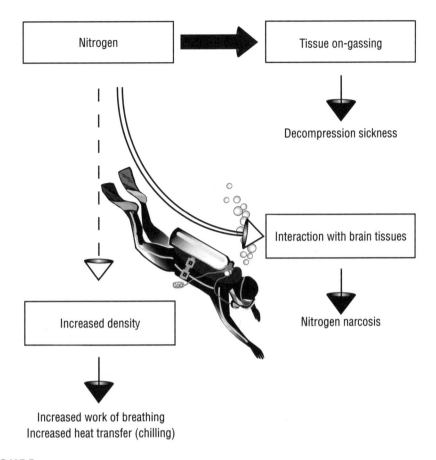

FIGURE 1.6   Side effects from nitrogen in the breathing gas. The deeper the dive, the more likely side effects will occur. The widths of the arrows indicate the significance for the sport diver.

gradient is too great, bubbles form in the tissues. This information forms the basis for understanding decompression sickness and is further discussed in subsequent chapters.

A second problem associated with the inert gas nitrogen is that it acts as a narcotic agent at increased pressures. Although many theories have been developed, the most commonly accepted mechanism of inert gas narcosis is that of interactions of the inert gas with nerve cell membranes (see chapter 14). The greater the pressure, the greater the narcotic effect of the nitrogen. At about a 750-FSW (229-MSW) depth, the effect is equivalent to being under general anesthesia for surgery. Obviously, during diving at depths of more than several hundred feet, nitrogen cannot be used as the inert, diluent gas to keep oxygen at a safe partial pressure for the diver. Helium is the inert gas most often used for deep diving because of its lack of narcotic effects. However, helium is not free of undesirable effects either (see chapter 14).

The high-pressure nervous system syndrome, manifested by tremors, occurs when helium–oxygen mixtures are breathed at great depths.

The final physiological effect associated with ventilation is that of the increased work of breathing from breathing gas at great pressures. For example, at a 1,000-FSW (305-MSW) depth, the breathing gas is more than 30 times as dense as it is on the surface. Although divers can function at these depths, their work capacity and endurance are greatly reduced because of the increased work of breathing the dense air. In addition, as discussed in the context of physical stresses, the increased density of gas at this pressure causes rapid chilling if the breathing gas is more than a few degrees cooler than the body temperature.

Orientation and Psychological Stresses

The aquatic environment is not a "friendly" place with respect to the sport diver's five senses or for rapid mobility. Vision and hearing are the two senses most notably affected. Sensation is diminished by the wearing of gloves and the chilling of the hands from cold water. For all practical purposes, in the underwater environment, smell and taste sensations are irrelevant. Movement through water is hampered by water's viscosity, and the water's density and buoyancy effect interferes with descent.

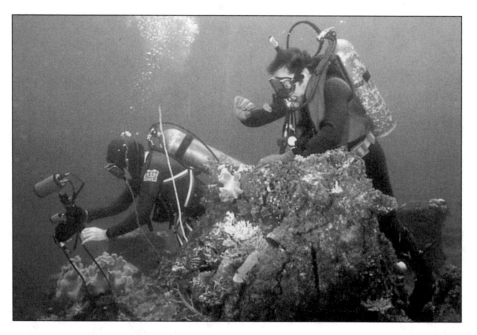

While underwater, divers are subject to physical (pressure and density effects), physiological (breathing gases under increased pressure), and psychological (limited vision, absence of voice communications) stresses unlike those found on land.

The Senses

Vision is the primary sense of orientation during diving. Vision is distorted underwater because of the difference in the refractive indexes of the cornea and the water at their interface. A diving mask mitigates this effect by interposing an airspace between these two media. However, a mask limits peripheral vision while creating a rigid-walled, air-filled cavity that is subject to face mask squeezes. Depth perception is altered by the dive mask faceplate-to-water interface with an approximately 33 percent magnification effect. For the unaccustomed diver, this can result in misses when reaching for objects underwater such as safety lines, game, and so on. The opacity of the water, which is highly variable due to turbidity, depth, obliquity of the sun's light rays, and plankton, limits distance vision. At night everything is "dark" except for the cone of light generated by the diver's underwater lantern.

With increasing depths, illumination and color recognition are progressively lost. Water filters out colors of the visible light spectrum. At the 30-FSW (9.1-MSW) depth, red disappears. By 75 FSW (23 MSW), yellow is lost. At these depths, all objects become a monotonous blue-gray. With loss of visual cues, the diver is subject to becoming disoriented as to direction. Any number of problems can arise when this occurs, including sinking deeper in the water when the diver thinks he or she is ascending. This may be compounded by negative buoyancy if the diver does not maintain neutral buoyancy to compensate for compression of the thermal protection suit and buoyancy compensator while descending. Likewise, the disoriented diver may swim in the wrong direction and become too exhausted from this extra effort to swim back to the dive platform or shore. Even more serious is the loss of equilibrium sensation from ear barotraumas, coupled with the losses of visual cues. In the disoriented state, divers may think they are ascending when in fact they are descending.

After vision, hearing is the sense that is most altered by the underwater environment. Although sound conduction in water is about 25 times as great as in air, the density of water results in impairment of auditory acuity. Intelligible speech is not possible without an air interface between the mouth and the surrounding water. A similar interface is needed between the water and the ear receiving the sound. Furthermore, ear barotraumas (squeezes), which are among the most frequently occurring medical problems of diving, can interfere with hearing due to fluid collections behind the eardrum. For communications while underwater, the sport diver may need to rely on hand signals and other methods of nonverbal communication such as rope pulls, tapping on metal objects, or underwater sound generators.

Other senses, such as taste, touch, and smell, are equally impaired by the underwater environment. Ordinarily these changes go unnoticed, however, due to the panorama of the underwater environment that the visual sense perceives so well. Although the rule for the sport diver is "look, but don't touch," wearing gloves is desirable for thermal protection of the hands and for protection from cuts and scratches in the marine environment. Often these minor injuries are unavoidable, for example, when a wave surge impales the diver into barnacle-encrusted rocks. Diving gloves, when very thick, markedly diminish tactile sensation and make safety maneuvers such as unsheathing a knife, adjusting a strap, or zipping up an exposure suit very difficult. When divers lose control in the water, they are likely to panic. Panic can lead to serious problems such as breath-holding during ascent and **arterial gas embolism,** which is a medical condition in which air bubbles introduced into arteries block their circulation (see chapter 15).

Mobility

Another psychological stress in the underwater environment is altered mobility. What may be a short step away on land can become an insurmountable distance in the water if the diver has to swim against a current. Conversely, altered mobility in the water with its buoyancy effect can be a source of relaxation that requires minimal efforts when underwater. For this reason SCUBA diving is not considered a good exercise for aerobic conditioning. If SCUBA divers do everything "right," by maintaining neutral buoyancy, drifting with currents, and breathing slowly and deeply while underwater, they should expend less energy than when resting on land. However, divers should be in good physical condition so as to have exercise reserves to meet the demands that an emergency might require.

Underwater Hazards

Encounters with underwater hazards are another potential stress for the diver. Examples include the sighting of sharks, entering sunken ships, entrapments in lines, swimming through pilings, and diving under stationary or moving vessels. Experience and dive planning help prevent these problems, which are often compounded by other physical or psychological stresses such as poor visibility and currents.

For Further Review

1. Describe the various units for measuring pressure and explain why each is used.
2. What are the theoretical advantages of fluid respiration?
3. Describe the body compartments as they relate to pressure.
4. Why does the majority of the human body tolerate elevations in pressure without difficulty?

5. Why is the partial pressure of oxygen more important than its percentage from a physiological point of view?

6. What is meant by the physiological range of oxygen partial pressures?

7. What effects do inert gases have on the body with respect to diving?

8. What are some of the psychological (orientation) stresses of the underwater environment?

TYPES OF DIVING, DIVE PROFILES, AND PHASES OF THE DIVE

Chapter Preview

- Types of diving
- Different ways in which the ventilation stresses of diving are met
- Concept of dividing a dive into four phases
- Types of dive profiles

Through technology and ingenuity, sport and commercial divers are able to meet the challenges of the underwater environment without undue risks of injury or interference with the enjoyment of the dive. Although minor injuries from diving occur commonly, they are probably no more frequent than the minor injuries that occur with terrestrial sports and probably no more serious. That is, medical attention rarely is required for their management. About one injury requiring medical attention occurs for every 1,000 SCUBA dives. Of these, about one-tenth require **recompression,** the method of treating decompression sickness and air embolism by placing the diver in a chamber and then pressurizing the chamber to reduce the size of bubbles. This is a testimony to the quality of equipment and the training of the diver. The major focus of this chapter is on the equipment used to meet the ventilation challenges of diving (see table 2.1). Other diving equipment is discussed in further chapters; for example, exposure suits are discussed in chapter 7. Descriptions of the phases of the dive and dive profiles are also included in the present chapter.

The distinction between the sport and the commercial diver today is no longer as clear as in the past, when commercial divers used equipment unavailable to the sport diver. Now equipment that was previously limited to the commercial diver is available to the sport diver who has the resources and motivation to purchase the equipment and undergo training for its safe use. Today, the main distinction is that the commercial diver gets paid while the sport diver does not. The scientific diver is a subcategory that encompasses aspects of both the commercial and the sport diver. As with the commercial

Table 2.1 Techniques to Meet the Ventilation Challenges of Diving

Type	Breathing equipment	Typical maximum depths	Advantages	Disadvantages	Comments
Breath-holding (free diving)	Snorkel	10-30 FSW (3-9.1 MSW)	Freedom; exercise challenge	Limited depth excursions; limited breath-hold time	Probably the largest number of participants
SCUBA (Self-Contained Underwater Breathing Apparatus)	Regulator and tank; open circuit[1]	Maximum depth recommendation 130 FSW (40 MSW)	Extending bottom time	Inefficient use of air supply; only about 5% of the oxygen in the SCUBA tank is used for ventilation	Most SCUBA diving is of this type
Nitrox (enriched air mixture)	Same as above	32%: 130 FSW 36%: 110 FSW (33 MSW)	Less chance of decompression sickness	Increased chance of oxygen toxicity	Less fatigue; less chance of decompression sickness
Rebreather	Closed circuit[2]	150 FSW (45 MSW) or more with mixed gas (helium–oxygen)	Prolongs underwater times	Many (>1,000) hours of training; increased hazards	Equipment costs about $10,000
Deep technical	Open or closed sequential gas mixtures	200 FSW (61 MSW) or more	Extends depths and duration of dives	Extended decompression	Technically demanding; divers may tote 5 tanks of gas, with additional tanks tied to decompression platforms
Surface supplied	Compressor on surface; gas by hose to divers	Air: 300 FSW Helium: 380 FSW (116 MSW)	Unlimited gas supply	Diver tethered to air hose	Commercial applications
Transfer capsules and habitats	SCUBA and/or tethered	1,000 FSW (305 MSW) or more	Bottom time to complete mission	May require days of decompression	Scientific, commercial applications

[1] Open circuit: After inhaling gas from the SCUBA tanks via the regulator, the diver exhales each breath into the water.
[2] Closed circuit: The gas supply recycles through breathing bags. Almost 100% of the oxygen in the SCUBA tank is used for ventilation.

diver, the diving activities of the scientific diver are usually mission oriented, as in marine archeology expeditions. Unlike the commercial diver, the scientific diver does not expect pay for scientific diving activities, although equipment and other expenses may be covered by funding sources. The technical diver is another subcategory of divers that use refined equipment to dive longer or deeper, as in explorations of caves or sunken ships in waters at depths greater than 130 FSW (40 MSW), the recommended depth limit for sport SCUBA divers.

Seven techniques are used to meet the ventilation challenges of diving. Of these seven techniques, tissue oxygen needs are met by one of four distinct methods: (1) breath-holding, (2) SCUBA with or without enriched air mixtures, (3) closed circuit, and (4) surface supplied. Each has its advantages and disadvantages, benefits and risks, special equipment requirements, and sport and commercial diving aspects. Each of these four methods will now be discussed from these perspectives.

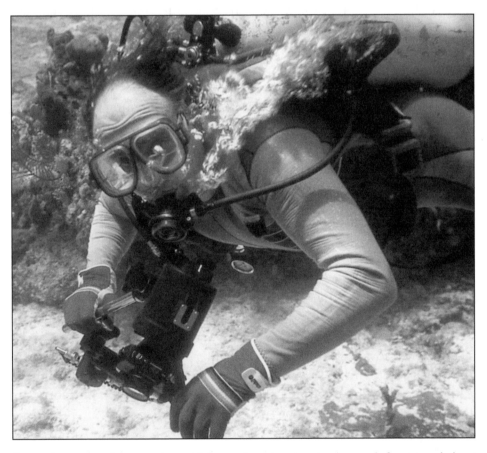

For underwater photography, which requires the time to descend, frame and shoot a picture, and then ascend, SCUBA diving is a better choice than is breath-hold diving.

Breath-Hold Diving

In **breath-hold diving,** as the name implies, one uses one's breath-holding abilities to remain underwater. Commonly breath-hold diving is referred to as skin diving (in contrast to SCUBA diving). This is a misnomer because skin diving implies that the diver is not using any type of thermal protection suit, which often is not the case. Free diving is yet another term used for this type of diving. **Snorkel diving** is a type of breath-hold diving in which a snorkel—a short breathing tube—is used to improve efficiency.

Breath-hold diving is the oldest of all diving techniques, dating back more than 5,000 years. It has played an important historic role in the search for food and treasure. Pearl divers of the South Sea Islands and female divers of Korea and Japan are among the better-known breath-hold divers. Breath-hold divers were also used in military operations in ancient times, as the Greek historian Thucydides reported. According to Thucydides, divers participated in an Athenian attack on Syracuse in which the Athenian divers cut through underwater barriers that the Syracusans had built to obstruct and damage the Greek ships.

Breath-hold diving approximates the type of diving done by diving mammals. The diver is unencumbered by tanks, hoses, regulators, bulky buoyancy compensators, or other devices that impede swimming—hence the term free diving. Repeatedly descending and ascending requires physical effort, thereby making breath-hold diving a good conditioning activity. Furthermore, depth excursions and breath-holding durations rapidly improve with practice. When snorkeling in waters with good visibility, the diver can cruise on the surface and view large expanses of the underwater panorama. The snorkel increases the diver's efficiency by eliminating the extra effort required to lift the head high enough to clear the mouth for breathing. Consequently, breath-hold diving can be a highly rewarding activity in terms of personal satisfaction, mobility, conditioning, and productivity. Since equipment requirements are minimal and this is largely a self-taught, self-acquired type of activity, there are minimal costs. Finally, those who are comfortable with breath-hold snorkel diving usually transition easily into SCUBA diving.

A major disadvantage of breath-hold diving is the limited time the diver can stay underwater. This is especially appreciated with underwater photography. Although taking pictures from the surface is not a problem, with snorkeling the time to descend, frame a picture, and wait for the marine life to "pose" for the picture may exceed the diver's breath-hold break point (i.e., the time before the diver has an irrepressible desire to breathe). If the dive is to depths more than 25 FSW (7.6 MSW), the descent and ascent consume much of the diver's air supply, thereby leaving little time to explore the bottom. Since each descent requires equilibrating pressures in the middle ear spaces (i.e., "clearing" the ears), ear barotrauma is much more likely to occur during a series of breath-hold dives than with a single descent for a SCUBA dive. The breath-hold diver is also at a greater risk of getting sunburned since much of the time is spent on the surface. Finally, as described in chapter 11, one can lose consciousness during breath-holding periods without the usual warning signs of air hunger.

Equipment Considerations

As the preceding information suggests, the equipment requirements for breath-hold diving are minimal. If the water is warm, fins, mask, and snorkel are the only equipment needed. Snorkels vary in quality and features. Prices range from less than $10 to over $30. Silicon rubber tubing, because of its flexibility, is preferable to plastic tubing. Soft rubber or silicon mouthpieces are much more comfortable than hard rubber or plastic ones. Airflow turbulence intensifies in and out of the snorkel with the increase of curves and their sharpness. While this may be a theoretical consideration, the curved portions of the snorkel also can hook onto kelp or other obstructions and become a hazard.

The snorkel is useful only for breathing on the surface. The pressure of water is so great that with only a few inches of descent, the diver lacks the inhalation force to suck in air from the surface. The snorkel need not be longer than one foot (0.3 meter), just enough for the end to be a few inches above the diver's head while the diver is on the surface. This allows the head to be in the water during breathing, thereby conserving energy and allowing uninterrupted vision of the bottom. The snorkel diameter need not be larger than the diameter of the diver's trachea, about three-fourths of an inch (two centimeters), in order for the diver to move air efficiently in and out for slower, deeper breaths and the hastening of recovery between breath-hold dives. Smaller-diameter tubes give the effect of breathing through a straw, while larger ones require more air volume for exchanging air and clearing water that has entered the tube. Although purge devices and valves to prevent water entry into the snorkel during the dive are a good idea, they are not always reliable. However, new technology has improved the reliability of the purge valve and "dry" snorkel technique such that snorkels with these devices are preferred by many free divers. The valves and purge devices also increase the resistance of moving through water. Aspiration (i.e., inhalation of water) is a potential hazard if the diver expects the snorkel to be dry when there is water in it. The best policy is to always assume that the snorkel has filled with water, whether or not it has a valve, and to save enough air to clear the snorkel upon reaching the surface. Discussion of fins and face masks is deferred to part II of the book.

Applications

There is no better way to explore a wide expanse of the ocean's bottom in clear, shallow, calm waters than breath-hold diving with a snorkel. Spearfishing, associated with breath-hold diving, is a recognized competitive sport. In addition, there is much interest in setting depth records for breath-hold dives. However, as discussed later, record depth-holding diving attempts are not without hazards. With the ease of application and minimal equipment requirements, we estimate that there are 10 times as many snorkel divers as SCUBA divers. But breath-hold diving is not limited to the sport diver. Three notable examples of professional divers using breath-holding techniques are the U.S. Navy Frogmen, the pearl divers in the South Sea Islands, and the diving women of Japan and Korea (Ama). Although the Frogmen (now designated as SEALS for the **S**ea, **A**ir, and **L**and missions) are trained in a variety of diving techniques, they use breath-hold diving for shoreline reconnaissance and obstacle clearing. The pearl divers in the South Sea Islands are noted for their deep dives and the Ama divers for their repetitive, shallower-water dives to collect food in colder waters. All three of these diver groups receive money for their breath-hold diving, thereby meeting the definition of commercial divers.

Snorkels are considered part of the diver's safety equipment. In fact, some states require that all divers carry a snorkel when SCUBA diving. Whenever one is swimming on the surface with SCUBA, use of the snorkel is recommended to conserve air supply in the SCUBA tank. If the SCUBA tanks are empty and the diver must swim back to shore or to the dive boat, the snorkel greatly reduces energy expenditures. The added effort of lifting the head out of the water to breathe while outfitted in SCUBA gear interferes with swimming and contributes to the diver's fatigue. As an alternative, divers may inflate their buoyancy compensators and swim in on their backs, thereby making swimming inefficient. They may fail to make headway even in mild currents. If a diver reenters the surf zone, it is necessary to return to the prone (i.e., facedown) position to avoid injury and maximize control.

SCUBA Diving (Open-Circuit Air and Nitrox)

SCUBA diving has become a popular sport. It is estimated that there are 5 million certified SCUBA divers in the United States, although the numbers reported vary from 3 to 15 million. SCUBA diving is also a safe sport with few serious problems. Two or three cases of decompression sickness occur for every 10,000 SCUBA dives. In 1943, two French inventors, Emile Gagnan and Captain Jacques-Yves Cousteau, demonstrated their "Aqua Lung," which used a demand intake valve drawing from two or three cylinders, each containing over 2,500 pounds per square inch (PSI) pressure. This apparatus was the forerunner of the modern open-circuit SCUBA regulator.

SCUBA diving offers the diver the freedom to stay submerged for extended periods of time and freedom of movement unencumbered by hoses tethered to the surface. The regulator and tanks are safe and reliable, with very few reports of accidents occurring due to mal-

Diving Physics: Air Supply Duration Versus Depth

Whereas a SCUBA diver on the surface may breathe from the regulator for more than one hour, at 99 FSW (30 MSW or 4 ATA) the air supply in the tank would last only one-fourth of this time. Since the pressure is four times greater at the 99-foot depth than on the surface, each breath at 99 FSW contains almost four times the number of gas molecules as on the surface. The result is that gas is consumed four times as rapidly. The regulator automatically accounts for the differences in ambient pressures between the surface and the 99-FSW depth.

functions. The nearly universal availability of compressors to refill SCUBA tanks makes it possible to dive in almost any exotic diving site. The compactness of the equipment facilitates airline flights to these areas. Most diving operators provide tanks and weight belts for their SCUBA diving clients. SCUBA diving is much "kinder" to the ears than breath-hold diving. The diver can spend as much time as needed to equilibrate pressures in the ears while descending without running out of breath. Likewise, with SCUBA diving, the dive profiles usually have only one descent and one ascent per dive. Achieving the same amount of time underwater with breath-hold diving might require 60 descents and ascents.

A major disadvantage of SCUBA diving is the inefficient use of the gas supply. During diving with air, approximately 79 percent of the tank's content is the inert gas nitrogen. Thus, each breath contains less than 21 percent oxygen. Since every exhalation contains about 16 percent oxygen, only 5 percent of the SCUBA tank's total gas contents is used for the body's ventilation needs, as summarized in table 2.2, which includes percentages for inhalation and exhalation of the gases found in air.

Approximately 95 percent of the tank's gas is exhaled to the surrounding water. This type of diving defines **open-circuit SCUBA;** each breath that is inhaled is then exhaled into the water after some oxygen is extracted from it and carbon dioxide added. Even with this inefficient use of gas, the SCUBA diver can stay underwater for considerable durations, but the durations are inversely related to the depth (see figure 2.1).

A second disadvantage of SCUBA diving with air is that it introduces the inert gas nitrogen to the body's tissues at the different ambient pressures of the dive (see chapter 3). The inert gas equilibrates with all the body tissues,

Table 2.2	Gas Composition of Inhaled and Exhaled Air		
Gas	Inhaled (percent)	Exhaled (percent)	Differences between inhalation and exhalation
Nitrogen	78.1	74.4	↓ 3.7%
Oxygen	20.9	15.8	↓ 5.1%
Carbon dioxide	0.03	3.6	↑ >100-fold
Water vapor	0.94	6.2	↑ >6-fold
Other gases*	Trace (<1%)	Trace (<1%)	Negligible

* Argon is the trace gas that is found in the highest concentration in the earth's atmosphere.

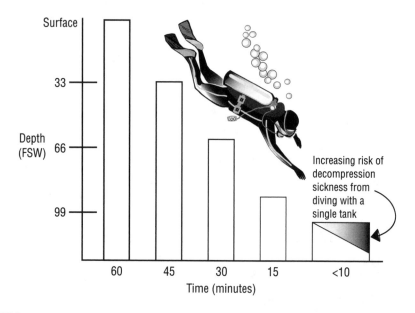

FIGURE 2.1   Approximate duration of a single 72-cubic-foot (2-cubic-meter) SCUBA tank relative to the depth of a dive. These estimates are based on normal breathing rates, depths at rest, and average-sized male divers. Durations for experienced, conditioned, and female divers may far exceed these estimates.

but at different rates. When the diver ascends, there is a reverse gradient for nitrogen to leave the tissues. If the gradient is too great, the inert gas forms bubbles. With coalescence of bubbles and enlargement with ascent, as described by Boyle's Law, the bubbles become large enough to distend tissues, block circulation, or both. This leads to decompression sickness, commonly referred to as "the bends" (see chapter 15).

Alterations in Nitrogen Levels

The percentages of gases in the SCUBA tank can be altered to reduce the amount of inert gas. During diving with pure oxygen, which is limited to about 33 FSW (10 MSW), no nitrogen will enter the tissues at the new ambient pressures of the dive. This depth limit is imposed because of the possibility of a seizure from oxygen toxicity. Is there a compromise between too much oxygen and too much inert gas? The answer is the use of enriched air **nitrox (enriched air) mixtures** in the SCUBA tank. The two most commonly used mixtures are 32 percent and 36 percent oxygen mixtures. Although these alterations do not eliminate nitrogen, the reduction decreases risks of decompression sickness so that divers can stay at depths (within a range of 60 to 130 FSW or 18 to 40 MSW) for longer periods (see table 2.3). Conversely, the increased oxygen percentages make the diver using nitrox mixtures more subject to oxygen seizures. With nitrox mixtures, the relative increase in oxygen percentage is over three times the relative decrease in nitrogen percentage.

Whereas the recommended maximum depth limitations for SCUBA diving with air are imposed by the nitrogen in the air, those for nitrox diving are imposed by oxygen limits. For example, the recommended depth limit for sport SCUBA divers using air is 130 FSW (40 MSW), with nitrogen being the limiting variable. Using nitrox-36 it is 110 FSW (33 MSW), with oxygen being the limiting variable. The theoretical depth limit for diving with air, based on the oxygen toxicity limit of 2 ATA for 30 minutes, is about 283 FSW (86 MSW). The risk of nitrogen narcosis (see chapter 14) and exhausting the air supply makes this limit largely a theoretical concern.

The inert gas in air presents an additional problem when breathed under increased ambient pressures. It leads to narcosis (i.e., sleepiness), analogous to the effect of an anesthetic agent. The narcotic effect of nitrogen for each 50 FSW (15 MSW) of descent is said to be equivalent to drinking one martini.

Table 2.3	Effects of Changes in Gas Compositions With Enriched Air (Nitrox) Mixtures*				
	Oxygen		**Nitrogen**	
Gas	**Gas percent**	**Relative % increase versus air**	**Gas percent**	**Relative % increase versus air**
Air	21	–	79	–
Nitrox-32**	32	52	68	14
Nitrox-36***	36	71	64	19

* All percentages rounded off to the nearest whole number; trace gases are disregarded.
** Enriched air nitrox—32% oxygen.
*** Enriched air nitrox—36% oxygen.

At a depth of 200 FSW (61 MSW), the narcotic effects would be equivalent to drinking four martinis. Diving with enriched air nitrox mixtures reduces but does not eliminate the likelihood that nitrogen narcosis will occur at an equivalent depth breathing air. To avoid this problem, helium, an inert gas that does not have narcotic effects, is used for deeper dives. Helium has three major disadvantages:

- It requires substantially longer times for gas elimination from tissues during ascent as compared to nitrogen.
- Tremors (i.e., the high-pressure nervous system syndrome [see chapter 14]) may occur during breathing at pressures greater than about 330 FSW (100 MSW).
- The decreased density of the gas causes almost unintelligible Donald Duck–like speech.

Because of the need for support staff and special equipment, diving with helium gas mixtures is primarily done by commercial and technical divers. These divers may switch gas mixtures, that is, use sequential gas mixtures, to avoid inert gas narcosis and possibly minimize decompression times. This requires the use of a separate tank for each gas mixture. Technical divers are noted for exploring sunken ships at great depths and for underwater cave explorations that may require many hours of bottom time.

One final consideration with SCUBA diving is the dehydration effect from the breathing of dehumidified air used to fill SCUBA tanks. Each exhalation on the surface after breathing from a SCUBA tank contains over six times the amount of water vapor as the air inhaled from the tank (see table 2.2). This effect is magnified in direct proportion to the diving depth. Dehydration, one of the precursors of decompression sickness, is given additional attention later in the book.

Equipment Considerations

The two essential equipment components of SCUBA diving are the regulator and the tanks. The three functions of the **regulator** are

- to reduce the high pressure in the tank to levels that will not injure the diver,
- to provide gas to the diver at pressures slightly greater than the ambient pressure, and
- to allow inhalation and exhalation on demand.

The first stage of the regulator performs the first two functions and is attached to the SCUBA tank. It has many connector plugs. Plugs with the larger-diameter holes connect via hoses to low-pressure devices, such as the second stage of the regulator, the buoyancy compensator, and the dry suit (if used). The smaller plugs reflect the pressure in the SCUBA tank and are used for connections to the tank pressure gauge and perhaps to other tanks (for providing additional air supplies).

The second stage of the regulator contains the mouthpiece and the exhalation port(s) for the third function. It is designed to equilibrate to the ambient water pressure so that a slight inhalation effort by the diver initiates the flow of air at a pressure slightly greater than the ambient pressure. Airflow stops when the diver ceases the inhalation effort. The diver exhales into the second stage of the regulator. A valve prevents water entry into the mouthpiece in order to keep it dry between breaths. During exhalation, gas bubbles are deflected to the side(s) of the diver's face by the port(s) so that the ascending bubbles will not interfere with vision.

Regulators vary in price from approximately $100 to over $600. Features that increase the price of regulators include the following:

- Manual adjustments to maintain a constant inhalation effort, regardless of depth
- Components that will not freeze up in icy waters
- Devices that help humidify the inhaled air
- The ability to work in the upside-down position
- Seals that prevent dirt and debris from entering the second stage of the regulator

Titanium is used for the more expensive first stages. All second-stage single-hose regulators have purge valves. While pressed, these allow a continuous flow of air to the regulator. This is very useful for clearing the second stage of water, for example, if the regulator accidentally gets dislodged from the diver's mouth and fills with water. If the second stage of the regulator is positioned more than a few inches higher than the first stage, air will flow continuously from it; this flow is termed "free flow." The sensitivity—that is, how much higher the second stage is in relation to the first stage to initiate free flow—can be adjusted by diving equipment repair shops. A spare regulator is another required safety item. Usually it is attached to a longer hose than the primary regulator to allow a buddy who needs an emergency air supply easy access to it. In these situations it is called an "octopus." Another alternative for the backup regulator is to integrate it with the oral inflation hose of the buoyancy compensator. This makes buddy-breathing more difficult than with an octopus regulator on a long hose. For additional safety, scientific and technical divers may attach two complete sets of regulators to their tanks or have a regulator for each gas mixture tank.

SCUBA tanks, available in many sizes and shapes, cost $100 to $300. Tank sizes are expressed as the volume of gas the filled tank can expand to when the gas in the tank is reduced to a pressure of 1 ATA. For example, a fully pressurized 72-cubic-foot (2-cubic-meter) tank would be able to fill a 72-cubic-foot balloon to a pressure of 1 ATA. The actual internal volume of the 72-cubic-foot tank is about 0.4 cubic foot (0.01 cubic meter). This equates to a change of about 180-fold or 2,600 PSI from unfilled to filled tank (another application of Boyle's Law). Tanks may be filled to a maximum designated safe pressure, for example, 2,250; 3,000; 3,500; or 4,500 PSI, which is embossed on the tank near its neck.

Enriched air mixtures are produced in one of two ways: mixing or denitrogenation. The latter technique is more commonly used. Mixing uses the technique of adding oxygen to an air tank until the desired percentage of oxygen is reached. With the denitrogenation technique, pumps with special nitrogen-permeable (but oxygen-impermeable) filters remove nitrogen from the air until the desired concentrations of nitrogen are reached. Because of the need for special equipment, nitrox tank fills are about 60 percent more expensive than air tank fills.

The two metals used for SCUBA tanks are steel and aluminum. Steel tanks are heavier than aluminum tanks. This can have some advantages for maintaining neutral buoyancy. For example, an 80-cubic-foot (2.3 cubic-meter) aluminum tank may have a 10- to 13-pound (4.5- to 6-kilogram) change in buoyancy from full to empty because the filled tank is 5 to 8 pounds (2.2 to 3.6 kilograms) negatively buoyant, whereas the empty tank has 5 pounds of positive buoyancy. This reflects the weight of the compressed air in the tank. Although weight changes occur between filled and empty steel tanks, the differences are usually about half the changes noted in aluminum tanks because of the increased weight of the steel tank. A 72-cubic-foot steel tank is about 8 pounds (3.6 kilograms) negatively buoyant when filled and 1 pound (0.5 kilogram) positively buoyant when nearly empty (500 PSI).

Tanks filled with nitrox mixtures have the word "Nitrox" or "Enriched Air Nitrox" stenciled on them and must also have one-inch (2.5-centimeter) yellow bands at their top and bottom borders. The

Diving Physics: The Increase of SCUBA Tank Pressure From Temperature Elevation

To what pressure would a SCUBA tank increase (without a burst plug) if the tank's pressure was 3,000 PSI at 72 degrees F (293 degrees absolute) room temperature but increased to 1,000 degrees F (811 degrees absolute) in a fire? With this information, the universal gas laws compute to a pressure increase of over 5,000 PSI. This would likely exceed the burst pressure of the tank and cause it to explode.

first stage of a regulator connects to one of two types of valves screwed into the SCUBA tank. For the "K" valve, the connection is made with an external clamp. Tank pressures for the "K" valve are limited to 3,000 PSI. The "Din" valve has a threaded female receptacle for the regulator connection. This type of valve has a pressure limit of 4,500 PSI. Both valve types have burst discs; that is, if the pressure exceeds a specified amount, the disc will "blow," and air will escape from the tank. Without this feature, the pressure in the tank could rise, for example, from a fire to the point of exploding.

Statistics regarding diving accidents reveal that the regulator is very reliable. Rarely has a regulator malfunction led to a diving accident. The regulator should have yearly inspections and necessary preventive maintenance. During the inspections, such functions as inhalation pressures and heights (between the first and second stage) to initiate free flow can be adjusted. The standard SCUBA regulator can be used interchangeably with air or nitrox mixes.

Tanks, like the SCUBA regulator, are very reliable. Nitrox tanks should never be filled with air and vice versa. Visual inspections of the tanks are required yearly. Hydrostatic (pressure) testing is required every five years. These standards are set by the U.S. Department of Transportation. The date of the pressure test is embossed on the tank near the neck. The dates of the visual inspections of tanks are noted on a waterproof label affixed near the bottom of the cylinder. Tanks should not be stored unpressurized with their valves open because of possible condensation of moisture in the tank, which leads to pitting and rusting. Likewise, if moisture enters, the tank must be dried out. Not only will moisture lead to pitting; the rusting process can also consume oxygen. This will decrease the oxygen partial pressure in the tank and cause the diver to dive with a hypoxic mix. The consequence could be loss of consciousness (see chapter 11). When tanks are stored for extended periods, they should be placed on their sides with the tank partial pressure reduced to 500 PSI. This will prevent condensation of moisture in the tank and eliminate the possibility of diving with a hypoxic mixture, since the tank will need to be filled before diving. Finally, the compressor intake source must be placed in a clean-air, exhaust-free environment. This essential requirement can be violated when wind shifts cause exhaust fumes from the gasoline compressor motor to be sucked into the intake valve. Although there are no constraints on purchasing equipment for SCUBA diving, SCUBA tanks are not filled at dive shops without a certification card verifying that the diver has completed a recognized training program.

Applications

The ability to stay submerged with a self-contained air supply adds a new dimension to our ability to enter the underwater environment. Most sport

SCUBA divers are content to visualize the underwater panorama in this fashion with the seeming ability to soar through the water as a bird would fly through the air. Others use SCUBA diving for underwater photography, game collection, and seeking buried treasures. For the scientific diver, SCUBA diving opens a world of opportunity for direct observation of the underwater environment.

Do the advantages of nitrox diving justify the added expenses for training and tank fills? In our opinion the answer is a "qualified" yes. Nitrox diving extends the safe time the diver can stay submerged while only slightly increasing the chances of oxygen toxicity. For example, 60 minutes is the maximum safe no-decompression time limit for a 60-FSW (18-MSW) dive using the U.S. Navy tables, whereas it would be 100 minutes using a 36 percent nitrox mixture. With deeper dives, the effects of enriched air mixtures are even more apparent, as table 2.4 shows. While nitrox mixtures can be used with air dive tables (thereby adding an even increased degree of protection from decompression sickness), the cut off (i.e., maximum) depths to avoid oxygen toxicity must not be exceeded. Commercial divers report that nitrox mixtures noticeably reduce fatigue after a day's diving and make them more productive for the next day's underwater work.

Table 2.4	No-Decompression Times (Minutes) With Air, Nitrox-32, and Nitrox-36 Gas Mixtures		
Depths in FSW (MSW)	**No-decompression times (minutes) (no-stop ascents)***		
	Air	**Nitrox-32**	**Nitrox-36**
40 (12)	200	310	310
50 (15)	100	200	200
60 (18)	60	60	100
70 (21)	50	50	60
80 (24)	40	50	60
90 (27)	30	40	50
100 (30)	25	30	40
110 (33)	20	30	30
120 (37)	15	25	Exceeds oxygen toxicity limits
130 (40)	10	20	
140 (43)	10	Exceeds oxygen toxicity limits	
150 (46)	5		

* Nitrox mixtures increase "no-decompression" stop bottom times; however, no-stop ascents do not eliminate the requirement for the 15-ft rest stop during ascent.

Closed-Circuit SCUBA Diving

Closed-circuit SCUBA (CCS) equipment offers an alternative to the inefficiency of open-circuit SCUBA diving, in which only a small percentage of the air in the tank is used for ventilation purposes. Using CCS is analogous to breathing into a plastic bag. But whereas the gas in the plastic bag rapidly becomes stale due to accumulation of carbon dioxide and the depletion of oxygen, the gas in CCS meets the requirements for sustained ventilation via (1) addition of oxygen at the rate it is consumed and (2) the removal of carbon dioxide as it is produced. The inert gas nitrogen remains relatively constant as it is breathed in, exhaled, and recycled in the breathing bags with each breath. However, with descent, additional inert gas must be added to the breathing system to maintain the gas in the breathing bags at the ambient pressure. This is accomplished through use of a second small tank filled with a diluent gas, usually air (for deep dives, helium can be used). These principles are also employed for atmosphere control in deep submersibles, as well as for submarines when submerged below snorkel depths. The basic components of the CCS rig are diagrammed in figure 14.1 (page 266).

The advantage of CCS equipment is that oxygen needs to be supplied only at the rate it is consumed, which is approximately *one liter (one quart) per minute.* A small cylinder of oxygen, about 1/10 the volume of a standard SCUBA tank, will supply enough oxygen to allow the diver to remain submerged for six hours or more at this utilization rate. In addition, a carbon dioxide–absorbing unit, about the size of a one-gallon (3.8-liter) cylinder, efficiently removes this gas from the CCS system for four hours or more. Thus, the gas supply for CCS diving is independent of depth. Remember, an open-circuit SCUBA diver consumes the gas supply onefold faster for each additional 33-FSW (10-MSW, 1-ATA) descent. The CCS system, since it utilizes oxygen completely (that is, at nearly 100 percent efficiency), is more than *20 times* more efficient in oxygen use than open-circuit SCUBA. Another advantage of CCS diving is that it nearly eliminates bubble production as long as the diver remains at a constant depth. This facilitates close observation of active marine life, a notable advantage for underwater photography, as well as allowing the diver to remain clandestine for military purposes.

The advantages of CCS must be paired with its disadvantages. Certification in CCS can require 100 hours of classroom instruction and 1,000 hours of diving practice. The special requirements for pure oxygen to fill the oxygen tanks and a supply of carbon dioxide absorbent (Baralyme) may pose logistic problems when diving in remote areas. Mixed-gas SCUBA equipment costs about $10,000. Also, there are special medical concerns associated with CCS diving (see chapter 14). The use of CCS equipment does not prevent decompression sickness; with the extended bottom times and depths this equipment allows, decompression from a dive may require hours. If oxygen is not added to the system at the required rates, the diver may lose consciousness without any sense of air hunger. If the carbon dioxide canister is not filled correctly, carbon dioxide buildup can lead to headaches and accelerate the onset of oxygen toxicity. If water enters the breathing system and wets the carbon dioxide absorbent, toxic fumes are produced that can burn the mouth and lungs.

Another disadvantage of the CCS system is the increased work of breathing it requires. Rather than inhaling air at a slightly positive pressure from the SCUBA regulator, CCS divers, through their own efforts, must move air in and out of the breathing bags. In essence the breathing bags are an extension of the diver's own lungs. Also, CCS diving is very demanding with respect to buoyancy control. With descent, the gas in the breathing bags compresses (as Boyle's Law shows), causing the diver to become negatively buoyant. To counteract this effect, additional diluent gas must be added to the breathing circuit. Naturally, the opposite occurs with ascent, and gas must be released to the water to allow the diver to remain neutrally buoyant. Finally, the diver must be highly cognizant of the oxygen concentrations in the CCS breathing circuit. This requires checking the oxygen monitors at intervals as frequent as each minute, although some monitors have automatic signaling devices.

Equipment Considerations

Most of the equipment considerations for CCS diving have been introduced. However, a few additional comments are necessary. A special mouthpiece is used with a manually operated valve to prevent water entry into the system when the mouthpiece is not in the diver's mouth. Three oxygen sensors constantly monitor the oxygen partial pressure in the circuit. The oxygen partial pressure is set at a predetermined limit, for example 0.8 ATA. If the sensor detects differences from this set level, oxygen flow from the oxygen tank is automatically adjusted to bring the level of oxygen in the breathing circuit to the set level. If one of the three sensors fails during the dive, the dive can still be completed per plan. However, if the failure is detected before the dive begins, the malfunction should be corrected before entering the water. If two sensors fail while underwater, the diver should terminate the dive as safely and expediently as possible. Dalton's Law is particularly applicable to the principles of CCS diving as illustrated in table 2.5.

On the surface, the oxygen partial pressure at the 0.8-ATA setting will be 0.8 ATA, and the corresponding nitrogen partial pressure 0.2 ATA. At 33 feet (10 meters), or 2 ATA, the oxygen partial pressure remains at 0.8 ATA, but the nitrogen partial pressure increases to 1.2 ATA in order to achieve an

Table 2.5	Dalton's Law and Closed-Circuit SCUBA Diving With a Constant Oxygen Partial Pressure			
Depths in FSW (MSW)	**Pressure in ATA**	**Partial pressure**		**Oxygen-nitrogen ratio**
		Oxygen partial pressure in ATA (%)	**Nitrogen PP in ATA (%)**	
Surface	1	0.8 (80)	0.2 (20)	4.0
33 (10)	2	0.8 (40)	1.2 (60)	0.66
66 (20)	3	0.8 (26)	2.2 (74)	0.36
99 (30)*	4	0.8 (20)	3.2 (80)	0.25
132 (40)	5	0.8 (16)	4.2 (84)	0.19
165 (50)	6	0.8 (13)	5.2 (87)	0.15

* This is the equivalent air depth (EAD). At 4 ATA (99 FSW or 3 MSW) the percentages of oxygen and nitrogen are essentially equivalent to those found in air.
** In closed-circuit SCUBA gear, oxygen percentage may be set from 0.2 to 1.6. In this table, 0.8 ATA is used. Since the oxygen partial pressures remain the same, oxygen toxicity is not a concern with increasing depth or duration of the dive.

ambient pressure of 2 ATA. With further descent, with the CCS system, the oxygen and nitrogen partial pressures become equal to those with breathing air. This depth is named the equivalent air depth (EAD). At depths less than the EAD, the diver is afforded protection from decompression sickness and nitrogen narcosis over that with air. At depths deeper than the EAD, there are increased risks of these problems because the nitrogen percentage is greater than that of air. Since the oxygen partial pressure is maintained at the set level (0.8 ATA as used in this example), the risk of oxygen toxicity during diving at deeper depths is no greater than at shallower depths. This of course is not the situation with nitrox diving, where the increased percentage of oxygen in the SCUBA tank makes oxygen toxicity a limiting factor for deeper dives.

This section has outlined most of the safety issues with CCS diving. There can be no compromises in following the maintenance requirements for this equipment. Equipment setup requires about 30 minutes. A checkoff sheet should be used so that no steps are overlooked. Once set up, the equipment can be used for several dives in one day without resetting up and dismantling, as long as the carbon dioxide absorbent has not been depleted and the gas supplies in the tanks remain sufficient. A checkoff sheet should also be used during dismantling. The breathing circuit, including the inspiration hose, the expiration hose, the mouthpiece, and the breathing bags, needs to be sanitized during the dismantling procedure since all of these components come in contact with the diver's expired air and upper airway secretions.

Malfunctions of the oxygen sensors, which have become increasingly more reliable, must always be addressed before the start of a CCS dive. Often, the support supplies for CCS include an additional oxygen sensor. Meticulous attention during setup must be given to the seals for the carbon dioxide absorber canister and the hose connections so that no water enters the breathing circuit.

Applications

For extended underwater activities, CCS equipment offers many advantages. For the sport diver, the investment in time, money, and logistics for this equipment must be considered within the context of the advantages that CCS equipment provides beyond open-circuit SCUBA diving. For the scientific diver and the deep technical diver, the advantages could be substantial. Presently, the major applications of CCS techniques are military. When only oxygen is used as the breathing gas, it is possible to make long shallow dives without the risk of air bubbles disclosing the diver's presence. The advantages of the pure oxygen rig (e.g., the Drager unit) over the CCS described earlier are the elimination of the second gas tank for the diluent gas and the elimination of the oxygen sensors. This makes the equipment lighter and more mobile, but the setup and sanitization requirements are analogous to those for other types of CCS equipment. Because of the added risk of oxygen toxicity during breathing of pure oxygen at greater than 1.6 ATA, CCS diving with pure oxygen is very limited by depth *and time*. Although the recommendations vary, a good guideline is to limit pure oxygen diving to 30 minutes at a pressure of 2 ATA (33 FSW or 10 MSW). At depths shallower than 15 FSW (4.5 MSW), the diver could exhaust the oxygen supply before oxygen toxicity would likely develop, since the oxygen partial pressure would remain below 0.9 ATA.

Surface-Supplied (Tethered) Diving

In surface-supplied diving (SSD) the diver's gas supply is provided by hoses connected to the surface. Techniques of SSD are listed in table 2.6. The hoses may connect directly to the diver's face mask (Jack Brown rig) or diving helmet (deep sea diving rig), or indirectly from a personnel transfer capsule. In the personnel transfer capsule technique, divers are transported to the bottom depth of the dive and then swim out of the capsule with gas provided to their diving rigs via umbilical lines from the transfer capsule. A variant of this technique is seen in habitat divers. The divers may remain pressurized in the habitat, usually at depths of 60 FSW (18 MSW) or less for days or weeks. They exit their habitat for scientific missions with scuba gear or tethered to umbilicals. There can be no compromises in the constraints

Table 2.6	Surface-Supplied Diving: Summary			
Type	**Depth limit in FSW (MSW)**	**Advantages**	**Disadvantages**	**Comments**
Recreational	30 (9.1)	Continuous air supply to a 30-ft depth	Diver must stay within close range of the air hoses	Risk of separation from air supply, causing the diver to swim to the surface breath-holding
"Jack Brown" (air hose connected to dive mask or helmet)	100 (30)	Mobility, sustained bottom times, minimal investments in equipment, minimal support staff	Diver tethered to the surface, usually limited to shallower depths	Used by commercial divers for bottom work such as abalone and sea urchin collecting
Deep sea (fully helmeted and suited)	350 (107)	Protection from the underwater environment since diving suit is pressurized with the surface-supplied gas	Markedly limits mobility; requires platforms for decompression from deep dives	Divers protected from the cold water and have phone communications with the surface
Personnel transfer capsule (PTC) and deck decompression chamber (DDC)	660 (201)	Pressurization and decompression in PTC; divers in water only for work activities; PTC can be brought to surface so decompression can be done in the DDC aboard the ship	Major equipment support and manpower requirements	Divers can remain at pressure and at the work site until the mission is completed; rest and eating done inside the PTC

imposed on depth excursions from the habitat depth in order to prevent medical problems of diving.

The principles of SSD are similar to those for other types of diving. Air or mixed gases may be used. Surface-supplied diving allows almost unlimited bottom times. Because of equipment requirements and support personnel, SSD diving is almost totally limited to the commercial diver. A recreational version of SSD uses a compressor resting on an inner tube–like float with hoses that carry air to divers below the surface. The hose lengths are limited to 30 feet (9.1 meters), supposedly to reduce the risk of diving problems. Surface-supplied diving has advantages for commercial and scientific divers because of the nearly unlimited bottom times, which may be particularly advantageous for work and scientific projects.

Phases of a Dive

All diving activities can be divided into four phases as portrayed in figure 2.2:

- Surface
- Bottom
- Descent
- Ascent and post-dive

Each phase has challenges that the diver must reconcile, as well as particular medical problems. Later in this book we use the phases of the dive as a format for discussing the medical problems of diving. The surface phase of the dive includes all activities from donning gear until the diver is ready to start the descent. The descent phase commences when the diver leaves the surface. The bottom phase reflects the time from completing the descent to the time of

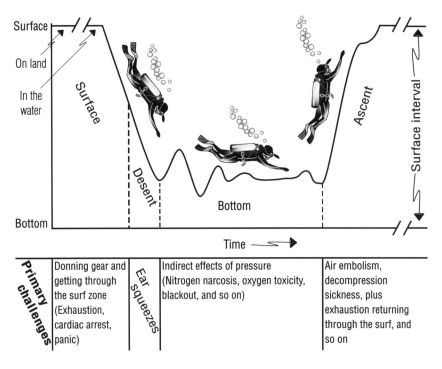

FIGURE 2.2   Phases of a dive and their primary challenges.

leaving the bottom. Most sport SCUBA divers make the ascent with stops at several depths as in the profile 60 FSW (18 MSW) for 30 minutes, 45 FSW (14 MSW) for 20 minutes, and 25 FSW (7.6 MSW) for 10 minutes. Are these stops part of the bottom phase of the dive or the ascent phase? As shown in the next chapter, the dive computer clouds this distinction while the dive tables do not. The ascent phase begins when the diver ascends to complete the dive. It is now recommended that all sport SCUBA divers perform a rest stop at 15 FSW (4.6 MSW) during the ascent before surfacing. Even with depth changes during the bottom phase, the phases of a dive are easily distinguished.

As shown in figure 2.3, exertional efforts and energy requirements are quite different for each phase. The surface phase is usually the most challenging because of the effort of carrying the diving gear to the diving site, donning the gear, and entering the water. Exceptional exertion efforts may be required to pass through the breaking waves of the surf zone if one is doing a shore-based dive. If underlying cardiac impairment or conditioning problems exist, complications such as arrhythmia or heart attack will most likely occur during the surface phase of the dive. The main challenge of the descent phase of the dive is the equilibration of pressure in the middle ear spaces (i.e., clearing the ears). Minimal exertion is required for descent if buoyancy is appropriately controlled. The diver may passively descend to the bottom depth if negatively buoyant. At the bottom depth, the buoyancy should

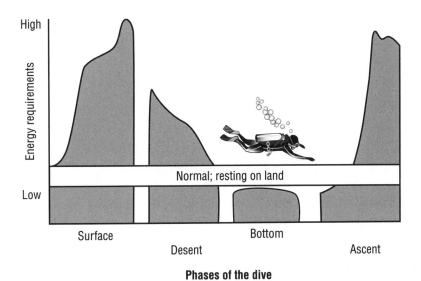

Phases of the dive

FIGURE 2.3 Exertional effects and energy requirements relative to the phases of a typical SCUBA dive. For the typical SCUBA dive, the energy requirements during the bottom phase are less than what they would be during resting on land. For this reason, SCUBA diving is not considered a good sport for conditioning.

Diving Physics: Buoyancy Changes With Ascent While Wearing a Buoyancy Compensator

Q: A diver is neutrally buoyant at a 99-FSW (30-MSW) depth with 0.1 cubic foot of air in his buoyancy compensator. What will the diver's buoyancy be when he reaches the surface if no air is exhausted from the buoyancy compensator during ascent? (Note: There is a fourfold [4 ATA to 1 ATA] decrease in pressure with ascent from 99 FSW to the surface.) The new volume of air in the buoyancy would approach 0.4 cubic foot. What is the buoyancy of 0.4 of a cubic foot of air?

A: Theoretically, the diver would have an additional 25 pounds (11.4 kilograms) of increased buoyancy from the expansion of air in the buoyancy compensator.

be adjusted to neutral. Here energy expenditures should be minimal, with the diver performing occasional slow flutter kicks or merely drifting with the current. For ascent, energy requirements again increase. A slow, controlled swimming ascent, at no more than 1.0 FSW (0.3 MSW) every two seconds, or 30 FSW (9.1 MSW) a minute, is recommended. Because gas expands with ascent and thereby increases buoyancy (Boyle's Law), the buoyancy compensator should be adjusted to maintain neutral buoyancy and to prevent uncontrolled ascent. In addition, due to gas utilization, the SCUBA tank may be 10 to 15 pounds (4.5-6.8 kilograms) lighter at the end of the dive than at the start.

Dive Profiles

A **dive profile** is the shape of a curve that is seen when the depth of the dive is plotted against the time progression of the dive. Although dive profiles are not functions of the type of diving equipment used, they often reflect the type of diving equipment used. Dive profiles are classified into five major types that are graphed in figure 2.4.

- Saw-toothed dive profiles are characterized by a surface interval, a rapid descent phase, a short bottom time, and a rapid ascent phase performed in a repetitive fashion. This profile describes the activities of a breath-hold diver.

- Rectangular dive profiles are seen in divers who spend almost their entire bottom time at one depth. This is the profile of divers who do projects on the bottom. For calculating bottom times when using U.S. Navy dive tables, all dives are considered to have rectangular profiles, even if the deepest depth was a bounce dive and the majority of the dive was spent at a shallower depth. The use of the rectangular profile to describe a dive (even if only a small portion of the time was actually spent at the deeper

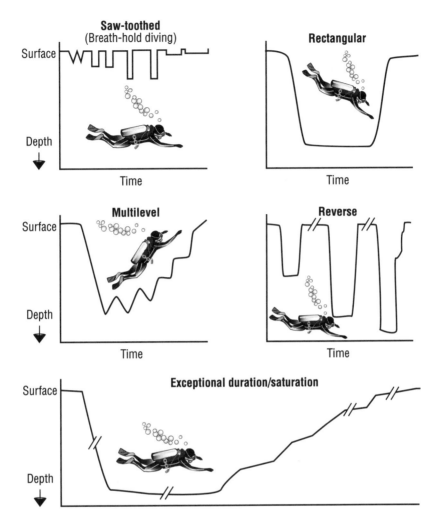

FIGURE 2.4 Dive profiles.

depth) adds an element of protection from decompression sickness, but shortens the actual allowable dive time.

- Multilevel diving profiles reflect the times the diver actually spends at each depth. Due to the sophistication of dive computers, reasonably accurate approximations of tissue gas saturations and safe ascent limits can be made. This greatly extends the dive time and affords the opportunity to do multiple dives each day.

- Reverse dive profiles describe a technique in which the deepest and longest dive of the day is reserved for the last dive. The depth limits needed for decompression stops and other elements are based primarily on this dive. In the past, this technique was considered anathema. However, with the ability of dive computers to show that the divers are in safe ranges and on the basis of observed outcomes (i.e., the avoidance of decompression sickness), people are questioning whether this is an acceptable diving technique rather than categorically rejecting it.

- Saturation dive profiles resemble rectangular dive profiles. However, rather than surfacing after each dive, the diver remains at depth—usually in a personnel transfer capsule or a habitat—until the mission is completed. Once all the body's tissues become saturated with inert gas, further time on the bottom does not impose any additional gas load for the diver. This technique has been used for underwater science studies and deep dive research projects. Once the project is completed, the diver ascends at very slow rates, for example 1.0 FSW (0.3 MSW) every 15 minutes. Whereas an ascent from a 1,000-FSW (305-MSW) dive with a 20-minute bottom time may require decompression of a week or longer, a saturation dive to this depth allows the diver to stay and work an unlimited amount of time at depth with about the same decompression requirements.

For Further Review

1. Name the main types of diving and the advantages and disadvantages of each.
2. What are the differences and similarities between sport, scientific, technical, and commercial diving?
3. Describe the different techniques that can be used for SCUBA diving.
4. What are the benefits and hazards of using nitrox mixtures?
5. What is the working principle of the regulator? Why is there a need for two stages?
6. What are the advantages and disadvantages of closed-circuit SCUBA?
7. How do exertion efforts vary during a dive? What challenges lead to increased exertion efforts?
8. Describe the different dive profiles and where they may likely be used.

CHAPTER

3

THE INERT GAS LOAD

The inert gas load is the "price" the SCUBA diver pays when diving with compressed gases. However, the "toll" is paid only after the diver starts to ascend. The inert gas load is the basis for the construction of decompression tables and the algorithms used in dive computers. Understanding the inert gas load makes it possible to understand why we dive as we do,

Chapter Preview

- Basic understanding of the principles of inert gas dynamics as they relate to diving
- Factors that lead to on-gassing and off-gassing of inert gases
- Recognition of the outcomes of decompression
- Basic concepts used to generate dive tables and algorithms used in dive computers
- Advantages and disadvantages of dive tables and dive computers
- Unorthodox diving practices

why decompression sickness occurs, and what we expect dive computers to do for us. For simplification purposes in this chapter, the only inert gas discussed is nitrogen; and with few exceptions, the only gas mixture discussed is air, with 79 percent nitrogen and 21 percent oxygen. The phrase "inert gas" can be substituted for nitrogen throughout this chapter. Again, for convenience, we most often use atmospheres absolute (ATA) to designate partial pressures but also use feet of seawater (FSW) and meters of seawater (MSW) when needed.

On-Gassing

For nitrogen gas dynamics purposes, the dive has two portions: (1) *on-gassing* and (2) *off-gassing* (see figure 3.1). When the partial pressure of nitrogen inhaled is greater than that of the tissues, inert gas is taken up by the tissues. This phenomenon is called tissue on-gassing, but other terms such as in-gassing, uptake, inert gas deposition, or in-diffusion are sometimes also used. When the partial pressure of nitrogen inhaled is lower than that of the tissues, inert gas is released by the tissues; this phenomenon is termed off-gassing. Other terms for this portion of nitrogen gas dynamics include inert gas out-gassing, elimination, release, and out-diffusion. The terms may have subtle differences in meaning whereby off-gassing implies the elimination of

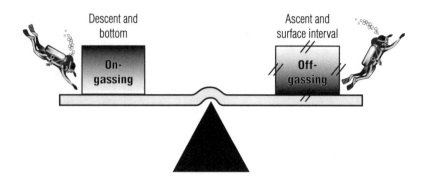

**FIGURE
3.1**   On-gassing and off-gassing as functions of the phases of the dive. // =
off-gassing takes longer than on-gassing.

nitrogen from the body while out-gassing suggests the movement of gas from
fixed body tissues to blood. However, the preferred terms used throughout
this book are on-gassing and off-gassing. Although the amount of off-gassing
will eventually equal the amount of on-gassing, the off-gassing portion of
the dive takes much longer to complete.

Tissue Nitrogen Saturation

At a constant ambient pressure for sufficient time, all tissues in the body
become fully saturated with nitrogen (see figure 3.2). On the surface of the
earth, all our tissues are fully saturated with nitrogen. However, the pressure
of nitrogen in these tissues, when fully saturated on the earth's surface, is not
1 ATA, but rather 0.79 ATA. This represents the partial pressure of nitrogen
(Dalton's Law). The other contributors to 1-ATA pressure are oxygen, water
vapor, carbon dioxide, and trace gases. When the diver descends (from the
earth's surface) to 33 FSW (10 MSW) breathing air, the new ambient pressure is 2 ATA. From Dalton's Law, the new nitrogen partial pressure is 1.58
ATA, which is two times the nitrogen partial pressure of 0.79. On-gassing
occurs at different rates among the tissues. Some tissues take up nitrogen
very rapidly, such as the lungs, which become fully saturated after one or
two breaths (a few seconds) at the new ambient pressure. Tissues like ligaments and joint capsules take up nitrogen very slowly, probably requiring
hours to become fully saturated. Muscles and other tissues take up nitrogen
at intermediate and variable rates.

For dive table and computer purposes, individual tissues are not considered.
Rather, the concept of tissue compartments, each with a specific tissue half-
time, is used. The uptake of nitrogen, as well as its elimination, is based on
an exponential (half-time) model describing events that cannot be measured
individually. The **tissue half-time** is the time it will take a particular tissue
to change its nitrogen saturation by 50 percent of the difference between its

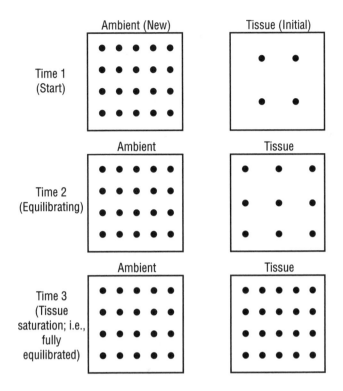

FIGURE 3.2 Tissue saturation (on-gassing) as a function of time at a new ambient pressure. ● represents molecules of nitrogen.

current saturation and the new ambient pressure. For example, a tissue that is saturated at 0.79-ATA partial pressure of nitrogen (room air) is exposed to a new ambient pressure of 1.58-ATA partial pressure of nitrogen. The time it takes to reach a partial pressure of 1.185 ([1.58 – 0.79]/2 = 0.395; 0.395 + 0.79 = 1.185) is its tissue half-time. The fastest tissue half-time (for dive table computation purposes) is 5 minutes. That means that after 5 minutes at the new ambient pressure, the tissue will be half saturated; at 10 minutes, another half or 75 percent; and so on (see table 3.1). Many tissue half-times are used for dive table computation, starting with 5 minutes and continuing to 10, 20, 40, 80 minutes, and so on. For a short, deep dive, the slow tissues will probably not take up enough nitrogen to cause any problems during ascent. The fast tissues, however, may be the limiting factor for the diver's ascent rate. Once the partial pressure of nitrogen in the tissue equals that in the ambient breathing gas, the tissue is said to be equilibrated or **saturated** with the inert gas at the new pressure.

Sequence of On-Gassing

The next question is, how does the inert gas get to the tissues from the outside (ambient) environment? It does so via the lungs and the circulatory

Table 3.1	Tissue Half-Times and Nitrogen On-Gassing (Percent of Tissue Saturation) at New Ambient Pressure				
	Tissue half-time (minutes)				
Time	**5**	**10**	**20**	**40**	**160**
Start	0	0	0	0	0
5	50%	25%	12.5%	6.3%	$\approx 0\ (1/2^{32})$
10	75%	50%	18.75%	9.4%	$\approx 0\ (1/2^{16})$
20	94%	75%	50%	25%	$\approx 0\ (1/2^{8})$
40	99.6%	94%	75%	50%	$6.25\%\ (1/2^{4})$
120	>99.9%	>99.9%	99.6%	94%	50%

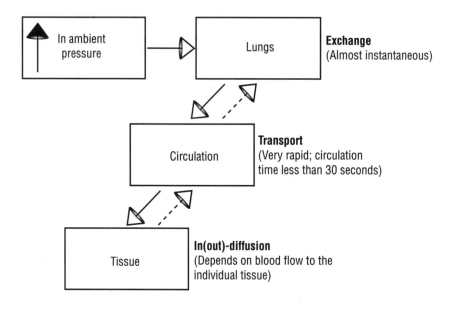

FIGURE 3.3   Sequence of on-gassing and off-gassing. If the ambient pressure increases (solid arrows), tissues on-gas. If it decreases (dashed lines), tissues off-gas.

system (see figure 3.3). Gas at the new ambient pressure is inhaled into the lungs. This tissue becomes saturated with nitrogen after one or two breaths, much faster than the fastest (five minute) tissue half-time used for dive table computations. The gas then diffuses across the exchange surfaces of the lungs (the alveoli) into the bloodstream, which takes about 0.25 second. Gas exchange is also very rapid between the blood and tissues. With a circulation time (the time it takes a blood cell to make one circuit through the body) of less than 25 seconds, blood has a tissue half-time that is much less than five minutes also. The blood, pumped by the heart, transports the physically dissolved nitrogen in the plasma (the liquid portion of the blood that does

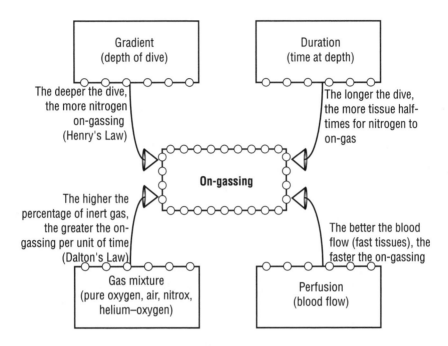

FIGURE 3.4 Factors determining the amount of nitrogen that on-gasses to tissues with increases in ambient pressure.

not include red or white blood cells) to the tissues. Because of the higher concentration of nitrogen in the blood as compared to the tissues, nitrogen diffuses (on-gasses) into the tissues.

Four factors determine how much nitrogen will get to each body tissue during the on-gassing portion of the dive (see figure 3.4):

- **Gradient** refers to the "driving force" for on-gassing. It reflects the difference between the ambient pressure of nitrogen and the tissue partial pressure of nitrogen. For example, at a 16.5-FSW (5-MSW, 1.5-ATA) depth, the gradient to move nitrogen into tissues is minimal at 1.185 ATA. At a 99-FSW (30-MSW, 4-ATA) depth, it is 3.16 ATA or 2.7 times as great. At equilibrium, for dives of the same duration at these depths, 2.7 times more nitrogen would enter the tissues at the deeper depth.

- *Duration* of exposure is the second factor that determines how much nitrogen diffuses into the tissues. For any given depth (i.e., gradient), a shorter time of exposure will result in less nitrogen entering the body's tissues and less chance for equilibration than a longer exposure.

- The composition of the breathing *gas mixture* also determines how rapidly the tissues will on-gas nitrogen. For example, with pure oxygen, no inert gas enters the diver and consequently there is no nitrogen on-gassing. Conversely, if the diver uses closed-circuit, constant oxygen partial pressure

SCUBA gear at depths deeper than the equivalent air depth (see chapter 2), higher nitrogen partial pressures are breathed than during diving with air at the same depth. The result is more nitrogen on-gassing per unit duration of exposure than during diving with air at the same depth. Gradient, duration, and gas mixture are reproducible and measurable; that is, their effects can be calculated precisely using gas laws and the tissue half-time concepts.

• **Perfusion** (blood flow) determines how much nitrogen enters tissues of the body during the on-gassing portion and is the only one of the four major factors that cannot be calculated precisely. Educated guesses must be made for this factor. The tissue half-time concept best explains how much nitrogen enters the tissues from the perfusion factor. On-gassing of nitrogen as a function of perfusion is imprecise because we are never quite sure of the actual blood distribution to the tissues of the body. The reason is that the five-quart (4.7-liter) blood volume in an average-sized human must be distributed through a vascular system that has an estimated potential capacity of about 100 quarts (95 liters). The potential capacity comes from venous compliance (24-fold ability to increase volume); alterations in muscle blood flow; venous reservoirs, sinusoids, and plexuses; arterial elasticity; and arterial–venous shunting. Consequently, the capacity (potential volume) of the vascular system exceeds the actual volume of blood in our bodies by a factor of 100 or more.

To summarize, the amount of on-gassing from the gradient, duration, and gas-mixture factors can be precisely calculated. The perfusion factor is variable and cannot be precisely calculated. This necessitates the use of tissue compartments with different half-times.

Controlling Blood Flow   The blood volume, limited as it is, must be carefully channeled in order to meet the tissues' metabolic needs for oxygen and nutrient delivery and waste removal, according to the tissue. The nervous system does this by controlling the sizes of the blood vessels (narrowing or vasoconstriction, and widening or vasodilatation) and altering the direction of blood flow (arterial–venous shunting). The signals—chemical in nature—that modify blood flow arise from local responses of the tissues to where the blood flows. Critical tissues like the brain and the heart must have constant, high blood flows. Less oxygen-sensitive (noncritical) tissues, like the muscles and the skin, have highly variable blood flows depending upon their metabolic activity. Muscle blood flow can increase 40-fold between rest and maximal exercise. Blood flow for a skin wound may have to increase 20-fold for healing to occur. Ligaments, tendons, joint capsules, and adventitious tissues (those covering and/or connecting nerves, muscles, organs, etc.) have very small requirements for blood flow. If specific tissues were assigned tissue half-times, these would be the slow ones, while the muscles, skin, internal organs, and

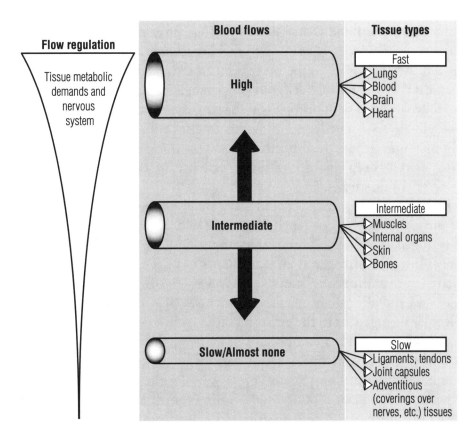

Flow regulation

Tissue metabolic demands and nervous system

Blood flows

High

Intermediate

Slow/Almost none

Tissue types

Fast
▷Lungs
▷Blood
▷Brain
▷Heart

Intermediate
▷Muscles
▷Internal organs
▷Skin
▷Bones

Slow
▷Ligaments, tendons
▷Joint capsules
▷Adventitious (coverings over nerves, etc.) tissues

FIGURE 3.5 Inert gas uptake versus blood flow to tissues. The limited blood volume (in comparison to the potential volume) of the vascular tree must be highly regulated. Blood flows in the intermediate tissues can change 20-fold or more depending on the tissues' metabolic demands.

bones would be the intermediate tissues (in which flow is highly regulated by the tissue's needs). The heart, lungs, brain, and blood would be the fast tissues (see figure 3.5).

Alterations in the finely adjusted blood flow patterns of the body can have serious consequences. For example, if a significant amount of blood is diverted from a critical tissue, such as the brain, to a noncritical tissue, loss of consciousness may occur. When alterations in the usual blood flow to tissues occur in the SCUBA diver, conditions may be set for bubbles to form in the tissues and lead to decompression sickness (see chapter 15). Except with sophisticated laboratory techniques, it is not possible to ascertain how much blood flows to any one tissue at a particular time. Likewise, activity level greatly alters blood flow. For these reasons, tissue half-times are used as a concept in contrast to exact measurements of tissue partial pressures of nitrogen during on-gassing.

Tissue Saturation and Other Factors   The diver is said to be saturated when on-gassing ceases, that is, when the diver's body is fully saturated with nitrogen. All the tissues in the body become saturated at the new ambient pressure if the diver remains at depth long enough, just as all the diver's tissues were fully saturated with nitrogen on the surface before the start of the dive. Once a tissue is saturated, extending the time at depth does not impose any additional nitrogen gas load for the diver. This is the concept of saturation diving, used for deep commercial diving activities, research, and underwater habitat scientific studies.

Other mechanisms may account for a small percentage of the nitrogen that enters the body's tissues, including tissue solubilities, temperature effects, and nitrogen–blood vessel lining interactions. First, fat tissues have five times more affinity for nitrogen than lean tissues have. This is why obesity is a relative contraindication for diving (see chapter 10). Nitrogen may enter the tissues and alter their metabolic processes (see chapter 14), although molecular nitrogen, as in the air we breathe, is not converted to elemental nitrogen, which is a component of many of the organic molecules in our bodies. Second, temperature elevations increase metabolism, which alters blood flow and on-gassing. Finally, molecular nitrogen may interact with the lining of blood vessels. This sets off a series of reactions that cause white blood cells to adhere to the blood vessel linings. The white cells then release toxic chemicals (superoxides and peroxides) that cause cessation of blood flow and tissue death. This sequence of events is termed **reperfusion injury.** This is a separate response from physical blocking of the blood vessel by the nitrogen bubble, but the nitrogen bubble may initiate the white blood cell adherence reaction. For the bubble problem itself, pressurization (i.e., Boyle's Law effect) in a hyperbaric chamber will reduce the size of the bubble and thus allow it to pass more easily through the circulation. The more quickly the bubble is dissipated, the less likely there is to be damage from obstructing circulation and the less chance the reperfusion injury will occur.

Off-Gassing

When a diver ascends, the effects are the opposite of on-gassing. There is a gradient for nitrogen to leave the tissues (i.e., out-gassing) and enter the bloodstream. The bloodstream then transports the nitrogen to the lungs, from which it is eliminated by exhalation to the ambient environment (see figure 3.3). If the partial pressures of nitrogen in the tissues remain below their saturation tensions during ascent, off-gassing is orderly and nitrogen bubbles are not expected to form in the tissues. There are five aspects of off-gassing that influence whether or not bubbles form in the tissues.

Diving Physics: On-Gassing of Nitrogen in a Slow Tissue During Ascent

The application of Boyle's and Dalton's Laws illustrates why tissues can on-gas during ascent (see table 3.2).

Table 3.2 On-Gassing of Nitrogen in a Slow Tissue During Ascent				
Depth in FSW (MSW, ATA)	**Ambient PP of nitrogen (ATA)**	**Nitrogen saturation in the tissue (%)**	**Tissue PP of nitrogen (ATA)**	**Gradient for nitrogen to in- or off-gas (i.e., column 2 minus column 4)**
Original depth: 99 (30 MSW or 4 ATA)	3.2	25	0.8	2.4 ATA (For nitrogen to off-gas from the tissue)
Depth after ascent: 33 (10 MSW or 2 ATA)	1.6	50	0.8*	-0.8 ATA (Nitrogen in-gasses to the tissues)

* Assumes no off-gassing occurs during ascent from 99 to 33 FSW.

First, ascents change the percentage of tissue saturation. If a tissue is 50 percent saturated at 99 FSW (30 MSW or 4 ATA), the amount of nitrogen in that tissue will be equivalent to 100 percent saturation at the 33-FSW (10-MSW or 2-ATA) depth. If the diver were to ascend very rapidly from 99 FSW to less than 33 FSW, the tissue would become more than 100 percent saturated, and bubbles would be expected to form. The ability to off-gas nitrogen is rate limited by perfusion (blood flow) and has two phases: (1) the dissolved gas phase in the tissues and (2) the free gas phase in the blood. The spontaneous formation of bubbles in the tissue phase is termed **autochthonous** (referring to bubbles originating spontaneously in the tissues in which they are found; pronounced aw-TOK-the-ness). The tissues in which the bubbles form produce symptoms of decompression sickness (DCS) such as pain in joints. When gas bubbles in inordinate amounts are present in the free gas phase in the blood, they lead to type 2 (serious) presentations of DCS such as those affecting the brain, spinal cord, and circulation (bends shock syndrome).

Second, while a **fast tissue** is off-gassing during a stop on the diver's ascent, a **slow tissue** may on-gas nitrogen at this same depth. As an example, a slow tissue may become 25 percent saturated at 99-FSW depth. The diver may then decide to spend the rest of his or her bottom time at a 33-FSW depth. The fast tissue will off-gas the nitrogen to the 33-FSW level. However, the slow tissue, being only 50 percent saturated, will on-gas nitrogen because the partial pressure of nitrogen at the 33-FSW depth is 1.6 ATA, while the nitrogen partial pressure in the slow tissue is 0.8 ATA at this depth. As summarized in table 3.2, a gradient of 0.8 ATA would exist for nitrogen to move into the slow tissue.

Halving the depth results in doubling the saturation, but the partial pressures of nitrogen remain the same in the tissue (assuming there is eventually no off-gassing of nitrogen from the slow tissue during the ascent from 99 to 33 FSW).

A third consideration is that the tissue that has the highest saturation may change with each level of the ascent. The tissue that assumes this status at each depth and time is defined as the **critical tissue.** During the initial portion of ascent, the fast tissues (e.g., tissues with half-times of 5, 10, or 20 minutes) are likely to be the critical tissues. After a few minutes at the new ascent level, the percentage of nitrogen saturation drops rapidly, and the slower tissues may become the critical tissues. For long deep dives, especially saturation dives (see chapter 2), the slow tissues become the critical tissues. Two different terms are used for defining the maximum amounts of nitrogen that the tissues can hold before autochthonous bubble formation is likely to occur. These are "tissue saturations," as explained previously, and "M-values." The **M-value** represents the maximum permitted level of supersaturation. The tissue saturation terminology is common in some of the models used in dive computers. The M-values are used in U.S. Navy dive tables and vary with the predicted speed of in- and off-gassing of the inert gas from tissues; being greater than 2:1 ratios for fast tissues and less than 2:1 ratios for slow tissues. Haldane proposed that the ambient pressures can be decreased by one-half without the risk of bubble formation in the tissue. This concept is referred to as the **Haldane 2-to-1 ratio.** Even though these ideas (tissue saturations, M-values, and ratios) are theory, they work well in the context of understanding the inert gas load and formulating ascents for dive computers and dive tables. The few studies available that test these models are in substantial agreement with the theories. The enormous numbers of diving experiences with minimal occurrences of DCS (two to three cases per 10,000 SCUBA dives) substantiate the validity of the theories.

Fourth, it is apparent that tissues, especially fast tissues like the blood, become supersaturated with nitrogen and form bubbles during ascent. This corresponds to bubble formation in the free gas phase in the bloodstream versus the dissolved gas phase in the tissues. Usually these bubbles are harmlessly filtered out in the lungs and exhaled to the ambient environment. In these situations, they are called **silent bubbles.** Silent bubbles are oftentimes detectable by Doppler ultrasound techniques. If the quantity of bubbles overwhelms this portion of the off-gassing process, bubbles move into the left side of the heart (instead of being filtered out in the lungs), causing bends, shock, or other serious presentations of DCS (see chapter 15).

A fifth and final consideration is the bubble evolution itself. Bubbles, once they form, evolve in a predictable fashion. Regardless of the additional knowledge that has been gained since bubbles were first observed during decompression, they remain fundamental to all explanations as to what occurs during a presentation of decompression sickness. Boyle (Boyle's Law) reported witnessing bubble formation in the cornea of a serpent's eye after he rapidly decompressed the snake from a pressurized container. This happened soon after Boyle invented the air pump in 1662. Autochthonous bubble formation is one theory, but many feel that it does not sufficiently explain the observed events. Many feel that bubble genesis takes place in nucleation sites that are microscopic foci of nitrogen, carbon dioxide, or other substances in the blood. These are felt to be ubiquitous with activities and not limited just to decompression. Whether or not they become clinically significant (i.e., cause symptoms of DCS) depends on how nitrogen interacts with them, their location, their growth, their coalescence, and how they interact with tissues (see figure 3.6). Venous gas emboli (detectable bubbles in the

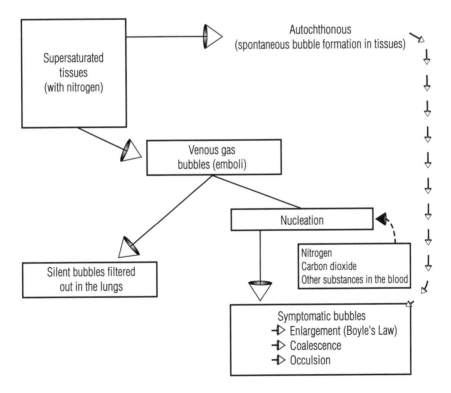

FIGURE 3.6 Bubble evolution. Whereas autochthonous bubble formation may be adequate to account for the less serious (pain only) presentation of DCS, the venous gas emboli–nucleation limb better accounts for the serious presentations such as paralysis and shock.

venous side of the systemic circulation), as mentioned previously, appear to be an almost universal consequence of off-gassing during the ascent phase of diving. Because these venous gas bubbles almost never cause symptoms, the term *silent bubble* is appropriate.

Summary of On-Gassing and Off-Gassing

With ascent, nitrogen off-gasses from tissues as a direct consequence of the decrease in ambient pressure. The increased gas load is transported to the lungs by the blood and exhaled to the ambient environment by the lungs. The factors (gradient, duration, gas mixture, and perfusion) that control on-gassing during the descent and bottom time portions of the dive are directly opposite to those that cause off-gassing during ascent and the surface interval. In contrast to on-gassing, whereby nitrogen can be added to the tissues with seeming impunity, the ability to off-gas nitrogen is rate limited and has two phases: (1) dissolved gas phase (in tissues) and (2) free gas phase (in blood). The consequences of exceeding the rate-limited endpoints of off-gassing in the tissues are autochthonous bubble formation in fixed tissues (joints, etc.) and intravascular (within the blood vessel) bubbles in the free gas, blood phase. During ascent, off-gassing and increased percentages of tissue saturation occur simultaneously (see figure 3.3). The challenge is to ascend at a rate that maximizes off-gassing yet does not allow tissues to exceed 100 percent saturation or their critical M-values.

Rate limitations for eliminating nitrogen are almost entirely a function of the circulation of the blood. For all but the most extreme gradients, off-diffusion of nitrogen from the tissues to the blood and exchange of nitrogen at the lungs with the ambient breathing gas are not rate limiting. In contrast, the venous blood has a limited capacity (rate limitation) for the transport of nitrogen to the lungs in the physically dissolved as well as free gas (silent bubble) states. Off-diffusion of nitrogen from the tissues appears to rely primarily on this rate-limited activity—"primarily" in that several other factors may contribute to the rate limitations. Fat tissue with its fivefold increased solubility for nitrogen as compared to tissue fluids may be one factor. The diffusion rate of nitrogen gas in and out of a bubble, a function of the nitrogen partial pressures inside and outside the bubble, may be another rate limiter. A third factor, especially in deeper dives, is that nitrogen may enter tissues, in addition to the brain, in a fashion similar to the mechanisms proposed for the cause of nitrogen narcosis (see chapter 14).

Outcomes of Decompression

For practical purposes, there are four permutations for the outcome of decompression from SCUBA (or other varieties of compressed gas) diving

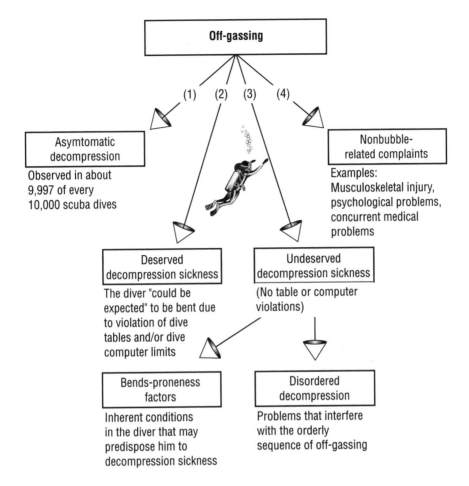

FIGURE 3.7 Outcomes of decompression.

(see figure 3.7). In the majority of SCUBA dives, the off-gassing of nitrogen is orderly, and the diver remains free of symptoms after the dive is completed. This appears to be the case in 9,997 to 9,999 of every 10,000 SCUBA dives. In the other one to three cases, symptoms of DCS develop. These cases are about equally divided between "deserved" and "undeserved" causes. **Deserved decompression sickness,** as its name implies, is attributed to the violation of dive computers or dive tables. However, violation of dive tables or dive computers, or both, does not correlate well with the occurrence of DCS (see "Unorthodox Diving Practices" later in the chapter). Location of symptoms is variable. Bubbling in the peripheral tissues before nitrogen is transported by the bloodstream to the lungs probably leads to pain, numbness and tingling, itching, fatigue symptoms, or some combination of these. If ascents are rapid, symptoms are likely to develop in the fast tissues such as the blood and nervous system. If gas exchange is overwhelmed at the lung level, probably associated with massive decompression or difficulties with ventilation, bubble formation occurs in the lungs and is termed **chokes.**

The other 50 percent of DCS occurrences are **undeserved decompression sicknesses,** meaning that there were no seeming violations of diving practices. In attempts to understand why DCS developed in these cases, we propose two causes: (1) bends-proneness factors and (2) disordered decompression. **Bends-proneness factors,** such as abnormal channeling of blood from the arterial to the venous side of the bloodstream or altered blood flow in scarred tissues from old injuries, are examples of conditions that predispose the diver to DCS. **Disordered decompression** refers to causes of DCS, usually one-time occurrences, that interfere with the orderly off-gassing of nitrogen from the body. As an example, applying a tourniquet to an extremity just before starting to ascend will interfere with the orderly off-gassing of nitrogen in the tissues distal to the extremity. Disordered decompression and bends-proneness factors are further discussed in chapter 15.

Dive Tables

With the background information just presented, the theory behind the dive tables becomes understandable. For each depth range and its time duration, the amount of nitrogen that has on-gassed to the tissue compartments is computed. The tables do not consider individual tissues but instead use the nitrogen saturations in tissues with half-times from 5 minutes to 160 minutes. The nitrogen saturations during ascent are computed at 10-foot (three-meter) increments. For the U.S. Navy tables, the ascents are designed to keep the tissue nitrogen saturations below the M-values, using the Haldane 2-to-1 ratio as the criterion for the maximum safe excursion of the ascent. That is, according to the Haldane ratio, halving the ambient pressure will not exceed the M-value. If the ascent would exceed the tissue saturation or M-value, then a decompression stop is required before the given depth to allow enough nitrogen to off-gas so that these criteria will not be violated.

Other tables are more conservative, using ratios less than 2 to 1. With the Haldane ratio, for example, a fully saturated tissue could be safely brought from the 99-foot (30-meter or 4-ATA) to the 33-foot (10-meter or 2-ATA) level without exceeding the ratio, whereas with a more conservative ratio of 1.8 to 1, the safe excursion would be to 40.3 feet (12.3 meters). When ratios more conservative than 2 to 1 are used, the 10-foot increment guidelines are not altered; rather the time at maximum depth is shortened. With the navy tables, for example, the maximum duration of a 60-foot (18-meter) dive without the need for decompression stops during ascent is 60 minutes.

With more conservative tables (Professional Association of Diving Instructors [PADI] tables), the maximum duration of a no-decompression dive to 60 feet is 50 minutes.

Safety Factors

At least seven safety factors are incorporated into U.S. Navy dive tables (NDT).

• All dive profiles are considered rectangular (see chapter 2). Hence, the maximum depth is considered to be the depth of the entire dive. This profile fits well with dives performed to complete a project at a particular depth, but it is usually not the profile of a sport SCUBA dive. The result is that the tables substantially reduce the "no-decompression" time limits (the period the diver can stay underwater without needing decompression stops) of a multilevel dive.

• When the maximum depth is between two 10-foot (three-meter) levels on the table, the next higher 10-foot depth level is used. For example, a maximum depth of 51 feet (15.5 meters) is considered a 60-foot (18-meter) dive.

• Analogous to the depth adjustment, bottom times are pushed up to the next longer time period on the table.

• Diving is limited to two dives in a 12-hour period.

• If the diver surfaces for less than 10 minutes and then resumes the dive, the surface time is considered part of the bottom time; that is, it is included in the sum of the time spent underwater before surfacing and after surfacing.

• The bottom time is considered the time from leaving the surface to the time of leaving the bottom for the ascent to the surface. If the diver delays descent, for example, because of difficulty clearing his or her ears, this is considered part of the bottom time. Likewise, the ascent is not intended to be interrupted by staying at shallower depths (except as required for decompression stops) as might be done with multilevel diving.

• After a dive is completed, the diver is assigned a residual nitrogen time. The **residual nitrogen time** is designated as a letter. The further down the alphabet, the more residual nitrogen in the diver's tissues. With time on the surface (surface interval), nitrogen is further off-gassed, and the letter designation moves toward the beginning of the alphabet. When the diver starts a second dive within a 12-hour period, the residual nitrogen is added to the bottom time. Even though this shortens the no-decompression time, it keeps the tissue saturations below the critical M-values during ascent from the second dive.

Risks of Dive Tables

Just as safety factors are incorporated into the NDT, use of the NDT has inherent risks as well. Consider the following:

• Only six tissue half-times from 5 minutes to 160 minutes are used. Faster tissues such as the lungs probably have much shorter half-times and slower tissues much longer ones. The rest stop at 15 feet (4.6 meters) for three minutes, to add an additional degree of protection from bubbling in fast tissues, is not a requirement of the NDT (but is strongly recommended).

• A 12-hour surface interval is probably too short for complete elimination of all residual nitrogen in the tissues.

• The tables are based on tissue nitrogen saturations only, without consideration for the free gas (silent bubble) phase in the bloodstream. Tissue half-times of less than five minutes would be needed to account for nitrogen in these very fast tissues.

• The tables were designed and tested for healthy, well-conditioned, young military men, who were paid to dive, which does not represent the spectrum of sport SCUBA divers.

• The ascent rate of one foot (0.3 meter) per second is twice the rate of current recommendations. If older editions of the NDT are used, the 60-foot-per-minute ascent is used. Newer versions of the tables, as included in this chapter, have ascent rates of 30 feet per minute.

• There are no provisions for interruptions during ascent (as is done with multilevel diving profiles), during which the slower tissues may accumulate nitrogen and become the critical tissues.

• Surveys indicate that the majority of sport SCUBA divers are not familiar enough with the NDT to use them correctly.

• The NDT are not adaptable for nitrox or rebreather gas mixtures; separate tables are required for these mixtures.

• The maximum depth and bottom time limits must be decided before the dive.

Use of Navy Dive Tables

The best way to understand how to use the NDT is to work through a few simple problems. The sport SCUBA diver must become familiar with a minimum of three tables in order to work out problems using this system: (1) "Unlimited, No-Decompression Limits and Repetitive Group Designation Table for Unlimited, No-Decompression Air Dives" (table 3.3), (2) a composite "Residual Nitrogen Timetable for Repetitive Air Dives" (table 3.4), and (3) "U.S. Navy Standard Air Decompression Table" (table 3.5).

Table 3.3 — Unlimited, No-Decompression Limits and Repetitive Group Designation Table for Unlimited, No-Decompression Air Dives

Depth (feet/meters)	No-Decompression limits (min)	A	B	C	D	E	F	G	H	I	J	K	L	M	N	O
10 3.0	Unlimited	60	120	210	300	797	*									
15 4.6	Unlimited	35	70	110	160	225	350	452	*							
20 6.1	Unlimited	25	50	75	100	135	180	240	325	390	917	*				
25 7.6	595	20	35	55	75	100	125	160	195	245	315	361	540	595		
30 9.1	405	15	30	45	60	75	95	120	145	170	205	250	310	344	405	
35 10.7	310	5	15	25	40	50	60	80	100	120	140	160	190	220	270	310
40 12.2	200	5	15	25	30	40	50	70	80	100	110	130	150	170	200	
50 15.2	100		10	15	25	30	40	50	60	70	80	90	100			
60 18.2	60		10	15	20	25	30	40	50	55	60					
70 21.3	50		5	10	15	20	30	35	40	45	50					
80 24.4	40		5	10	15	20	25	30	35	40						
90 27.4	30		5	10	12	15	20	25	30							
100 30.5	25		5	7	10	15	20	22	25							
110 33.5	20			5	10	13	15	20								
120 36.6	15			5	10	12	15									
130 39.6	10			5	8	10										
140 42.7	10			5	7	10										
150 45.7	5			5												
160 48.8	5				5											
170 51.8	5				5											
180 54.8	5				5											
190 59.9	5				5											

* Highest repetitive group that can be achieved at this depth regardless of bottom time.
Reprinted, by permission, from United States Navy/Best Publishing Company, 1993, *US Navy diving manual*, vol. 1 (Falgstaff, AZ: Best Publishing Company), 7-35.

Table 3.4 Residual Nitrogen Timetable for Repetitive Air Dives

Locate the diver's repetitive group designation from his previous dive along the diagonal line above the table. Read horizontally to the interval in which the diver's surface interval lies.

Next, read vertically downward to the new repetitive group designation. Continue downward in this same column to the row which represents the depth of the repetitive dive. The time given at the intersection is residual nitrogen time, in minutes, to be applied to the repetitive dive.

* Dives following surface intervals of more than 12 hours are not repetitive dives. Use actual bottom times in the Standard Air Decompression Tables to compute decompression for such dives.

** If no Residual Nitrogen Time is given, then the repetitive group does not change.

Repetitive group at the beginning of the surface interval

Repetitive group	Z	O	N	M	L	K	J	I	H	G	F	E	D	C	B	A
A																0:10 12:00*
B															0:10 3:20	3:21 12:00*
C														0:10 1:39	1:40 4:49	4:50 12:00*
D													0:10 1:09	1:10 2:38	2:39 5:48	5:49 12:00*
E												0:10 0:54	0:55 1:57	1:58 3:24	3:25 6:34	6:35 12:00*
F											0:10 0:45	0:46 1:29	1:30 2:28	2:29 3:57	3:58 7:05	7:06 12:00*
G										0:10 0:40	0:41 1:15	1:16 1:59	2:00 2:58	2:59 4:25	4:26 7:35	7:36 12:00*
H									0:10 0:36	0:37 1:06	1:07 1:41	1:42 2:23	2:24 3:20	3:21 4:49	4:50 7:59	8:00 12:00*
I								0:10 0:33	0:34 0:59	1:00 1:29	1:30 2:02	2:03 2:44	2:45 3:43	3:44 5:12	5:13 8:21	8:22 12:00*
J							0:10 0:31	0:32 0:54	0:55 1:19	1:20 1:47	1:48 2:20	2:21 3:04	3:05 4:02	4:03 5:40	5:41 8:50	8:51 12:00*
K						0:10 0:28	0:29 0:49	0:50 1:11	1:12 1:35	1:36 2:03	2:04 2:38	2:39 3:21	3:22 4:19	4:20 5:48	5:49 8:58	8:59 12:00*
L					0:10 0:26	0:27 0:45	0:46 1:04	1:05 1:25	1:26 1:49	1:50 2:19	2:20 2:53	2:54 3:36	3:37 4:35	4:36 6:02	6:03 9:12	9:13 12:00*
M				0:10 0:25	0:26 0:42	0:43 0:59	1:00 1:18	1:19 1:35	1:36 2:05	2:06 2:34	2:35 3:08	3:09 3:52	3:53 4:49	4:50 6:18	6:19 9:28	9:29 12:00*
N			0:10 0:24	0:25 0:39	0:40 0:54	0:55 1:11	1:12 1:30	1:31 1:53	1:54 2:18	2:19 2:47	2:48 3:22	3:23 4:04	4:05 5:03	5:04 6:32	6:33 9:43	9:44 12:00*
O		0:10 0:23	0:24 0:36	0:37 0:51	0:52 1:07	1:08 1:24	1:25 1:43	1:44 2:04	2:05 2:29	2:30 2:59	3:00 3:33	3:34 4:17	4:18 5:16	5:17 6:44	6:45 9:54	9:55 12:00*
Z	0:10 0:22	0:23 0:34	0:35 0:48	0:49 1:02	1:03 1:18	1:19 1:36	1:37 1:55	1:56 2:17	2:18 2:42	2:43 3:10	3:11 3:45	3:46 4:29	4:30 5:27	5:28 6:56	6:57 10:05	10:06 12:00*

NEW GROUP DESIGNATION

Repetitive dive depth feet	meters	Z	O	N	M	L	K	J	I	H	G	F	E	D	C	B	A
10	3.0	**	**	**	**	**	**	**	**	**	**	**	797	279	159	88	39
20	6.1	**	**	**	**	**	**	917	399	279	208	159	120	88	62	39	18
30	9.1	†	†	469	349	279	229	190	159	132	109	88	70	54	39	25	12
40	12.2	257	241	213	187	161	138	116	101	87	73	61	49	37	25	17	7
50	15.2	169	160	142	124	111	99	87	76	66	56	47	38	29	21	13	6
60	18.2	122	117	107	97	88	79	70	61	52	44	36	30	24	17	11	5
70	21.3	100	96	87	80	72	64	57	50	43	37	31	26	20	15	9	4
80	24.4	84	80	73	68	61	54	48	43	38	32	28	23	18	13	8	4
90	27.4	73	70	64	58	53	47	43	38	33	29	24	20	16	11	7	3
100	30.5	64	62	57	52	48	43	38	34	30	26	22	18	14	10	7	3
110	33.5	57	55	51	47	42	38	34	31	27	24	20	16	13	10	6	3
120	36.6	52	50	46	43	39	35	32	28	25	21	18	15	12	9	6	3
130	39.6	46	44	40	38	35	31	28	25	22	19	16	13	11	8	6	3
140	42.7	42	40	38	35	32	29	26	23	20	18	15	12	10	7	5	2
150	45.7	40	38	35	32	30	27	24	22	19	17	14	12	9	7	5	2
160	48.8	37	36	33	31	28	26	23	20	18	16	13	11	9	6	4	2
170	51.8	35	34	31	29	26	24	22	19	17	15	13	10	8	6	4	2
180	54.8	32	31	29	27	25	22	20	18	16	14	12	10	8	6	4	2
190	59.9	31	30	28	26	24	21	19	17	15	13	11	10	8	6	4	2

Residual nitrogen times (Minutes)

† Read vertically downward to the 40/12.2 (feet/meter) repetitive dive depth. Use the corresponding residual nitrogen times (minutes) to compute the equivalent single dive time. Decompress using the 40/12.2 (feet/meter) standard air decompression table.

Reprinted, by permission, from United States Navy/Best Publishing Company, 1993, *US Navy diving manual*, vol. 1 (Falgstaff, AZ: Best Publishing Company), 7-36.

Table 3.5 U.S. Navy Standard Air Decompression Table

Depth feet/meters	Bottom time (min)	Time first stop (min:sec)	Decompression stops (feet/meters) 50 15.2	40 12.1	30 9.1	20 6.0	10 3.0	Total decompression time (min:sec)	Repetitive group
40 / **12.1**	200						0	1:20	*
	210	1:00					2	3:20	N
	230	1:00					7	8:20	N
	250	1:00					11	12:20	O
	270	1:00					15	16:20	O
	300	1:00					19	20:20	Z
			Exceptional Exposure						
	360	1:00					23	24:20	**
	480	1:00					41	42:20	**
	720	1:00					69	70:20	**
50 / **15.2**	100						0	1:40	*
	110	1:20					3	4:40	L
	120	1:20					5	6:40	M
	140	1:20					10	11:40	M
	160	1:20					21	22:40	N
	180	1:20					29	30:40	O
	200	1:20					35	36:40	O
	220	1:20					40	41:40	Z
	240	1:20					47	48:40	Z
60 / **18.2**	60						0	2:00	*
	70	1:40					2	4:00	K
	80	1:40					7	9:00	L
	100	1:40					14	16:00	M
	120	1:40					26	28:00	N
	140	1:40					39	41:00	O
	160	1:40					48	50:00	Z
	180	1:40					56	58:00	Z
	200	1:20				1	69	72:00	Z
			Exceptional Exposure						
	240	1:20				2	79	83:00	**
	360	1:20				20	119	141:00	**
	480	1:20				44	148	194:00	**
	720	1:20				78	187	267:00	**
70 / **21.3**	50						0	2:20	*
	60	2:00					8	10:20	K
	70	2:00					14	16:20	L
	80	2:00					18	20:20	M
	90	2:00					23	25:20	N
	100	2:00					33	35:20	N
	110	1:40				2	41	45:20	O
	120	1:40				4	47	53:20	O
	130	1:40				6	52	60:20	O
	140	1:40				8	56	66:20	Z
	150	1:40				9	61	72:20	Z
	160	1:40				13	72	87:20	Z
	170	1:40				19	79	100:20	Z

* See No Decompression Table for repetitive groups
** Repetitive dives may not follow exceptional exposure dives

Reprinted, by permission, from United States Navy/Best Publishing Company, 1993, *US Navy diving manual*, vol. 1 (Falgstaff, AZ: Best Publishing Company), 7-3.

For the following scenarios, it is assumed that the diver precisely follows the NDT without consideration for a rest stop or the new 30-foot- (9.1-meter) per-minute ascent rate.

DIVING SCENARIOS

SCENARIO 1

A sport SCUBA diver wants to know the maximum duration at 60 feet (18 meters) for the first dive of the day without having to stop for decompression during the ascent.

Answer: From the table "Unlimited/No-Decompression Limits and Repetitive Group Designation Table for Unlimited/No-Decompression Air Dives" (table 3.3), the maximum bottom time for a 60-FSW dive is 60 minutes. When the diver completes the dive, "J" amount of residual nitrogen remains in the diver's tissues. (Note: This is the dive table designation for the amount of nitrogen yet to off-gas in the diver's most critical tissue [that is, the compartment that has the highest saturation] at the time the dive is complete.)

SCENARIO 2

After a one-hour surface interval, how long can the diver stay at 60 FSW, having a residual nitrogen time "J" at the end of the first dive?

Answer: Five steps and two tables are required! First, "J" is entered on the "Residual Nitrogen Timetable for Repetitive Air Dives" (table 3.4), and the horizontal row is followed to the right until it intercepts the time range (0:55 to 1:19 hours:minutes) in which one hour lies. Second, this line is then followed vertically downward (move down the column) to give the new (i.e., after the one-hour surface interval) residual nitrogen time letter designator "H." This means the diver has off-gassed two alphabet letters (J to H) of nitrogen during the surface interval. Remember, the closer to the beginning of the alphabet, the less residual nitrogen in the tissues. Third, the time equivalent of "H" amount of residual nitrogen, 52 minutes, is found for the 60-FSW depth. (Note: This means that the diver has 52 minutes of remaining nitrogen before starting a second dive to the 60-FSW depth after a one-hour surface interval.) Fourth, look at table 3.3 ("Unlimited/No-Decompression Limits and Repetitive Group Designation Table for Unlimited/No-Decompression Air Dives") and find the maximum no-decompression time for a dive to 60 FSW, which is 60 minutes. Fifth, the 52-minute residual nitrogen time is subtracted from the 60-minute no-decompression time to give an 8-minute bottom time for the second dive to 60 feet.

SCENARIO 3

Upon learning that only an eight-minute bottom time is allowed for a second dive to 60 FSW, the diver decides to limit the maximum depth of the second dive to 50 FSW (15 MSW). What will be the no-decompression time?

Answer: The first three steps are the same as those described for scenario 2. With "H" amount of residual nitrogen, the "Residual Nitrogen Timetable for Repetitive Air Dives" (table 3.4) is reentered. For a dive to a maximum depth of 50 FSW, the residual nitrogen time is 66 minutes. This number subtracted from 100 minutes (the maximum no-decompression time limit for a 50-foot dive; see table 3.3) allows a 34-minute no-decompression bottom time at this shallower depth. (Note: By going to a shallower depth for the second dive, the diver gains an additional 26 minutes of bottom time [i.e., 34 minutes for 50 FSW vs. 8 minutes for 60 FSW].)

SCENARIO 4

The SCUBA diver decides to spend 60 minutes at the 50-FSW depth on the initial dive and then dive to 60 FSW after a one-hour surface interval to the endpoint of the no-decompression limit. What would the no-decompression bottom time be for the second dive?

Answer: At the end of a 60-minute dive at 50 FSW, the residual nitrogen time would be letter "H." After the one-hour surface interval, the new residual nitrogen designator is "G." The residual nitrogen time at the "G" level for a 60-foot dive is 44 minutes. This means that the no-decompression limit for the second dive would be 16 minutes (i.e., 60-minute no-decompression time at 60-FSW depth minus 44 minutes of residual nitrogen time). Note: This is an example of a reverse dive profile, in which a subsequent dive of the day is deeper than the first. Compared to the no-decompression time for the previous example (scenario 2), the no-decompression time for this scenario is 18 minutes shorter (34 minutes for the previous scenario vs. 16 minutes). Although reverse profile dives were considered anathema a few years ago, with dive computers they seem to be gaining acceptance as a routine for repetitive (same day) dives.

SCENARIO 5

The sport SCUBA diver decides to violate the no-decompression stop rule and stay at 60 feet for 60 minutes for the second dive (conducted after an hour surface interval), realizing the need for decompression stop(s) during ascent. What decompression stop(s) will be required?

Answer: The new dive time in terms of nitrogen loading in the tissues is the sum of the 52 minutes of residual nitrogen time from the first dive plus the 60 minutes of bottom time for the second dive, for a total of 112 minutes. The "U.S. Navy Standard Air Decompression Table" (table 3.5) is required. For a depth of 60 feet, the bottom time that is next greater than 112 minutes is 120 minutes. The table directs that a 26-minute decompression stop be done at 10 FSW (3 MSW) before surfacing.

Admonitions About Planning Dives With Decompression Stops

Sport divers are advised to plan dives that do not require decompression stops. Although decompression stops may seemingly be easy to do in clear, calm waters, challenges can arise. These include exhausting the SCUBA tank air supply before decompression is completed, the need to maintain prescribed depths (swells and surges can accidentally bring the diver to the surface), hypothermia associated with inactivity, the need for an anchor line to maintain position, and depth control and buoyancy problems due to increasingly positive buoyancy as the air in the SCUBA tank is depleted. To meet these contingencies, as in commercial diving activities, a surface support crew with placement of a diving stage in the water, surface-supplied air, heavy-duty exposure suits, and a means of communication between the divers and the surface, if not absolutely required, are highly recommended.

SCENARIO 6

Extending the no-decompression stop bottom time for scenario 2, the diver still desires to return to the 60-foot depth but for longer than an eight-minute safe bottom time

(continued)

(continued)

while not violating the sport diver no-decompression stop rule. What suggestions can be given to the diver to meet these objectives?

Answer: The easiest solution is to increase the surface interval time. For example, if the diver extended the surface interval to six hours, the new residual nitrogen designator would be "B" rather than "H." With a "B" residual nitrogen letter, the diver would have an 11-minute residual nitrogen time for a 60-foot dive. The no-decompression bottom time would then be 49 minutes (i.e., 60-minute no-decompression time minus the 11-minute residual nitrogen time). If the diver extended the surface interval to over 12 hours, the second dive would be considered a new day's dive according to the NDT, and the full 60 minutes could be spent at the 60-foot level. A few techniques, such as breathing pure oxygen on the surface, using nitrox mixtures, performing light exercise, or rebreather diving with oxygen partial pressures greater than 0.21 ATA, could also add to the "safe" bottom time for the second dive. Unfortunately, at present, our knowledge is limited as to how to use these latter techniques and what their effects are on tissue nitrogen saturations after an initial air dive. With the development of tissue sensors for nitrogen that have practical applications for the diver, this information may be forthcoming.

Other Diving Tables

Other navy dive tables (see table 3.6) have special applications but are not likely to be used by the sport SCUBA diver. Other countries, as well as different diving certification agencies, have also developed their own tables. These utilize the concepts described earlier in this chapter but tend to alter the Haldane 2-to-1 ratio such that they are either more or less conservative (e.g., by limiting the no-decompression time as compared to the NDT for a 60-FSW (18-MSW) dive to less than 60 minutes, or by extending the time to greater than 60 minutes). The majority of sport divers do not use dive tables. They use their dive computers or rely on the diving guide and the dive supervisor, or do both, to keep them from having "bubble trouble." From the examples presented in the previous section, it is apparent that the use of dive tables, although not complex, can be tedious and subject to errors, such as misreading a number or jumping a line in a matrix of numbers. With all the choices of dive tables that are available, it is apparent that no single table is right for everyone. The fact that there are so many choices indicates that the algorithms (variations of the Haldane 2-to-1 and M-values/tissue saturations) used for the tables belong to the realm of art as much as science. The reason is that the critical factor of blood flow (perfusion) to the tissues is so variable.

Dive Computer

The dive computer has done more to change sport diving than anything else since the development of the SCUBA regulator. Whereas the regulator

Table 3.6	Examples of Other Dive Tables		
Name	**Purpose**	**Depth range in FSW (MSW)**	**Comments**
Equivalent air depth	Nitrox diving	36 to 167 (11 to 51)	For nitrox mixtures from 28% to 40%; from the equivalent air depth, standard air decompression tables are used.
Exceptional exposure	Deep air dives	40 to 300 (12 to 91)	Less than 10% incidence of decompression sickness. A 300-FSW dive for 180 min requires 19 hr and 20 min of decompression!
Nitrox (enriched air nitrox-32 and nitrox-36)	Standard nitrox mixtures	15 to 130 (4.6 to 40)	Similar in format to navy diving tables; includes surface interval and residual nitrogen times.
Saturation	Shallow-water versus deep-water research studies and commercial activities	Usually 60 (18) or less for marine biology studies	For deeper saturation dives, ascent rates may be 1 ft every 15 min with daily rest stops for 6 to 12 hr.
Standard helium	Deep surface-supplied helium–oxygen diving	40 to 380 (12 to 116)	Oxygen partial pressure range from 15% to 55%.
Surface decompression	Allow about 2/3 of the decompression to be done out of water	40 to 190 (12 to 58)	Transfer to surface decompression chamber at either the 20- or 10-ft water stop; oxygen or air alternatives; surface intervals must be less than 5 min.

has allowed us to mediate the ventilation stresses of sport diving, the dive computer has allowed us to radically change our concepts about repetitive, multilevel, and multiday diving. With the dive computer, we feel comfortable diving three, four, or more times a day while making deep, brief depth excursions without having to adhere to the severe diving time restrictions of a rectangular dive profile. The rectangular dive profile has all but become an anachronism for the sport SCUBA diver, who likely changes depths continuously during the dive. Furthermore, with the recognition that the five-minute tissue half-time is too long a time period to use to describe the dynamics of nitrogen off-gassing, transport (free gas phase), and exchange in the very fast tissues, tissue half-times of two and one-half minutes, and even one minute, are utilized in the algorithms of the later-generation dive computers. The consequences of this recognition are the recommendations for slowing ascent rates, from one foot (0.3 meter) a second to one foot every two seconds and the incorporation of a three-minute rest stop at the 15-FSW (4.6-MSW) depth for every dive.

Dive computers rely on the same theories that are used in constructing dive tables. The majority are based on the Haldane tissue saturation model. This model, of course, considers only tissue saturation. Some computers also take into consideration the free gas formation that occurs in the bloodstream as venous gas emboli (silent bubbles). This adds an additional margin of protection from DCS. Using ambient pressure ratios less than Haldane's 2-to-1 ratio offers additional protection. The disadvantage of using these safety factors is that they shorten the no-decompression (nonstop) bottom times. For the rectangular dive profile, this can substantially limit bottom time. However, for the multilevel dive profile, as most commonly used by the sport SCUBA diver, the advantages of the dive computer compensate for the shortened bottom times, the slower ascent rate, and the three-minute 15-FSW rest stop. The net result is longer times underwater and more dives per day.

Advantages and Limitations of the Dive Computer

The advantages of the dive computer include the following:

- The dive computer measures the actual time spent at each depth. Consequently, if the diver spends only a couple of minutes at the maximum depth, the dive computer records on-gassing only for that period of time.

- It uses actual times and depths rather than rounding upward to the next time segment and deeper depth increment as required with the use of the dive tables. The upward-rounding, although a safety factor, further limits the bottom times when one is using the dive tables.

- In most cases the dive computer has built-in alarms to signal the diver that the ascent rate is greater than one foot (0.3 meter) every two seconds.

- It provides additional versatility to the dive plan. If the diver deviates from the original dive plan, for example, by making a bounce descent for an inspection or gear retrieval, the computer accounts for this depth excursion. With the dive tables, new bottom times would need to be computed. To do so while underwater not only would be cumbersome, especially for a second dive (see scenario 2), but also would violate the dictum that dive table computations should not be done when breathing compressed gases.

- The computer also indicates when a diver is approaching the point when a decompression stop will be required, the "yellow" zone, as well as the time and depth for which actual stops are needed, the "red" zone. The diver should not ascend further until the computer readout is no longer in the red zone. In association with this information, some dive computers signal the diver when to begin the 15-FSW (4.6-MSW) rest stop and count down the time until it is over.

- Some dive computers also have personal adjustment modes to alter the bottom times and depth limits to make them more or less conservative. The diver adjusts these based upon fitness, age, diving experience, and so on.

- Most dive computers also have indicators to show when it is safe to fly after SCUBA diving.

- Some dive computers have modes that may be used for altitude diving and mixed-gas diving.

- The dive computer utilizes a wider spectrum of tissue compartments than the NDT. Some computers make computations for as many as nine compartments, whereas the NDT use six.

The dive computer also has some limitations, and reliance upon the computer does not ensure protection against DCS. In about half the recorded cases of DCS in which dive computers were used, the computers did not indicate violations in ascent rates and decompression. The dive computer's main limitation, as with the dive tables, is that it cannot account for alterations in blood flow (perfusion) to different tissues. For example, increased activity associated with an emergency while underwater may change blood flow to the critical tissues and alter the expected on- and off-gassing rates. Likewise, the computer is unable to account for the effects of blood vessel blockages, tissue injury, tissue compression (e.g., from constricting bands from exposure suits), obstruction of circulation from falling asleep in a contorted position during the surface interval, changes in hemoconcentration (thickening of blood), changes in blood composition, or possible reactions of blood vessel walls with the nitrogen bubbles.

Other Considerations Regarding Dive Computers

Other features that dive computers of the future might consider include the diver's age, diving experience, level of fitness, pre-dive status (in terms of hydration, alcohol use, fatigue, circadian [sleep] rhythm alterations, new injuries, residuals of old injuries, medication usage, and so on), the challenges of the dive such as work effort and coldness of the water, and anticipated activity level after the dive. Exercise activity during ascent and after a dive may have mixed benefits. On the positive side, it increases blood flow to muscles and joints, accelerating the off-gassing of nitrogen from these tissues.

Negative effects include the production of waste products that may act as bubble nucleation sites and the shunting of blood from other tissues, which would adversely affect their ability to transport their off-gassed nitrogen.

Dive computers require familiarity to be used safely and effectively. The main components are the computer chip with its embedded algorithm and ability to integrate time and pressure inputs, a pressure (depth) sensor, a timekeeping device, and a readout dial. With mode and operation adjustments, a single wrist-sized dive computer can contain as many as 50 different types of input and readout/output information. Another very desirable feature is the ability of dive computers to transfer information to personal computers (see figure 3.8). From the transferred dive profile information, tissue saturations for any point in the dive (e.g., at the beginning and at the end of the dive as in the figure), maximum depths, average depths, gas consumption, water temperature, and surface intervals can be recorded. In addition, a variety of inputs such as dive site, purpose of the dive, weather conditions, and visibility can be added to the record. As with other diving equipment, there are many options for purchasing dive computers. Prices can range from $250 to over $1,000.

Other features that add to the versatility and costs of dive computers include the following:

- Number of readouts
- Alarm systems for maximum depth, dive duration, ascents, and 15-foot (4.6-meter) rest stop
- Compactness
- Size of memory (i.e., the number of dives the computer can contain in its storage capacity)
- Ability to interface with a personal computer
- Ability to adjust for diver skill
- Modes for altitude and mixed-gas diving
- Readout for remaining air supply duration based on gas consumption rate and depth
- Backlighting for night diving
- Remote (hoseless) monitoring of tank air pressure

Unorthodox Diving Practices

Several noteworthy unorthodox diving practices have evolved that seem contrary to the principles we have discussed regarding prevention of complica-

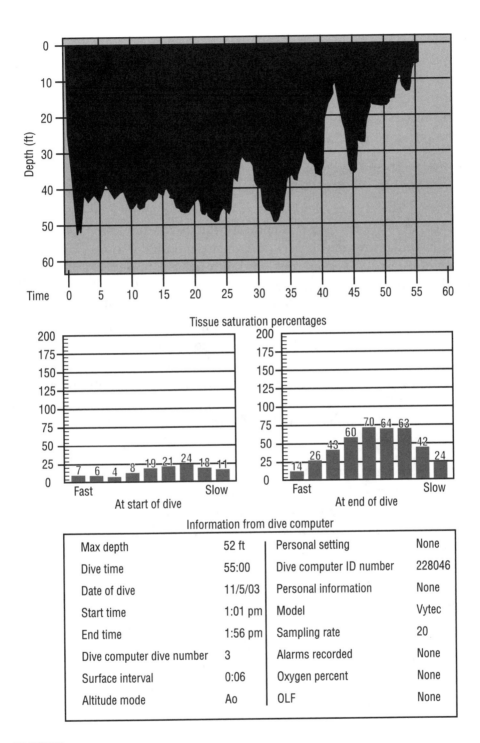

FIGURE 3.8 Computer printout of multilevel dive. At the start of the dive, compartment seven (from fast to slow) was the critical tissue with a 24% saturation level. At the end of the dive, compartment five was the critical tissue with a 70% saturation level.

tions of the inert gas load. In these situations, decompression schedules have been determined empirically, that is, by experience rather than science. The driving force for these practices has been economic. The divers developed their diving practices to gain as much bottom time as possible to collect pearls, black coral, and food products while minimizing "lost" time spent decompressing from these dives.

Okinawa Pearl Divers

Incredible diving profiles are done by divers from Okinawa seeking pearls off the coastal waters of northern Australia. Their profiles include repetitive air dives to 300-FSW (91-MSW) depths for summated durations, as long as an hour, twice daily, six days a week, over many-month durations. Such diving practices using NDT would require hours of decompression each day. To avoid these decompression requirements, the divers use deeper decompression stops and shorter decompression times. If DCS develops, the diver returns to a 30-FSW (9.1-MSW) depth and breathes pure oxygen for 30 minutes at this depth if the symptoms are mild and for an hour if the symptoms are severe. The effects of pressure, to reduce bubble size, and of oxygen, to wash out the nitrogen, complement each other. The immediate institution of these interventions appears to prevent permanent tissue damage from blockage of circulation by the bubble, as well as the interaction of the bubble with the lining of the blood vessel.

Diver Fishermen of Hawaii

The diver fishermen of Hawaii have developed similar diving practices. They may make as many as a dozen dives a day with the deepest depths greater than 350 FSW (107 MSW). Each succeeding dive is at a shallower depth. The last three to four dives are made at depths less than 60 FSW (18 MSW). Comparisons from computations with NDT indicate that these divers may omit as many as four hours of decompression time each day with their dive profiles. These divers also have developed their own techniques to manage DCS. If symptoms appear, divers are immediately returned to the water and taken to a depth where symptoms are relieved. Air is used as the breathing medium. From the depth of relief, the divers are gradually brought to the surface. From personal communications we have learned that when a diver is stricken with quadriplegia (total body paralysis), a regulator is placed in his mouth and he is pulled downward by a diving buddy to whatever depth is necessary to relieve the symptoms. From this depth, the diver is gradually brought to the surface. While these techniques have proven effective, reports from Hawaiian recompression chamber facilities show that some divers have residual symptoms and require conventional treatment in a recompression chamber.

Bends Resistance Factors

Just as factors described previously are known to increase the likelihood that DCS will occur, other factors, in addition to the diving profiles, may contribute to the Okinawan and Hawaiian divers' **bends resistance.** These factors include the following:

• Male sex: Some observations suggest that the incidence of DCS is slightly increased in females, in both divers and inside tenders for hyperbaric oxygen treatments.

• Diving in warm waters: Warm water diving is not as stressful on the body's heat-conserving mechanisms. It does not require as much (or any) thermal protective gear or the extra weight to keep the diver neutrally buoyant while wearing the protective gear (see chapter 7).

• Young age: With increasing age the ability to perform athletic feats decreases. These changes are multifactorial and include decrease in cardiac reserves, circulation efficiency, oxygen diffusion into tissues, time available for conditioning, lifestyle (e.g., walking to classes as a college student might vs. being chauffeured to all one's activities as might be the case for an executive), gain in weight, decreases in muscle strength and joint mobility.

• Experience: With repeated diving experiences, efficiency and improvement in gas consumption and energy expenditures are noted. This may reduce on-gassing to tissues such as muscles and joints that are required for activity.

• Race (Indo-Pacific origins): Just as some races seem adapted to heat exposure and running performance, persons of Indo-Pacific origins may have racial adaptations for bends protection.

• Prophylactic use of aspirin: Aspirin prevents red blood cells from sticking together. This may afford protection from DCS since the opposite effect, sludging, is associated with this medical problem of diving. Also, aspirin may decrease the inflammatory response of nitrogen bubbles and the linings of the blood vessels.

• Conditioning: Conditioning improves dive performance by generating lower oxygen deficits, providing more energy reserves for the stresses of diving, decreasing the time for recovery, and improving the efficiency of off-gassing.

Probabilistic Modeling

Although much is known about the inert gas load and the various ways to effectively deal with it, bends cannot be prevented in all situations. Evolving techniques, such as slower ascent rates and rest stops, have lessened the chances of the occurrence of bends. A day's rest after several days of repetitive diving or before flying is another measure for preventing DCS. The dive computer adds a new dimension for extending the underwater time for multilevel dives, thereby eliminating the constraints of the rectangular dive profile.

With the recognition that DCS has a certain probability of occurrence, the U.S. Navy has developed the concept of "probabilistic modeling." For no-decompression dives or those dives with minimal decompression, the predictable incidence of DCS is less than 2.5 percent. For dives with longer decompression requirements, the incidence is less than 5 percent. For dives with exceptional exposures and long decompression time requirements, the probabilistic modeling incidence is 10 percent. While these numbers seem higher than the incidence rates (two to three cases per 10,000 SCUBA dives) reported for DCS in the sport diver, they support the observations that shallower, no-stop dive limits are safer than deeper dives that require decompression stops.

For Further Review

1. What is meant by the inert gas load in diving? Why is it a concern to the diver only during the ascent, surface interval phase of the dive?

2. What factors determine the amount of on-gassing that occurs in a diver?

3. Why is the concept of tissue compartments, rather than the actual measurements of nitrogen in the tissues, used for constructing dive tables?

4. What is meant by the term "critical tissue"? Why may different tissues become the critical tissue during ascent?

5. Why could one diver get bent (DCS) while the dive buddy (diving the same profile) remains free of symptoms?

6. What is meant by "bends-proneness" and "disordered decompression" factors? Give examples.

7. What safety factors are inherent in the use of dive tables? What disadvantages are there to use of these tables?

8. What are the advantages of using the dive computer?

9. Why do divers get bent (DCS) even though they have not violated the dive computer or the dive table?

10. What is "probabilistic modeling"?

11. What are some of the ramifications of nitrogen off-gassing in the "dissolved gas" and the "free gas" phases during ascent?

12. Describe how "unorthodox" diving practices differ from practices using the dive computer and dive tables.

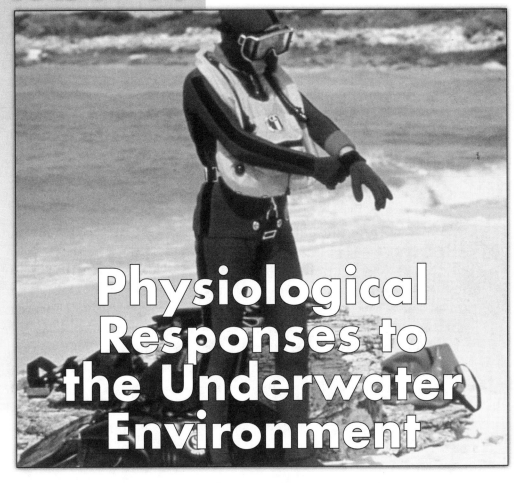

PART II

Physiological Responses to the Underwater Environment

Diving mammals are remarkably adapted to the underwater environment. The human diver's responses to this environment are of several types:

- Physiological—automatic adjustments that the diver's body makes. These improve performance and do not harm the diver. The elevation of heart rate with exercise is an example of a physiological response to activity.

- Acclimatizations—temporary changes that improve performance and occur as a result of practice or continuing exposure to the activity. High-altitude exposure leads to acclimatizations to this environment. Acclimatizations are temporary, disappearing soon after the activity is stopped.

- Adaptations—permanent changes that improve performance. These changes are inherited. The shapes of diving mammals represent adaptations that improve swimming speed and tolerance to cold water.

- Pathological—changes that cause harm to the diver.

The first three types of responses are associated with positive feedback. They help the human or mammalian diver to better perform in the underwater environment. This part of the book explores these responses from six different perspectives: cardiovascular (chapter 4), respiratory (chapter 5), blood and muscle tissue (chapter 6), thermal (chapter 7), propulsion (chapter 8), and orientation (chapter 9). Each chapter begins with a discussion of the pertinent anatomy and physiology and then compares the adaptations found in diving mammals to the responses that occur in the human diver. Many of the adaptations have counterparts in the human diver. In other cases, practice and experience result in the diver's making acclimatizations to meet the challenges of the underwater environment. Each chapter concludes with a discussion of the equipment the diver uses to meet these challenges.

Diving and diving mammals have been a source of fascination for humans since the beginnings of recorded history. Poseidon, the god of the sea in Greek mythology, is mentioned in Homer's *Iliad*. Herodotus' writings also attest to the long-standing interest humans have had in the underwater environment. Aristotle recognized that the porpoise was a mammal that made adaptations to the aquatic environment. About 2,200 years later, in the 1870s, Paul Bert studied diving vertebrates. Approximately 70 years after that, Irving, Scholander, and Elsner generated classic papers on the adaptations of seals and other diving mammals to the water environment. More recently, Kooyman supplemented our knowledge of diving with his study of Weddell seals using remote sensors. Part II of this book uses

Table II.1	Breath-Hold Diving Abilities in Aquatic Animals	
Animal	**Breath-hold times (minutes)**	**Maximum recorded depth in excursion feet (meters)**
Human	2.5 (15)[1]	120 (37); 500 (152)[2]
Porpoise	6	1,000 (305)
Killer whale	12	Not available
Beaver	15	Fresh water
Manatee	30	Fresh water
Sea lion	30	500 (152)
Weddell seal	60	1,000 (305)
Sperm whale	75	3,300 (1,006)
Bottle-nosed whale	120	2,700 (823)

[1] After breathing pure oxygen for 15 min.
[2] Passive descent with weighted sled-like device (chapter 5).

specific citations sparingly and only when the information is unique to one author or set of investigators. All the references are included in a single listing at the end of the book.

In general, when sources are cited, they are the classical references on the subject and appear as valid today as when the information was first published. For more contemporary information, the reader is referred to the recommended readings list, also at the end of the book.

Table II.1 compares the diving abilities of humans with those of porpoises, whales, and other aquatic animals in terms of depths and durations of the dive. Most of this information is of the observation type of the diving mammals in their natural environments. Like records in competitive sport, these are expected to improve with time and advances in methods of monitoring. Nevertheless, the information demonstrates a spectrum of responses and, even with limited observations, remarkable diving feats. With technology, the human diver is able to "compete" with the diving mammals, but the downside is the risk of medical problems of diving when the stresses lead to negative feedback and harm to the organism, addressed in part III. In contrast, part II focuses on positive feedback, that is, the physiological responses to the underwater environment of both human and nonhuman mammalian divers.

ADAPTATIONS OF THE HEART AND VASCULAR SYSTEM FOR DIVING

Special **cardiovascular** (heart and blood vessel) adaptations occur in diving mammals. These not only extend the animals' ability to dive but also help protect them from the medical problems of diving. Many of the adaptations are extensions of the universal oxygen-conserving mechanism that is found in almost all animals as a response to anoxia (interruption of the

> **Chapter Preview**
>
> - Important anatomical components of the cardiovascular system
> - Basic physiology of the cardiovascular system
> - Three cardinal components of the diving reflex
> - Significance and magnitude of the diving reflex in diving mammals
> - Counterparts of the diving reflex in humans
> - Universal nature of the oxygen-conserving reflex

oxygen supply). The **diving reflex,** which is a finely tuned counterpart of the universal oxygen-conserving reflex observed in diving mammals, has three major components:

- Bradycardia (slowing of the heart)
- Peripheral vasoconstriction (narrowing of blood vessels)
- Anaerobic metabolism (energy production without oxygen)

Apnea (breath-holding) and immersion appear to be the stimuli that initiate the diving reflex. Each component of the diving reflex is highly developed in the diving mammal, but counterparts of all three are also found in the human breath-hold diver.

Anatomy and Physiology

The important components of the anatomy and physiology of the cardiovascular system are relatively easy to understand. In essence the system consists of a pump (the heart) and conduits to carry the blood (the blood vessels). The heart is a remarkable pump that works by contracting its muscles. It can speed up or slow down to meet the body's blood flow demands. Even though blood flow is continuous, the heart chambers themselves fill passively during two-thirds of each heartbeat and actively by muscle contraction during the remaining third. The heart does an incredible amount of work. At rest it pumps about five quarts (4.7 liters) of blood a minute. This is termed the **cardiac output.** In a week the heart pumps enough blood to fill a railroad boxcar. Over a 70-year life span, this equates to pumping about 46 million gallons (184 million liters) of blood. The cardiac output is able to increase by a five- to sixfold factor through tripling of the heart rate and doubling of the filling capacity. In a period of 24 hours the heart beats over 85,000 times, and over a year, almost 32 million times. This level of function, which continues for the lifetime of the individual, is incredible. No other mechanical pumping system can even come close to approaching the function, efficiency, and durability of the human heart.

Heart

The muscles of the heart are arranged into four chambers: two receiving chambers termed atria and two pumping chambers termed ventricles as diagrammed in figure 4.1. Valves situated between the atrial and ventricle chambers and at the outflows of the ventricle chambers keep blood flowing in a forward direction. Blood is received in the right atrium from the two great veins (the superior and inferior vena cavae). The venous pressure in the vena cavae, although only about 1/20 of the arterial pressure, is ample for filling the right atrium. This pressure is enough so that 75 percent of the blood flowing into the right ventricle does so passively from the right atrium. For the right atrium this is an energy-conserving mechanism. The remaining 25 percent of the blood flow to the right ventricle arises from contraction of the right atrium. The pressure generated from the right atrial contraction is only one-quarter of that generated from the contraction of the right ventricle.

Blood from the pumping action of the right ventricle flows through the pulmonary arteries to the lungs. As blood passes through the lungs, oxygen is taken up by the red blood cells, and the pulmonary veins carry the oxygenated blood to the left atrium of the heart. Consequently, the pulmonary arteries carry deoxygenated blood while the pulmonary veins carry oxygenated blood, the only blood vessels in the body that normally do so. Analogously to what happens on the right side of the heart, on the left side the blood flows passively and is also actively pumped into the left ventricle. The left ventricle has the most forceful contractile ability of any of the chambers of the heart. It normally pumps blood into the arteries with a force of 120mmHg or more. This pressure determines the **systolic blood pressure,** the highest point of the blood pressure, which coincides with the end of systole. The blood pumped into the arteries distends their elastic walls. The elasticity of the arterial walls forces blood downstream through the arteries. The aortic valve, which separates the left ventricle from the major outflow vessel of the heart, the aorta, prevents backflow into the left ventricle. The pressure of the elastic recoil of the arteries averages about 80mmHg during **diastole** (relaxation phase of the heart; this defines **diastolic blood pressure**). The valve system and elasticity of the arteries are a major reason that the heart muscles do not actively contract for two-thirds of each heartbeat, thereby helping to make it possible for this organ to function for a lifetime.

A variety of problems can interfere with the normal function of the heart. One, in particular, a patent (open) foramen (communication) between the right and left atria, has particular significance for the sport SCUBA diver, as depicted in figure 4.1. The medical term for this condition is patent **foramen ovale** (PFO). The PFO allows venous gas emboli, a usual occurrence with ascent from a SCUBA dive (see chapter 3), to short-circuit from the right atrium to the left atrium and so bypass being filtered out and exchanged with the ambient air in the lungs. Once bubbles are in the left atrium, they enter the left ventricle and then are pumped into the arterial circulation. If the bubbles are carried to the brain or the other vital organs, they may occlude the circulation, resulting in loss of function and eventually death of the oxygen-deprived tissues. According to one report, about one-third of the divers who were treated for serious symptoms of decompression sickness had this heart problem (Moon, Camporesi, and Kisslo 1989). Normally, PFOs are observed in one-quarter to one-third of the population. This observation points to one reason some divers are more likely to get decompression sickness than others, and PFO is considered a bends-proneness factor (see chapter 15).

Arteries and Capillaries

Arteries carry blood to all parts of the body. They divide into smaller and smaller segments until they eventually become capillaries (figure 4.2). Capillaries facilitate the exchange of oxygen, carbon dioxide, and nutrients with tissues. As blood moves more distally through the arterial tree, the systolic pressure decreases progressively. By the time blood reaches the capillary level, the pressure has dropped to about 30mmHg or one-fourth the original systolic pressure. This pressure is termed the capillary perfusion pressure. There are about 10 billion capillaries in the peripheral (extremities and skin) circulation, and it is estimated that there are an equal number in the core (head,

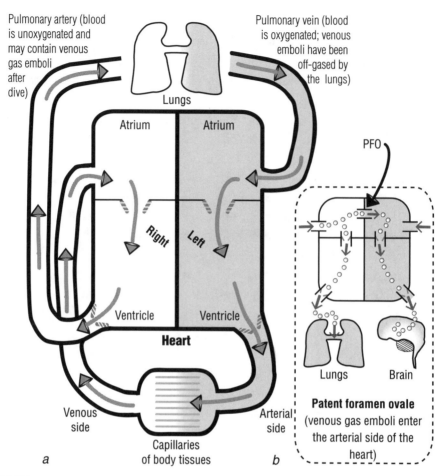

Pulmonary artery (blood is unoxygenated and may contain venous gas emboli after dive)

Pulmonary vein (blood is oxygenated; venous emboli have been off-gased by the lungs)

Lungs

Atrium   Atrium

PFO

Right   Left

Ventricle   Ventricle

Heart

Lungs   Brain

Venous side   Arterial side

Capillaries of body tissues

Patent foramen ovale (venous gas emboli enter the arterial side of the heart)

a   b

FIGURE 4.1   Heart anatomy and blood flow: *(a)* normal heart; *(b)* patient with foramen ovale. Shading represents oxygenated blood.

neck, and trunk deep to the skin) circulation (Guyton and Hall 2000). Whereas the aorta, the largest artery in the body, has a diameter of about three-fourths of an inch (two centimeters), the diameter of the capillary is about 1/4000th of that, or five micrometers. The length of a capillary is about 100 times its width.

Since red blood cells are 7.5 micrometers in diameter, they must undergo elongation (termed red blood cell deformability) in order to pass through the capillary. When the blood thickens and blood flow slows, red blood cells tend to adhere to one another and no longer are able to pass through the capillary. This problem is termed **sludging.** Sludging, associated with serious forms of decompression sickness (see chapter 15), interferes with flow through the capillaries and deprives tissues of oxygen. There are many potential causes of slowing and sludging of red blood cells as listed in table 4.1.

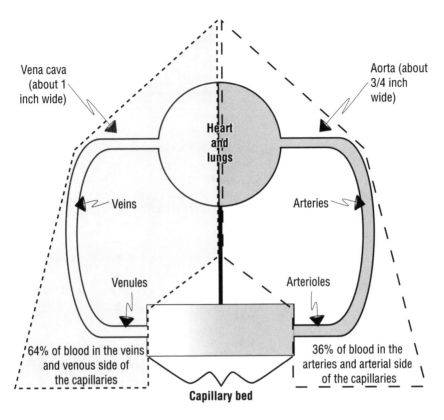

FIGURE 4.2 Systemic circulation.

Table 4.1	Causes of Sludging
Condition	**Contributing factors and effects**
Dehydration	Insensible losses from the lungs, increased urine production
Fluid shifts	Immersion
Hypothermia	Likely to occur especially in the hands and feet during diving in cold water
Impairment in blood flow	May result from tight bands on diving exposure suits
Posture	Falling asleep with joints tightly bent (crush syndrome)
Sepsis (infection)	Loss of ability of red blood cells to deform and pass through the capillary
Low oxygen tensions	Same as for sepsis

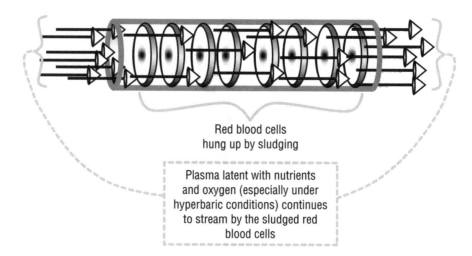

Red blood cells
hung up by sludging

Plasma latent with nutrients
and oxygen (especially under
hyperbaric conditions) continues
to stream by the sludged red
blood cells

**FIGURE
4.3**   Sludging of red blood cells in the microcirculation (arterioles, capillaries, and venules) and streaming of plasma through the areas of stasis.

Even though there may be cessation of the flow of the cellular elements of the blood (red and white blood cells), the fluid portions of the blood (plasma) tend to stream through the area of sludging as depicted in figure 4.3. With **hyperbaric oxygen therapy** (breathing pure oxygen in a pressurized chamber at approximately 2.4 ATA), enough oxygen is forced into the plasma to supply resting tissue oxygen needs without red blood cell–carried oxygen. Subsequent chapters present more information about hyperbaric oxygen.

Capillaries are differentiated from arteries by the lack of muscle in their walls and are only a single cell thick. This cell, named the **endothelial cell,** forms the lining of every blood vessel. All exchange of oxygen, nutrients, and waste products between the tissues and the blood occurs at the capillary level. The exchange takes place through pores and channels between the endothelial cells. The total exchange surface area of the capillaries is estimated to be about one-quarter the area of a football field or about 1,330 square yards (1,112 square meters). Almost every cell in the body (except for fingernails and hair) is within 25 to 30 micrometers (about five to six capillary diameters) of a capillary. This is the maximum distance that oxygen and nutrients can diffuse through tissue fluids to the cells. Hyperbaric oxygen treatments increase the diffusion distance threefold.

Blood flow to capillaries is highly regulated by the muscles around the arteries and arterioles (the smallest division of arteries and the segment of the arterial tree that just precedes the capillary). The regulation is directed by the oxygen demands of the tissues and mediated by the nervous system. When at rest, noncritical tissues such as skin, muscles, and the bowel have

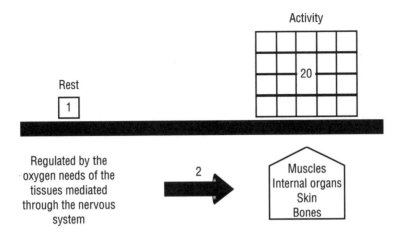

Activity

Rest

20

1

Regulated by the oxygen needs of the tissues mediated through the nervous system

2

Muscles
Internal organs
Skin
Bones

**FIGURE
4.4**   Difference in oxygen requirements and blood flow of noncritical tissues between rest and activity. Activity includes functions such as muscle contraction/ relaxation, digestion, repair of injuries, and fighting infections. Increases come from diversion of blood flow from one tissue to another.

very low oxygen demands and receive almost no blood flow. As seen in figure 4.4, during activity and repair, blood flow may need to increase 20-fold or more. This ability to highly regulate flow conserves energy and body mass. If all the tissues in the body had to be supplied by their maximum possible blood flow, we estimate that the blood volume would need to increase 100-fold (based on the potential volume of the vascular system). If the regulatory system is disrupted, for example, by injury to the brain or other parts of the nervous system, the distribution of blood flow is also disturbed. Blood flow from critical tissues, such as the heart and brain, may be diverted to noncritical tissues, thereby providing an environment for bubbles to form in critical tissues. We consider this a "disordering event," and it provides an explanation for the occurrence of undeserved decompression sickness (see chapter 15).

Venous System

Blood is returned to the heart through the venous system. Capillaries connect to venules, the smallest division of the venous system, which progressively enlarge until they form the superior (returning blood to the heart from the head, neck, and upper extremities) and the inferior (returning blood from the trunk and lower extremities) vena cavae. The vena cavae may be an inch (2.5 centimeters) or more in diameter. Veins are thin-walled vessels. Consequently the normal pressure in the venous system is about 10 percent of the systolic arterial pressure. Normally 64 percent of the blood in the body is in the venous system while 20 percent is in the arteries and arterioles (small arteries). This means that the volume of blood flow in the venous system needs to be 10 times (because of 1/10 the flow rate) that of the arterial system in order to keep the flow in the arterial and venous sides of the vascular system in balance.

The presence of bubbles in the venous circulation due to nitrogen off-gassing from the tissues (see chapter 3) during ascent appears to be a normal occurrence. Ordinarily the bubbles are transported harmlessly to the lungs where the gas is exchanged with the outside environment. In spite of the slow flow of blood in the veins, venous gas emboli usually do not cause symptoms of decompression sickness unless the flow is slowed so much that the bubbles coalesce, enlarge with ascent, or are so extensive from overwhelming gradients that they occlude the circulation. Venous sinuses and plexuses are structures that act as storage reservoirs for blood (and oxygen in diving mammals). Subsequent chapters in this part of the book present further discussion of how these structures contribute to diving ability and protection from injury.

Endothelial Cell

The endothelial cell is an additional blood vessel structure that has relevance to the diver. As already suggested, the endothelial cell is far more than a lining to keep fluid in the bloodstream. When it is perturbed by noxious substances, problems arise. One noxious substance that causes problems in diving is the nitrogen bubble. The bubble not only acts as a mechanical blockage for blood flow but also interacts chemically with the endothelial cell wall. The result is that white blood cells attach to the irritated endothelial cell wall and release the same chemicals that kill bacteria. This causes blood vessels to contract to such an extent that no blood flows through them (the "no-reflow" phenomenon), as well as causing irreparable damage to the blood vessel linings. Whereas intravascular (inside the blood vessel) bubble occlusion is thought to be a transient phenomenon, the damage from the chemical reaction is permanent and helps to explain why full recovery does not always occur with treatment of decompression sickness.

Bradycardia

Bradycardia (slowing of the heart rate) during breath-holding immersion is observed in all diving mammals and to some extent in the human diver, as shown in table 4.2. Seals demonstrate the greatest bradycardia changes of all diving mammals. They are able to slow their heart rates abruptly to 10 percent of their normal resting rates. When diving, porpoises gradually slow their heart rates over a 30-second interval to about 50 percent of normal. The bradycardia reflex in human divers appears to be independent of sex, swimming ability, or familiarity with the water. Heart rates may decrease by as

Table 4.2	Bradycardian Response to Immersion in Diving Mammals and Humans		
Animal	Resting pulse	Immersion pulse	Percent (decrease)
Seal	100	10	90
Whale	100	18	82
Porpoise and killer whale	60	30	50
Human	75	45	40

much as 40 percent, but anxiety and frantic activity override the bradycardia reflex in the human diver.

Initiation

The bradycardia reflex is initiated by stimulation of the **trigeminal nerve,** one of the 12 major nerves emanating from the brain. It functions to transmit sensations from the face to the brain. Facial immersion in water is the stimulus for the bradycardia reflex of diving. This occurs through the branch of the nerve that receives sensations from inside the nose. Once the nerve impulse from facial immersion is received in the brain, it is processed and a message is transmitted through the **vagus nerve,** another of the 12 facial nerves that innervates (transmits messages from the brain to) the gut, heart, and larynx, to slow the heart. **Atropine,** a drug known for its ability to block message transmission of the vagus nerve, abolishes the bradycardia reflex.

Characteristics and Influences

Several observations help to further explain the characteristics of the bradycardia reflex. First, in humans, the effect is much more evident if the subject is breath-holding with the face immersed in water rather than breath-holding in air. The response is not obliterated by controlled, nonfrantic swimming activity. This has important ramifications in that if the response were obliterated by exercise, the breath-hold time would be markedly shortened with underwater activity. Also, the bradycardia reflex is independent of pressure. For example, it is not initiated by breath-holding in a hyperbaric chamber that has been pressurized with air. However, water temperature does influence the bradycardia reflex. The colder the water temperature is, the slower the heart rate. The heart rates of the female divers of Japan (Ama divers) are 20 percent slower during diving in the colder, winter-season waters than in warmer waters during the summer months. A similar effect is observed with facial immersion in waters of different temperatures.

Subconscious brain activity may influence the bradycardia reflex also. Fainting from the sight of blood is an example of subconscious brain activity that influences the heart and blood vessels, although the effect on the blood vessels is the opposite of that observed with the bradycardia reflex. Nonimmersion laboratory conditioning techniques do not decrease the heart rates in seals. With ascent, the bradycardia responses in seals gradually terminate. However, if the seal approaches the surface and descends again without breathing, the heart rate slowing resumes.

Heart Rhythm Consequences

Electrocardiograms of diving mammals while underwater indicate that they tolerate the slowing of their heart rates well. The changes observed on the **electrocardiogram** (i.e., the recording of the electrical activity of the heart on a moving strip of paper) in both human and nonhuman divers include a prolonged resting phase (diastole), widening of the pumping phase **(systole)** of the heartbeat, and a progressive lengthening of the time from initiation of the electrical activity of the heart to the time the pumping action actually occurs. This latter change has also been observed in world-class endurance athletes. Even with these changes, the heart rhythm remains regular. However, not all the heart rhythm changes in the human breath-hold diver are benign. Irregular heart rhythms are commonly observed in humans during breath-hold dives; these may be associated with the slowing of the heart to the point that heartbeats are omitted. One study indicated irregular heart rhythms in 75 percent of the human divers examined (Olsen, Fanestil, and Scholander 1962). The heart rhythms promptly normalized after the divers surfaced. Irregular heart rhythms are exaggerated by immersion in cold water. When seals dive with their airways blocked, irregular heart rhythms are also observed.

Vasoconstriction and Shunting of Blood

The second major component of the diving reflex is the shunting of blood from the extremities and noncritical organs to the great blood vessels, heart, lungs, and brain. This is achieved through vasoconstriction (narrowing of blood vessels). Shunting of blood from the extremities allows the oxygen in the blood to be used to supply exclusively the heart and the brain. The bradycardia response slows the heart rate, thereby reducing the heart's oxygen requirements. However, the brain's oxygen requirements remain steady regardless of the activity. To illustrate this, one can use the example of oxygen requirements in the seal. At rest, harbor seals consume oxygen at a rate of 300 milliliters (0.634 pint) a minute. Of this amount of oxygen, 40 to 50 milliliters (0.085-0.106 pint) per minute are required to supply the brain and maintain the seal's normal level of consciousness. The blood oxygen stores of the seal are about 1,000 milliliters (2.1 pints). If no shunting occurred, the maximum dive duration would be slightly over three minutes (1,000 milliliters of oxygen stores divided by an oxygen utilization rate of 300 milliliters a minute). After initiation of the oxygen-conserving reflex with blood shunting to the core circulation, the oxygen in the blood would be capable of supplying the brain's oxygen requirements for almost 25 minutes. This corresponds closely with the maximum observed diving times of the harbor seal. Shunting is uniformly observed in diving mammals.

Effectiveness
Shunting of blood associated with vasoconstriction during the dive in diving mammals is so complete that blood almost ceases to flow in the vasoconstricted areas. Incisions through muscles and skin do not bleed while the diving mammal is submerged. During dives, temperatures in the extremities of diving mammals decrease to a degree comparable to that associated with a tourniquet applied to these areas at the surface. Dye injection studies in blood vessels of seals indicate that vasoconstriction is so complete that the effect is as if the area were surgically removed from the animal during the dive (Murdaugh et al. 1965). There is also arrest of blood flow to the kidneys with cessation of urine production during the period of vasoconstriction. It is noteworthy that atropine does not block this effect as it does for slowing of the heart rate, which suggests that the shunting mechanism is different from the bradycardia reflex mechanism. In addition, during the vasoconstriction response in seals, blood flow to the abdominal organs ceases. In humans, limb blood flow was observed to fall nearly to zero during breath-hold dives (Elsner and Scholander 1963). The effect was almost nonexistent with breath-holding in air. Electrical stimulation of an area adjacent to the **hypothalamus** (i.e., a portion of the brain that lies beneath the thalamus and secretes substances that regulate metabolism) in the elephant seal results in vasoconstriction responses similar to those observed in the diving reflex, suggesting that this is the area of the brain where the reflex is initiated (Van Citters et al. 1965).

Blood Flow to the Brain and Heart
Uninterrupted blood flow to the brain and heart is essential to maintain consciousness during the dive. Without changes in the distribution of blood flow to these organs during the period of bradycardia, one would lose consciousness due to insufficient oxygen delivery. A moment's interruption of oxygen availability to the brain can result in loss of consciousness (see chapter 1). Changes occur in the pattern of blood flow during the diving reflex. Although the average (systolic plus diastolic divided by 2)

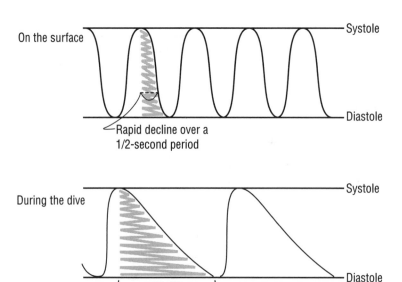

On the surface — Systole

Diastole

Rapid decline over a
1/2-second period

During the dive — Systole

Diastole

Gradual decline over
a 6-second period

**FIGURE
4.5**   Blood pressure patterns on the surface and during the diving reflex in the seal.

blood pressure remains the same on the surface and during the dive, the lapse between systole and diastole contractions is extended from 1 second to over a 5- to 10-second time period during the diving reflex as diagrammed in figure 4.5. This ensures a continuous, uninterrupted blood flow to the brain between heartbeats.

This effect occurs because of several structural changes in diving mammals' blood vessels. First, the blood vessels to the heart and brain are very elastic. During systole they are stretched out like a rubber band. During the prolonged interval from systole to diastole, they contract from the elastic (rubber band) effect so that there is a continuous flow of blood as the blood pressure decreases during the heart cycle. The elasticity is so great that there is a transient reversal in the forward direction of blood flow in the abdominal aorta (major artery to the abdomen and lower extremities). The vasoconstriction is so complete that blood flow is totally occluded distal to the abdominal aorta. This contributes to ensuring a constant supply of blood to the brain. Second, a secondary "passive" (i.e., no active muscle contraction) pumplike expansion just beyond the outflow of their hearts have been observed in diving mammals. They are characterized by a near doubling of the size of the aorta. The effect of this elastic-walled reservoir is to provide continuous blood flow to the brain during the nonsystolic portion of the slowed heart cycle.

Anaerobic Metabolism

Anaerobic metabolism (without oxygen) is the third component of the diving reflex. It allows muscles to function in the absence of an oxygen supply. Ordinarily, oxygen is required for all metabolic processes including muscle contraction (see chapter 8). The energy for metabolism comes from the **oxidation** (combining of oxygen with a fuel-like substance) of glucose, a sugar. This is analogous to the requirement for oxygen to burn fuel in the automobile engine. The initial stage of energy release from the glucose molecule is by glycolysis. It is the anaerobic phase of glucose metabolism. **Glycolysis** produces products (pyruvic acid), which are later oxidized (pyruvic acid conversion and in the citric acid cycle) to produce energy. The **citric acid cycle** is the aerobic phase of metabolism.

Energy Production From Metabolism

Aerobic metabolism (oxygen utilization) of glucose provides 285 kilocalories of energy in the formation of 38 high-energy adenosine triphosphate (**ATP;** a high-energy phosphate compound present in all living cells that serves as the primary energy source for many metabolic processes) molecules for each unit (mole or gram molecular weight) of glucose oxidized. This number is subject to variation with changes in temperature and concentrations of the substrates. The 285 kilocalories represent a 45 percent efficiency rate for energy production. The other 55 percent of the energy is lost as heat, explaining why heat generation is associated with muscle activity. The other by-products of aerobic metabolism are carbon dioxide and water.

In contrast, during anaerobic metabolism, only two molecules of ATP are produced for every mole of glucose utilized. This generates only 15 kilocalories of energy, which is equivalent to about a 2 percent efficiency rate for utilization of the total energy potential in the glucose molecule; the energy production from anaerobic metabolism is thus one-fifth as efficient as the energy production from aerobic metabolism. The end product of anaerobic metabolism is **lactic acid.** It is produced from pyruvic acid when oxygen is not available for completing the metabolism of glucose in the citric acid cycle. However, when oxygen again becomes available, as in mediation of the oxygen deficit, additional energy is produced from metabolism of the lactic acid by conversion of lactic acid back to pyruvic acid. Without oxygen, further metabolism of lactic acid and energy production is halted. When lactic acid leaves the tissues and enters the circulation after termination of the shunting reflex (or if the shunting reflex is incomplete as in the case of human divers), an **oxygen deficit** (an older term referred to it as an "oxygen debt") occurs. Symptoms of an oxygen deficit include elevations of heart and breathing rates, irrepressible desire to breathe, and muscle cramping. It appears that because of the completeness of the shunting reflex, diving mammals do not experience the symptoms of an oxygen deficit. The oxygen deficit is resolved during the recovery phase when shunting is terminated and oxygen delivery to the muscles is resumed.

Tolerance of Anaerobic Metabolism

During the diving reflex, the muscles of diving mammals are able to function under anaerobic conditions for the duration of the dive. In humans, such as short-distance sprinters in running or swimming races, anaerobic metabolism is tolerated for only brief periods, typically on the order of seconds. The diving mammal's ability to tolerate anaerobic metabolism for sustained periods of time has three elements:

- Increased tolerance of carbon dioxide levels in the blood
- Increased tolerance of lactic acid in the muscle tissues
- The ability of lactic acid to leak out of the muscle into the tissues surrounding the muscle. This effect prevents high accumulations of lactic acid that would block further anaerobic metabolism. This mechanism also may prevent muscle cramping during activity of oxygen-deprived muscles.

Conditioning and experience improve human breath-hold divers' and other athletes' abilities to tolerate elevated carbon dioxide and lactic acid levels while still being able to do the activity (see chapter 5). In diving mammals, recovery from the oxygen deficit appears to be very rapid, perhaps within seconds, as witnessed in their quick resumption of diving activities. In humans, the recovery period for a significant oxygen debt is longer; as measured by return to resting pulse and breathing rates, recovery may take minutes or even hours.

Noncritical tissues such as the skin, bone, ligaments, and tendons are able to tolerate long periods without oxygen. However, this process is different from anaerobic metabolism. These tissues are at rest and their metabolic state could be considered a form of suspended animation or hibernation. Consequently, no significant oxygen deficit is incurred from these tissues during the diving reflex. The kidneys of diving mammals also act in this fashion during the dive.

Universal Nature of the Oxygen-Conserving Reflex

Bradycardia, peripheral vasoconstriction, and anaerobic metabolism are the three cardinal components of the diving reflex. This is a universal response in animals to oxygen deprivation. In the human it is observed in the fetal distress syndrome, which is typically characterized by slowing of the heart rate, and in the victim of near-drowning. In the absence of struggling, the diving reflex can be very profound and can add an enormous margin to the preservation of brain function. In an isolated report of a miscarriage, a fetus that was discarded into a toilet bowl and then recovered and resuscitated after a two-hour immersion survived with normal brain function. There are many reports of full recovery of near-drowning victims in cold water with immersion times of 30 minutes or longer. A very illustrative study of the effects of the diving reflex was done with ducks, which are diving birds (Andersen 1966). A duck strangulated with a noose around its neck survived for 4 minutes in room air. When immersed in water under the same circumstances, the survival time increased to 15 minutes due to the diving reflex.

Technology to Meet the Cardiovascular Challenges of the Aquatic Environment

Technology has allowed us to surmount the challenges of providing an oxygen supply to the heart, brain, and other tissues of the body during SCUBA diving activities. This is, of course, through the use of compressed gas and utilization of the SCUBA regulator to provide the compressed gas at a safe breathing pressure, regardless of the depth (see chapter 3). Equally important, knowledge of the anatomy and physiology of the cardiovascular system and its responses to diving provides an understanding of the reasons for medical problems of diving and a basis for their prevention (see part III).

Although SCUBA gear allows the human diver to stay underwater, on par with diving mammals with respect to time, it does not provide the flexibility for the deep dives, the freedom from decompression sickness, or the rapid recovery and quick return to diving observed in the diving mammals. As technology is developed, these obstacles may be surmounted. For example, rebreather gear has extended the bottom times of divers regardless of depth. Saturation diving makes it possible for human divers to descend to extraordinary depths, but with greatly reduced work capacity (due to the density of the breathing gases under such great pressures) and enormous requirements for decompression. Fluid respiration would eliminate most of these problems since oxygen would be "carried" to the lungs in a noncompressible fluid, on-gassing and off-gassing of inert gas would be eliminated, and repetitive diving would be simply a matter of when the diver feels rested enough to return to the water.

For Further Review

1. What are the main components of the cardiovascular system?
2. What are the main components of the diving reflex? How does each complement the others?

3. How does the diving reflex differ between humans and diving mammals?

4. What factors contribute to making the heart an efficient pump while allowing it to continue working for a lifetime?

5. How are the volumes and proportions of blood flow to various parts of the body regulated in the human?

6. How does energy production compare between aerobic and anaerobic metabolism?

7. What is an oxygen deficit? How does it occur? How is it resolved?

8. How has technology mediated the cardiovascular challenges of the underwater environment?

THE RESPIRATORY SYSTEM IN DIVING

The respiratory systems of diving **mammals** (warm-blooded animals that possess hair, have bony vertebral columns, breathe air, and breast-feed their young) have adaptations that improve their swimming and diving abilities. In contrast to the diving reflex, many of the respiratory adaptations in diving mammals do not have counterparts in the human breath-hold diver. With repetitive diving activities, the respiratory systems of

Chapter Preview

- Anatomy and physiology of the respiratory system
- Mechanisms of gas exchange (oxygen, carbon dioxide, and nitrogen) in the lungs
- Medical problems of the respiratory system that may occur in the human diver
- Comparison and contrast of how the respiratory systems of the human diver and diving mammals function during a dive
- Breath-hold diving abilities improved with conditioning
- Buoyancy compensator

human divers make temporary changes in response to the aquatic environment. These changes, referred to as acclimatizations, disappear after the diving activity is stopped. Acclimatizations are associated with conditioning for competitive sport, general fitness, and high-altitude activity. Although humans are mammals who dive, in this part of the text "diving mammals" refers to nonhuman divers while "breath-hold divers" refers to the human counterparts.

Anatomy and Physiology

The mammalian respiratory system consists of five major components as diagrammed in figure 5.1.

- Conduits are connecting structures from the air in the ambient environment to the **alveoli** (the air-exchanging structures of the lungs). Air enters the conduits through the mouth and nose. Then it passes through the pharynx, the back of the mouth and throat, to the **trachea** (windpipe). The **larynx** is at the top of the trachea. At its upper edge is the epiglottis, the valvelike structure that closes when food and liquid are swallowed to prevent their passage into the airways. The larynx has a very important role in preventing

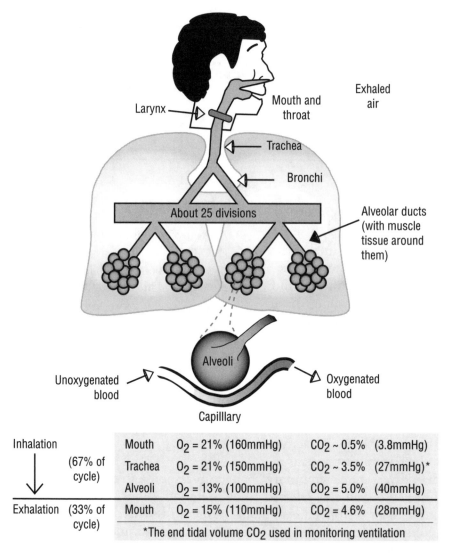

Larynx — Mouth and throat — Exhaled air — Trachea — Bronchi — About 25 divisions — Alveolar ducts (with muscle tissue around them) — Alveoli — Unoxygenated blood — Oxygenated blood — Capilllary

Inhalation					
(67% of cycle)	Mouth	O_2 = 21% (160mmHg)		CO_2 ~ 0.5% (3.8mmHg)	
	Trachea	O_2 = 21% (150mmHg)		CO_2 ~ 3.5% (27mmHg)*	
	Alveoli	O_2 = 13% (100mmHg)		CO_2 = 5.0% (40mmHg)	
Exhalation (33% of cycle)	Mouth	O_2 = 15% (110mmHg)		CO_2 = 4.6% (28mmHg)	
	*The end tidal volume CO_2 used in monitoring ventilation				

FIGURE 5.1   Structures of the respiratory tree. O_2 = oxygen; CO_2 = carbon dioxide.

complications from near-drowning as discussed later (see chapter 16). The trachea splits into two tubes named **bronchi.** The two bronchi further divide into smaller and smaller tubes, eventually becoming bronchioles and terminating in alveolar ducts. There are about 25 divisions of the airway from the trachea to the alveolar ducts. The sum volume of air in these conduits is labeled the **dead space.** No exchange of oxygen or carbon dioxide occurs in this portion of the respiratory system. In humans an average dead space volume is about one-fifth of a quart (one-fifth liter). With inefficient breathing patterns, like those that may be associated with panic or with lung disease such as emphysema, most of the air only moves in and out of the dead space.

When this occurs, exchange of oxygen and carbon dioxide becomes insufficient to meet the body's ventilation requirements.

• The alveoli are the structures budding from the alveolar ducts where gas is exchanged from the lungs to the bloodstream. The exchange area of the alveoli is enormous, with a total surface area equivalent to that of a tennis court or about 300 square yards (250 square meters). The smaller airway tubes are encircled with muscles. When the muscles relax, as is the usual situation, air easily moves through these passageways. When they constrict, airflow is restricted, causing a problem that interferes with breathing, as in people with **asthma,** a disease causing reversible narrowing of the bronchi (lung passageways). Since inhalation is an active process, it is easier to get air into the alveoli than out of them. The failure of air to move out of the alveoli blocks ventilation at the microscopic level. With the inability to provide a new oxygen supply to the alveoli and remove carbon dioxide, the normal physiological ranges of these gases are altered in the bloodstream. These changes generate the symptoms of shortness of breath ("air hunger").

• The capillaries, the gas and nutrient transfer segments of the circulatory system, exchange gases with the alveoli. During ventilation, oxygen moves from the alveoli with their higher concentration of oxygen (partial pressure of about 160mmHg) to the capillaries with their lower concentration of oxygen (partial pressure of about 46mmHg). Likewise, carbon dioxide moves from the capillaries with a partial pressure of about 46mmHg to the alveoli with a partial pressure of about 40mmHg. The exchange is passive and is a response to the gradients (the differences in concentrations) of the gases on either side of the walls of the alveoli. Like the terminal branches of the respiratory tree, the noncapillary blood vessels of the lungs are encircled with muscle. When constricted, they limit flow distal to the areas of constriction. Insults to the lungs, such as **aspiration** (inhalation) of water, may cause vasoconstriction (narrowing of blood vessels) in portions of the lung circulation. While these portions may not have blood flow (perfusion), the alveoli may still have air coming into and going out of them. In other areas of the lung, the opposite may occur due to bronchial constriction from the aspirated water. The result is inequalities of air exchange and blood flow. The medical term for this is "ventilation/perfusion inequalities," which can become life threatening since oxygen is not being added to the blood and carbon dioxide is not being removed from it. Ventilation/perfusion inequalities are among the major complications of near-drowning (see chapter 16).

• The chest wall portion of the respiratory tree consists of skin, muscles, bones, and connective tissues. It provides a semirigid structure in which the lungs reside (lung cavity). Increases in the internal volume of the cavity cause the lungs to expand and draw in air. The chest wall increases about

20 percent in front-to-back thickness with a maximal inspiration effort. This is an active process that requires muscle effort. Since the lungs (primarily the alveoli) and the chest wall are elastic structures (i.e., they have the ability to stretch and then return to their initial size), once the muscle effort is relaxed, the lung cavity returns to its original volume without muscular effort. This property is termed elastic recoil. Whereas inhalation of air is an active process requiring muscle effort, exhalation is passive. Elastic recoil explains why mouth-to-mouth artificial respiration (positive pressure ventilation) is so much more efficient for air exchange in the lungs than the older techniques whereby attempts were made to force air out of the lungs and then allow air to passively flow into the lungs.

• The respiratory muscles include the **diaphragm** (the thin muscle below the lungs and the heart that separates the chest from the abdomen and is the main muscle used for inspiration of air into the lungs) and the accessory respiratory muscles of the chest wall and neck such as the intercostal (between the ribs) and the sternocleidomastoid muscles. When they contract, they increase the volume of the lung cavity. This creates a negative pressure in the lung cavity and causes air to be inhaled. The stimulus to breathe arises in the breathing center of the brain. Input to the brain comes from receptors in blood vessels to alterations—primarily to elevated carbon dioxide levels but also, to a lesser extent, to low oxygen levels. This information in the form of nerve impulses is then conducted to the diaphragm by the **phrenic nerve,** which comes off the upper level of the spinal cord (cervical nerves C-3 to C-5). For normal breathing activities, at rest, the movements of the diaphragm provide sufficient air exchange. With hyperventilation during exercise or other situations requiring increased ventilation efforts, the accessory muscles of respiration aid in increasing the amount of chest expansion and the volume of air inhaled.

Lung Volumes and Capacities

Very specific terms refer to the different quantities of air that the lungs hold, as illustrated in figure 5.2. The maximum amount of air the lungs can hold at the end of the fullest possible inhalation is termed the total lung capacity (TLC). In an average-sized man this is about five quarts (4.7 liters). The amount of air that is exchanged with each breath is termed the tidal volume (TV). At rest this is about half a quart (one-half liter). With activity demands the tidal volume can increase eightfold. The residual volume (RV) is the amount of air remaining in the lungs after the fullest possible exhalation. This volume is about one quart (one liter). Any further reduction of the lung volume beyond the residual volume will cause injury

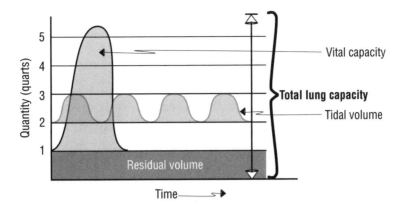

FIGURE 5.2 Lung volumes and capacities. Volumes represent a single lung measurement; capacities consist of two or more volumes. Volumes and capacities vary with a person's size, sex (decreased in females), age, and medical conditions.

to the lung. This does not occur on land but is a possible risk in breath-hold divers (see chapter 13).

The vital capacity (VC) is the amount of air that can be exhaled from the lungs after a maximal inhalation. It is the largest amount of air that can be moved with a single breath, and it is the most important measurement made with simple lung function tests. Measurements of these volumes are about 20 percent less in females than in males. Other terms relate to lung volume and capacity (two or more volumes) designations, but the terms just defined have the most pertinence to the breath-hold diver.

Immersion in water has several effects on the lungs. First, immersion to the neck level increases the diffusing capacity of gases in the lungs. Blood moves from the extremities to the blood vessels of the lungs due to the hydrostatic pressure gradient that occurs with a vertical position in water. There is more pressure at the foot level to force blood out of the lower extremities than at the chest level. This increases the amount of blood in the lungs and reduces their vital capacity. A second effect is blackout during deep breath-hold dives due to the use of the lungs for oxygen storage. As the ambient pressure increases during descent with breath-hold diving, oxygen and carbon dioxide tensions in the lungs and the blood change. By the 50-FSW (15-MSW) depth, there is a shift of carbon dioxide from the lungs to the bloodstream. The higher pressures increase oxygen partial pressures in the blood so that the breath-hold times tend to increase. During ascent the reverse processes occur, resulting in an influx of carbon dioxide and oxygen into the lungs from the bloodstream. This may reduce the stimulus to breathe and may dangerously lower (to the point of causing loss of consciousness) oxygen tensions during ascent (see chapter 11).

Respiratory Adaptations in Diving Mammals

The preceding chapter demonstrated the importance of the blood as an oxygen storage reservoir. The question now is, how important are the lungs as oxygen storage reservoirs for breath-hold dives? In contrast to what human breath-hold divers do, diving mammals dive after full exhalation of air from their lungs. After full inhalation, the pulmonary oxygen stores in diving mammals would account for only one-third to one-half of their oxygen requirements during a dive. In contrast, human breath-hold divers use their lungs for oxygen storage during a dive. Since the lungs of diving mammals do not act as oxygen reservoirs, what respiratory adaptations have they made for diving and what counterparts exist in human divers? Four such adaptations in diving mammals have been identified and include those that protect them from thoracic squeeze, enable them to avoid decompression sickness, alter sensitivities to respiratory gases, and increase their efficiency of ventilation.

Protection From Thoracic Squeeze

Thoracic squeeze is an extremely rare medical problem in breath-hold divers (see chapter 13). It occurs when the increased pressure of a deep breath-hold dive compresses the volume of the gas in the lungs to less than the residual volume (see figure 5.3). Fluid leakage and bleeding into the lungs result when this threshold is exceeded. For an average-sized human breath-hold diver, the calculated thoracic squeeze threshold after a maximal inhalation is 120 FSW (37 MSW).

Diving mammals have been observed to dive to extraordinary depths; why do these animals not get thoracic squeezes? At least three adaptations in the respiratory systems of diving mammals protect them from thoracic squeeze:

- First, the lungs of seals and whales are able to collapse completely without causing injury. This contrasts to the situation with the human lung, which becomes injured if compressed below its residual volume. When these mammals dive, the only air in their respiratory systems is in the dead spaces. Consequently, the exchange of oxygen and carbon dioxide at the alveolar level is nil. This is consistent with the information that gas stores in the lungs are not important for determining the breath-hold time in diving mammals. Even though the lungs in these mammals collapse fully during the dive, they do not separate from the chest walls as might be seen with a collapsed lung (pneumothorax) in the human. Upon surfacing and resumption of breathing, the lungs re-expand without incident.

- The second adaptation in diving mammals for protection against thoracic squeeze is seen in the shape and flexibility of their chest walls, which are more

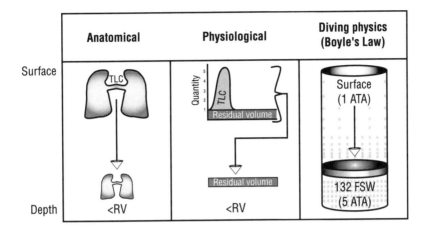

	Anatomical	Physiological	Diving physics (Boyle's Law)

FIGURE 5.3 Methods to describe thoracic squeeze (theoretical) threshold in the human breath-hold diver. TLC = total lung capacity; RV = residual volume; ATA = atmosphere absolute; FSW = feet of seawater.

cylindrical and more elastic than the chest walls of humans. These changes allow reduction in the chest cavity volume as pressure increases during descent. This lessens the pressure differentials between the inside (lung cavity) and outside (chest wall) of the chest and may be another protective mechanism against thoracic squeeze. In this manner, the chest wall and lung cavities begin to approximate the liquid-filled structures of the body that transmit pressure equally and undiminished so that no pressure gradients develop, in contrast to what happens with rigid-walled, air-filled cavities (see chapter 1).

• The third adaptation is seen in the use of venous reservoirs to replace, at least partially, the cavities created by the collapsed lungs during the dive. Seals have venous sinuses

Diving Physics: Computation of Thoracic Squeeze Threshold

Q: If the TLC of five quarts (4.7 liters) is compressed by the effects of hydrostatic pressure with descent to the residual volume of one quart (one liter), what would the depth threshold for thoracic squeeze be for this diver? We assume that the air-filled lungs compress like a balloon filled with air as predicted by Boyle's Law.

A: This represents a fivefold decrease in lung capacity. According to Boyle's Law, a fivefold increase in pressure would be required to achieve this decrease. This is equivalent to a change in pressure from 1 ATA to a pressure of 5 ATA. Since each ATA of pressure equals 33 FSW (10 MSW), the depth would be 5 × 33 = 165 feet (50 meters) of absolute pressure. Remember that this number needs to be converted to gauge pressure by subtracting 1 ATA (33 FSW) to give a thoracic squeeze threshold of 132 feet (40 meters) for this diver.

that become reservoirs in the venous system, storing large volumes of blood. They are located adjacent to the inferior vena cava, the large vein in the body that collects the blood from the trunk and lower part of the body before entering the heart. The diaphragm acts as a valve mechanism to prevent outflow of blood from the sinuses during the dive. The blood in the sinus helps to compensate for the space created by the collapsed lungs. Since blood is a noncompressible liquid that transmits the ambient pressure uniformly and undiminished (Pascal's principle), no pressure differentials arise in the lung cavity displaced by the venous reservoir.

Some counterparts to these adaptations are found in the human diver. Enormous discrepancies are noted in the depth records set by breath-hold divers as compared to their theoretical thoracic squeeze thresholds. For example, the most recent record, set in August 2002, was 525 FSW (160 MSW) by a female diver. Unfortunately, this diver died during a subsequent attempt to break her own record. The cause of death was not revealed, but several possibilities include blackout, drowning, and oxygen-induced seizure as well as thoracic squeeze. In studying the holder of a previous breath-hold dive record (Schaefer et al. 1968), the authors noted that about a quart (one liter) of blood shifted into blood vessels in the thoracic cavity during a dive to 90 FSW (27 MSW) and even more during a dive to 130 FSW (40 MSW). This blood displaced a corresponding amount of air in the lung cavity and apparently afforded additional protection against thoracic squeeze.

This effect has also been observed in the female divers of Japan. During their breath-hold dives, about one-fifth of a quart (200 milliliters) of blood shifts into the blood vessels of these divers' lung cavities (Rahn 1965). This adds another 15 FSW (4.6 MSW) to their theoretical thoracic squeeze depth threshold. After surfacing, the Ama always breathe slowly and whistle during the exhalation phase of respiration. The Valsalva-like effect (breathing against resistance) of the whistling may help return the blood that shifted into the blood vessels of the lung cavity back to the systemic circulation. The breathing pattern that the Ama use during recovery may also protect them from blackout associated with hyperventilation and gas diffusion (see chapter 11) during their relatively deep 60- to 75-FSW (18- to 23-MSW) breath-hold dives.

Another acclimatization that offers protection from thoracic squeeze is the increase in lung capacities that occur with breath-hold diving training. After repeated breath-hold dives, TLCs increase significantly while residual lung volumes decrease relatively (Schaefer 1963). This acclimatization increases the thoracic squeeze depth threshold.

How can the enormous discrepancies between the world record breath-hold dives and their theoretical thoracic squeeze thresholds be reconciled?

There are several possible explanations for the ability of these divers to tolerate depth well below what should be possible.

- First, the elasticity of the lung tissue itself may add an increased margin of tolerance so that damage does not occur until well beyond the theoretical threshold.

- Second, the effects of increased pressure on compressing the air-filled chest wall during a breath-hold dive may be more significant than previously believed, allowing the chest itself to reduce in size along with the lungs.

> ### Diving Physics: Effect of Increasing Total Lung Capacity on the Theoretical Thoracic Squeeze Threshold
>
> **Q:** After repetitive breath-hold dives over the course of a month, a diver has increased his TLC by 10 percent, from five quarts (4.7 liters) to five and one-half quarts (5.2 liters). His residual lung volume (RV) remains the same at one quart (one liter). How does this change his thoracic squeeze depth threshold?
>
> **A:** *From the previous problem, the diver's thoracic squeeze depth threshold was 132 FSW (40 MSW). The new threshold [(new TLC/RV × 33) – 33] is 148.5 FSW (45 MSW). The 10 percent improvement in TLC resulted in an additional 16.5-foot (5-meter or 12.5 percent) increase in the theoretical thoracic squeeze depth threshold.*

- Third, deep breath-hold divers say that they are able to "hyperinflate" (i.e., add further air) to the lungs or "pressurize" their lungs by further inhalations after their maximal inhalation.

- Fourth, the deeper the dive, the greater are the shifts of blood from the blood vessels of the extremities to the chest cavity. This blood may compensate for the decreased volume of the compressed lungs, which is analogous to the effect observed from the venous reservoirs in seals as described earlier.

- Fifth, congenital or developmental anomalies may increase the diver's TLCs. For example, the diver who held an earlier world breath-hold dive record had an abnormally large TLC, which he attributed to the effects of childhood asthma.

- Sixth, female divers may have hereditary factors that increase their resistance to thoracic squeeze. The current world record breath-hold dive is held by a female.

Protection From Decompression Sickness

In the past, it was believed that human breath-hold divers could not get "bent" (decompression sickness). A statement like "Decompression sickness is virtually impossible for the skin diver because he can not take up a troublesome amount of nitrogen—unless he has access to a supply of air at depth" (NAVMED 1956) summarizes the thinking before 1965. Challenging this opinion, Paulev (1965) showed that it is possible for decompression sickness to occur in breath-hold divers. In his study, four experienced, well-conditioned, highly trained divers participated in a series of repetitive breath-hold dives. Their dive profiles involved rapid descents to 65 FSW (20 MSW), and bottom times approached two minutes. Surface intervals varied from a few seconds to a maximum of two minutes so that the accumulated time spent underwater was greater than the accumulated time of the surface intervals. After five hours of diving, which included about 60 dives, signs and symptoms of decompression sickness appeared while the divers were on the surface. The diagnosis was confirmed when the signs and symptoms were resolved with recompression in a hyperbaric chamber. When Paulev (1967) calculated the amount of nitrogen accumulation in tissues with these dive profiles, he found that the tissue nitrogen tensions exceeded maximum tissue saturations (i.e., M-values; see chapter 3) and thereby verified that decompression sickness can occur with breath-hold diving.

Polynesian pearl divers of Tuamotu have become paralyzed after repetitive, deep breath-hold dives (Cross 1965). They call their symptoms *taravana*, which translates into the "falling syndrome." Symptoms occur after four to five hours of breath-hold diving to depths as great as 165 FSW (50 MSW) with very short surface intervals. Unfortunately, many of these divers remained permanently paralyzed due to lack of a recompression chamber on their island. Had their symptoms resolved with recompression therapy, the diagnosis of decompression sickness would have been confirmed in these cases. This problem was not observed in divers on an adjacent island who descended to equivalent depths but had surface intervals two to three times the durations of the Tuamotu divers.

These observations raise the question of why diving mammals do not get decompression sickness with their long, deep dives. From deep buoyancy-assisted submarine escape training exercises, it is known that decompression sickness will occur upon surfacing if the ascent is not started within a few seconds of pressurization at the 500-FSW (152-meter) submarine escape depth. The sperm whale and the Weddell seal (see introduction to part II) would surely incur decompression sickness after ascending if they initiated their dives with their lungs filled to capacity. They and other diving mammals apparently avoid decompression sickness by descending after full exhalation. As the lungs collapse, the residual air in the alveoli is forced into the nondiffusable portions of the respiratory tree (trachea, bronchi, bronchioles, and so on).

By the time a depth of 100 FSW (30 MSW) is reached, all of the residual gas in the alveoli of the lungs will have in-gassed to the tissues. Thus, there will be no further in-gassing of air into body tissues with descent beyond this point. During ascent the expansion of air that was forced into the nondiffusible portions of the respiratory tree (dead space) could be a factor in re-expansion of the lungs. Why diving mammals instinctively exhale before descent is an interesting behaviorism. Exhalation may help initiate the diving reflex. Buoyancy reduction from exhalation undoubtedly helps with descent.

Not all human breath-hold divers descend after full inhalation. For example, the Ama divers of Japan inhale to 80 percent of their TLC before starting their descent (Elsner 1969). Further inhalation may cause discomfort as well as making descent more difficult. However, because of the dive profiles of the Ama, it is not likely that this modest decrease in full inhalation at the start of the dive is empirically based to prevent decompression sickness. In summary, the same adaptations that prevent thoracic squeeze from occurring in diving mammals also protect these mammals from decompression sickness.

Alterations in Sensitivities to Respiratory Gases

A third respiratory adaptation observed in diving mammals is their decreased sensitivity to low blood and lung oxygen concentrations and high carbon dioxide levels. In the seal, the resting lung (alveolar) carbon dioxide tensions are higher and oxygen tensions are lower than in the human. In comparison to humans, diving mammals have a depressed breathing response to elevations in carbon dioxide and reductions in oxygen. These are undoubtedly adaptive mechanisms to increase the ability to tolerate anaerobic metabolism and oxygen deficits to extend the durations of their dives. As shown by Andersen (1966), though, diving vertebrates are not insensitive to elevated carbon dioxide levels. Andersen demonstrated increased breathing responses in the animals when they breathed gas mixtures with elevations of carbon dioxide, but the responses were not as great as those observed in humans. In muskrats and beavers, also aquatic mammals, 10 percent concentrations of carbon dioxide (330 times the normal amount) in the gas they breathed caused only minimal increments in their breathing responses (Irving 1938).

With practice, according to one study, human breath-hold divers developed respiratory acclimatizations that were not observed in a control group of non-divers (Schaefer 1963). Four acclimatizations were noted:

- Significantly decreased ventilation responses ("air hunger") to breathing 10.5 percent carbon dioxide
- Improved oxygen utilization, that is, more extraction of oxygen from the blood without loss of consciousness

DIVING SCENARIO

THE EMPHYSEMA PATIENT—THE ULTIMATE IN TOLERANCE TO ELEVATED CARBON DIOXIDE TENSIONS

It is ironic that the greatest acclimatizations to elevated carbon dioxide levels are seen in patients who have chronic obstructive airway disease (**emphysema;** disease condition in which the alveoli lose their elasticity and no longer passively move the air within them to the bronchial tubes for exhalation) with carbon dioxide retention. Their breathing receptors have become so desensitized to chronically elevated carbon dioxide levels that this gas no longer stimulates breathing. Their respiratory drive (desire to breathe) becomes entirely dependent on low oxygen tensions in the blood. If the blood oxygen tensions are increased, for example, with hyperbaric oxygen, the patient may stop breathing.

- Tolerance to larger oxygen deficits without having to stop the exercise activity
- Increased tolerance to elevated tissue carbon dioxide levels

These responses disappeared three months after diving was discontinued, which is consistent with their classification as acclimatizations rather than adaptations. However, there are natural differences in human tolerance to breathing elevated levels of carbon dioxide that are consistent with adaptations. Schaefer (1954) reported that a lower-ventilation-response group of subjects uniformly had larger tidal volumes, lower respiratory rates, and improved tolerances to elevated alveolar carbon dioxide tensions than a higher-ventilation, less tolerant group. The Ama divers of Japan demonstrate similar respiratory adaptations as compared to their non-diving counterparts (Elsner and Scholander 1965).

In summary, alterations in sensitivities to respiratory gases are observed in both mammalian and human breath-hold divers. These changes improve their abilities to tolerate exercise and the effects of anaerobic metabolism (see chapter 4). The changes include decreased breathing responses to elevated levels of carbon dioxide, both in the breathing gas and in the body tissues, and improved ability to tolerate and function with low oxygen tensions in their tissues. While the changes that occur in humans are acclimatizations, with the possible exception of ventilatory responses to elevated levels of inhaled carbon dioxide, those in the diving mammals are probably adaptations. Conversely, the need for diving mammals to dive in order to survive in the aquatic environment may reflect a conditioning response to elevated carbon dioxide and lowered oxygen levels, just as observed in human breath-hold divers.

Efficiency of Ventilation

A fourth group of changes observed in the respiratory systems of diving mammals includes improvements in the efficiency of ventilation and reductions in the recovery time after a breath-hold dive. The human respiratory exchange function, in comparison to that in diving mammals, is relatively inefficient as indicated in table 5.1. Although body masses as compared to lung capacities are similar in humans, seals, and porpoises, the latter two diving mammals have markedly slower respiratory rates, higher oxygen utilization percentages, and larger tidal volume to total lung capacity ratios than humans do. Whales, although much larger, show even greater changes.

As tidal volumes (amount of air exchanged with each breath) approach TLCs, ventilation becomes increasingly efficient. The effects of these changes are fourfold:

• First, lower respiratory rates and larger volumes of air exchange with each breath reduce the energy expenditures required for ventilation. A secondary benefit of a lower respiratory rate includes less insensible fluid losses from the lungs. In humans, about 20 percent of body fluid losses are from the lungs (see chapter 1). When respiratory rates are reduced from 12 to 15 breaths per minute to 1 or 2 breaths a minute, the insensible fluid losses from the lungs are proportionally reduced.

• Second, higher percentages of oxygen utilization increase the efficiency of each breath. Oxygen utilization in the lungs of diving mammals is about twice that of humans. This reduces the need to increase the respiratory rate to maintain the same level of oxygenation of the blood. Highly trained human breath-hold divers demonstrated improved efficiency of breathing as compared to non-divers (Carley et al. 1955). Their vital capacities were 14 percent higher than would be predicted by age, gender, and height. Significantly increased tidal volumes, inspiratory reserve volumes, and TLCs

Table 5.1	Comparison of Respiratory Functions in Aquatic Mammals and Humans		
Animal	Resting breathing rate (breaths per minute)	Oxygen utilization (percent)	Relative* tidal volume to relative lung capacity (percent)
Human	15 (100%)**	4-5 (100%)**	20 (100%)**
Seal	3-4 (23%)	5-7 (133%)	36 (180%)
Porpoise	1-4 (17%)	8-10 (200%)	83 (415%)
Whale	1-2 (10%)	8-10 (200%)	87 (435%)

* Relative refers to liters per 100 kilograms of lung tissue.
** Compared to humans, using the human value as 100% and averaging the ranges.

accompanied the increases in vital capacity in these trained divers. With increases in TLC, there is also a relative decrease in residual volumes. This improves the efficiency of ventilation as well as the thoracic squeeze depth threshold.

• Third, fully inflated lungs assist in buoyancy. With improved buoyancy, swimming movements are minimized during recovery from a dive on the surface. This reduces energy expenditures and hastens recovery. The importance of utilizing the lungs for buoyancy is apparent in porpoises. These animals spend time on the surface in a semiconscious state, probably analogous to sleep, breathing one to four times a minute. When a breath is needed, they roll to their sides, make several apparently reflexive movements of their pectoral fins in order to clear their blow holes above the surface of the water, exhale, quickly inhale, and then resume their former semiconscious nonbreathing state.

• A final effect of improved efficiency in breathing is associated with conservation of body heat, which is discussed in chapter 7.

While alterations in sensitivities to oxygen and carbon dioxide are adaptations in diving mammals, changes to improve the efficiency of ventilation, for the most part, occur with conditioning (acclimatizations) in the human breath-hold diver. These changes are probably little different from those seen in athletes who train for endurance events or mountain climbing.

Technology to Meet the Respiratory Challenges of the Aquatic Environment

Chapter 2 described the SCUBA regulator and tanks. These two pieces of equipment have greatly mediated the ventilation stresses of the underwater environment and require no additional discussion here. Since the lungs assist the diving mammal and the sport diver in fine-tuning buoyancy, in this section we discuss the buoyancy compensator (BC) as a technological development for the respiratory system.

In the past, the rule was "If you are in trouble, first drop your weight belt," because the modified life preservers, which were inflated with a carbon dioxide cylinder, provided adequate buoyancy only on the surface. Therefore, many divers elected not to use them. When underwater, the capacity of the carbon dioxide cylinder often was not sufficient to improve buoyancy enough to bring the diver to the surface. This inability to provide buoyancy at depth in these circumstances is explained by Boyle's Law (see chapter 1). In addition, the carbon dioxide inflation mechanisms were notoriously unreliable. One observation revealed that the majority were not operational as a consequence of corrosion or expended carbon dioxide cartridges. When inflated on the surface, they functioned like a life preserver, which interfered with swimming.

Today's BCs are another major technological improvement for the SCUBA diver. Although bigger and bulkier than the legendary UDT (Navy Underwater Demolition Team—Frogmen) swimmer vest, the modern BC does much more. It allows the diver to maintain neutral buoyancy easily at any depth. This is done with an inflator hose that has a connection to a low-pressure port on the primary stage of the SCUBA regulator. Consequently, the diver can add air to the BC by manual inflation (from air in his or her lungs) or from air in the SCUBA tanks. The oral inflator hose in many BCs can be connected to a second stage regulator, for emergency backup, similar to an octopus regulator.

Air is released from the BC through an exhaust valve at the end of the inflator tube. To allow air to exit from the BC, the diver raises the end of the inflator tube above the air bladders and presses the exhaust valve. This allows a controlled release of air from the BC. At the beginning of the descent, while on the surface, air in the BC is released to provide negative buoyancy to lessen the effort to descend. During ascent, air may need to be released to compensate for the increased buoyancy associated with expansion of gas in the BC (Boyle's Law). In the head-down position, a second exhaust valve with a toggle release at the bottom of the vest (when in the vertical position) also can be used to release air from the BC. The connectors for the inflator tube and the exhaust valves use large-diameter, threaded screw fittings. This makes their disassembly, for cleaning the insides of the air bladders, and their reassembly easy.

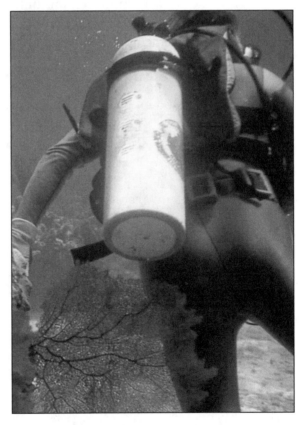

The SCUBA tank stores an air supply to allow one to meet the challenges of the underwater environment.

Another advantage of the modern BC is its vertical stability when inflated. Some of the older models tended to put the diver in the horizontal, facedown position or to bend the neck and obstruct the airway (or both) when inflated fully. All current BCs have pressure relief valves, usually in combination with the exhaust valve at the lower portion of the BC. These prevent overinflation and possible rupture of the BC when gas inside the bladders expands with ascent (Boyle's Law)—which could be lifesaving. With a ruptured BC, the unconscious diver could sink if negatively buoyant, or could aspirate water on the surface without the BC to prop his or her head out of the water. If in panic and struggling to stay on the surface, the diver may overlook other buoyancy-improving interventions such as dropping weights. Buoyancy compensators range in price from about $200 to $500. The more expensive models have larger capacities and an increasing array of features as described in table 5.2.

The disadvantages of the modern BC are few in comparison to its advantages. The BC is a requirement for virtually all SCUBA diving activities, especially when others assume responsibility for the dive, such as diving boat operators. Modern BCs cannot be worn with closed-circuit SCUBA gear since they impede movement of the breathing bags and there are no adaptors for

Table 5.2	Features That Add Costs to the Modern Buoyancy Compensator (BC)
Feature	**Comment**
Weight integrated	Slide-out pockets in the front of the BC that allow a maximum of 6 to 10 lb (2.7 to 4.5 kg) of weight to be added to each side near the diver's center of gravity
Swivel buckles	Facilitate adjustments and connecting of straps
Pockets	Have Velcro or zipper closures; useful for carrying a backup knife, food snack (foil wrapped), and emergency signal tube
D-rings	For attaching dive knives, catch bags, and so on
Padded back	For increased comfort, especially during carrying of equipment on land
Octopus regulator integrated with oral inflator	Streamlines equipment; not as versatile for buddy breathing as the long hose-length octopus; adds more than $100 to the cost of the BC
Compensating waistband	Usually elastic-neoprene with Velcro closure; is easy to don and keeps BC secure on diver's back
Chest and abdominal straps	Further secure BC to the diver; straps are adjustable with quick releases
Cordura covering	Provides increased strength, durability, and resistance to rubs, punctures, and ruptures

connections to the BC inflator tube. In these situations, horseshoe-like collars are required with the old-style carbon dioxide inflators. The BC, although a potential air-containing cavity, is not useful as an emergency air source, since even if inflated it would provide only a few breaths of air. The loss of buoyancy resulting from "breathing" the gas used to inflate the BC may put the diver in more jeopardy than the benefit of using it for an emergency air supply. Finally, the inflated BC makes swimming on the surface difficult and slows swimming underwater due to drag. If one is swimming on the surface in the facedown position, using a snorkel is highly recommended, since much effort is required to lift up the head and clear the mouth for breathing.

Buoyancy compensators require the same meticulous care and maintenance that other pieces of diving equipment do. When packing, one must prevent punctures or rubs (abrasions) from other equipment in the dive bag. After the dive, the components of the BC, including the insides of the air bladders, need to be rinsed with fresh water and allowed to dry thoroughly. Before the BC is stored, it should be inflated fully and observed for leaks, for example, by noting if the BC remains firm a few hours later. Finally, during storage of the BC, the material of the air bladder must not be sharply creased; this could lead to a stress point in the air bladder when inflated at a later time.

For Further Review

1. What are the main components of the respiratory system? What are their functions?

2. What is the theoretical limit for breath-hold diving in humans? Why is it significantly different from the world record?

3. What protective mechanisms do diving mammals have against thoracic squeeze?

4. How can decompression sickness occur in breath-hold divers?

5. How are diving mammals protected from decompression sickness?

6. What acclimatizations are found in conditioned breath-hold divers?

7. How do the efficiencies of respiratory functions differ between human divers and diving mammals?

8. What are the desirable features of the modern buoyancy compensator?

CHAPTER 6

ADAPTATIONS IN BLOOD AND MUSCLE TISSUES TO IMPROVE OXYGEN CARRYING AND STORAGE

There are changes in the oxygen-carrying and storage ability of blood and muscle tissues that complement the diving reflex and further help to extend the breath-hold times of diving mammals. These changes are mostly unique to the diving mammal. Although some counterparts are observed as acclimatizations in human populations living at high altitudes, they are not observed in the human breath-hold diver.

Chapter Preview

- Physical structures in diving mammals that increase their oxygen storage capacities
- Relationship of blood volume to oxygen storage capacity
- Comparison of the red blood cells of diving mammals and humans
- Role of myoglobin in the storage of oxygen
- Biochemical changes in the blood that influence oxygen utilization
- Basic mechanisms of hyperbaric oxygen therapy

Anatomy and Physiology

Blood is a complex mixture of cells, fluids, and substances dissolved in the fluids. Ordinarily **red blood cells** carry 97.5 percent of the oxygen in the bloodstream in their hemoglobin, as diagrammed in figure 6.1. **Hemoglobin** is an iron-containing molecule found in red blood cells that binds oxygen in the presence of high oxygen concentrations and releases it when surrounded by tissues with lower oxygen concentrations. The oxygen-binding and -releasing characteristics of hemoglobin make it possible for higher life forms to meet their oxygen demands. The deadly gas carbon monoxide attaches 250

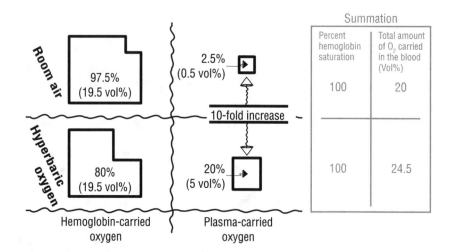

FIGURE
6.1   Oxygen transport (%) hemoglobin versus plasma in room air and with hyperbaric oxygen.

times as firmly to the hemoglobin molecule as oxygen does (see chapter 14). Consequently, very small concentrations of carbon monoxide can have devastating effects on oxygen delivery to tissues. The remaining 2.5 percent of oxygen transport in the blood is from physically dissolved oxygen in its fluid portion. The amount of oxygen physically dissolved in the plasma equates to about the same percentage as found in seawater. This amount of oxygen is sufficient to meet the oxygen demands of lower life forms such as fish (which have gills to extract oxygen) but not those of humans and mammalian divers.

Oxygen binding to the hemoglobin molecule occurs in the lungs, where the oxygen tensions from breathing the inspired air are high. Then the oxygen-laden red blood cells are carried by the bloodstream throughout the body. At the capillary level, the oxygen moves from the hemoglobin molecule to the tissues in response to the lower oxygen tensions in the tissues. The tissues then utilize the oxygen for metabolic purposes. The oxygen-depleted hemoglobin then returns to the lungs to on-load additional oxygen and repeat the circulation cycle. Several factors, such as the acid content and the temperature of the blood, influence how much oxygen can be off-loaded at the tissue level. Normally, the oxygen off-loaded at the tissue level is only about 25 percent of the total amount of oxygen carried by the red blood cell after the hemoglobin becomes fully saturated in the lungs, as illustrated in figure 6.2.

All cells in the body require oxygen in order to survive and carry out their metabolic functions. There are great variations in the oxygen requirements of various types of tissues. Brain tissues require a constant, uninterrupted

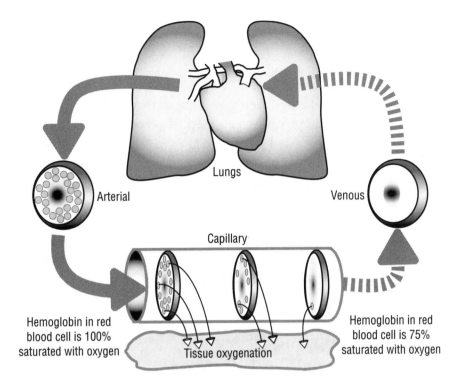

FIGURE
6.2   Oxygen utilization from the hemoglobin molecule. The oxygen extraction (arterial–venous oxygen difference) is 5 volume percent. Thus, hemoglobin normally off-loads only 25 percent of the total oxygen it is carrying. With hyperbaric oxygen, an amount equal to the off-loaded oxygen can be physically dissolved in the plasma.

supply of oxygen. A moment's interruption in the oxygen supply to the brain will result in loss of consciousness. Heart muscles are the tissues that are the next most sensitive to oxygen deficits. In contrast, connective tissues such as ligaments, tendons, and joint capsules have minimal requirements for oxygen and can survive long periods without oxygen. It is not by coincidence that the diving reflex ensures adequate provision of oxygen to the two most critical tissues in the body, the brain and the heart, during the breath-hold dive (see chapter 4).

In humans, red blood cells normally comprise 35 to 45 percent of the blood volume. When the amount of red blood cells is too low (**anemia**), the oxygen transported to tissues may be insufficient to meet the metabolic requirements of the tissues. When the red blood cell amount becomes too high, blood flow is slowed by the increased viscosity from the greater mass of cells. This places an added stress on the heart and makes the red blood cells more subject to sludging when passing through the capillary circulation (see chapter 4). Sludging blocks the flow of red blood cells, and the consequence is oxygen deprivation to tissues. Sludging of red blood cells is observed in decompression sickness (see chapter 15) and several disease conditions.

In an average-sized human, the blood volume is about five quarts (4.7 liters). When the optimal blood volume decreases, there is a reduced capacity to supply the body's tissues with oxygen. Reduction of blood volume occurs with bleeding. However, it is more frequently associated with thickening of the blood from movement of the fluid portions of the blood into tissues **(dehydration)** as a consequence of sweating, insensible losses from the lungs, and diuresis (excretion of urine). Infection, malnutrition, drugs, or combinations of these may also reduce the blood volume. The cellular elements, the red blood cells and the white blood cells (for fighting infections), remain in the bloodstream. SCUBA and breath-hold diving lead to dehydration in humans. Diving mammals have physiological and anatomical characteristics that prevent this problem.

Oxygen Carrying and Storage in Diving Mammals and Humans

Diving mammals have a 50 percent greater oxygen-carrying and storage capacity than terrestrial mammals of corresponding size (Irving et al. 1935). This is attributed to five anatomical and physiological changes in their blood, which include

- larger relative blood volumes,
- higher percentages of oxygen-carrying red blood cells,
- better oxygen storage capacities in muscles,
- oxygen extraction from venous blood, and
- greater oxygen extraction from hemoglobin.

Blood Volumes

Diving mammals have larger blood volumes than non-diving mammals. When blood volumes are expressed as percentages of body weight, diving mammals have twice the blood volume of their non-diving counterparts (Andersen 1964). The diving mammals maintain their blood volumes during diving by several techniques. First, during breath-holding, diving mammals (as well as human breath-hold divers) do not incur fluid losses through their lungs. In SCUBA divers, fluid losses increase in direct proportion to the depth of the dive (see chapter 1). However, during the recovery phase of breath-hold dives, human breath-hold divers lose relatively more fluid through breathing than the diving mammals. This is attributable to the decreased efficiency of our ventilation responses as compared to those of the diving mammals (see chapter 5). Blood volumes are maintained in diving mammals by three mechanisms: minimizing fluid shifts, decreasing urine production, and reducing insensible fluid losses.

Minimizing Fluid Shifts   Fluid shifts from the **periphery** (the portion of the body outside the core; typically, this refers to the appendages [arms and legs] and the skin and subcutaneous [below the skin] tissues of the core) to the **core** (the central portion of the body; refers to the structures contained within the thorax, abdomen, head, and neck) during immersion are minimized in diving mammals due to the effectiveness of shunting associated with the diving reflex. In the human diver, shifts of blood to the core circulation initiate reflexes that cause increased urine formation. The increased blood volume in the core results in an increased venous return. This slightly distends the right atrium, the receiving chamber in the heart for blood from the body. The distended right atrium initiates a reflex to increase blood flow to the kidneys, which results in increased production of urine. The fluid for urine production comes from fluid in the blood. Ordinarily, the amount of fluid lost through this mechanism is insignificant. However, when coupled with respiratory fluid losses, this loss can contribute to dehydration and sludging. In diving mammals, blood flow to the kidneys ceases during the dive as a consequence of the diving reflex so that no fluid is lost through this route. In experiments, the effect is so strong that it persists even in the presence of drugs that otherwise would terminate the diving reflex.

Decreasing Urine Production   Another cause of fluid loss is involuntary excretion of urine. With repetitive breath-hold dives, as the endpoints of breath-holding are approached, comes an increasingly stronger desire to pass urine. Similar effects have also been reported in SCUBA divers. This effect is probably due to a combination of factors including psychological factors, fluid shifts, elevations in blood carbon dioxide levels, and cooling. This virtually uncontrolled need to pass urine is termed **involuntary diuresis.** These effects do not appear to occur in diving mammals, since urine is not produced during their dives. In addition, diving mammals have the ability to increase the concentration of urine so that less fluid is needed to excrete waste products of metabolism through the kidneys. This is associated with the fact that the only source of fluid for diving mammals is from the food they consume.

Reduction of Insensible Fluid Losses   Sweating is a cause of insensible fluid loss in humans. Sweating may not be appreciated during diving because of immersion in water; but with activity, especially in very warm (greater than 90 degrees F or 32 degrees C) water, body fluids may be lost through sweating. However, a more likely cause of fluid loss occurs during the surface intervals after diving in warm, tropical environments. Like canines, diving mammals do not have sweat glands; nor do whales and porpoises spend their surface intervals out of the water as humans do. Insensible fluid loss from the lungs is magnified by breathing dehumidified gasses under pressure, as discussed in chapter 1.

Red Blood Cell Alterations

Two differences in red blood cells are noted in diving mammals as compared to humans. First, the red blood cells of diving mammals are smaller than those of humans. This morphological change (alteration in shape or structure) may be a factor in protecting diving mammals from decompression sickness and may increase the ability of red blood cells to transfer oxygen to tissues. The smaller the size of the red blood cell, the better it will be able to pass through the most narrowed portions of the circulation, the capillary bed, without risk of stasis or sludging. The smaller size may also allow a higher portion of oxygen to be off-loaded to the tissues. This would improve oxygen utilization during breath-holding and help to extend the diving mammals' bottom times.

The second difference is in the quantity of red blood cells. The percentage of red blood cells (the **hematocrit**) in diving mammals' blood is in the 50 percent range. This is about 20 percent higher than in humans. The higher the red blood cell percentage, the greater the oxygen-carrying capacity of the blood. World-class athletes attempt to increase the oxygen-carrying capacity of their blood by training at high altitudes. This represents acclimatization to the hypoxic environment.

The smaller red blood cell size in diving mammals presumably helps to avoid some of the complications associated with increased red blood cell percentages that have been observed in humans, such as sludging, blood clotting, and blockage of circulation to body parts such as the brain, heart, and bones.

Oxygen Storage in Muscles

Myoglobin is a variant of hemoglobin that is found in muscle tissues. Like hemoglobin it is a storage reservoir for oxygen. Diving mammals have greater stores of myoglobin than non-diving mammals. Myoglobin binds oxygen more firmly than hemoglobin does. This means that there has to be a greater difference between the oxygen levels attached to the myoglobin and the oxygen levels in the muscle tissue before myoglobin off-loads its oxygen to the muscle tissues.

DIVING SCENARIO

BLOOD DOPING TO INCREASE THE OXYGEN-CARRYING CAPACITY OF BLOOD

Blood doping is a generic term referring to what are generally regarded as illegal methods to increase the oxygen-carrying capacity of blood. The two most common methods of blood doping are blood transfusions and use of agents to stimulate the production of red blood cells. The latter method is by administration of recombinant (synthesized in the laboratory from ribonucleic acids) erythropoietin. Erythropoietin is a substance normally produced by the kidneys to stimulate the body's production of red blood cells.

About 50 percent of the total amount of oxygen storage in the bodies of diving mammals at the beginning of a dive is in the myoglobin (Andersen 1964). Oxygen transfer from hemoglobin (with its lower affinity for oxygen) to myoglobin (with its higher affinity for oxygen) does not occur as the myoglobin oxygen stores are depleted. The reason is shunting of blood from the muscles during the diving reflex. Consequently, the oxygen attached to the hemoglobin in the core circulation remains available to supply the brain and the heart. After the first three to four minutes of the breath-hold dive, the oxygen stored in seals' myoglobin is exhausted while the arterial oxygen saturation in the core is still greater than 50 percent (Scholander, Irving, and Grinnell 1942a). At that time muscle energy production switches to anaerobic (energy production without oxygen) metabolism. This creates lactic acid and other products of anaerobic metabolism in the muscle tissues. The waste products are cleared when the diving mammal surfaces, terminates the diving reflex, resumes breathing the surface air, and corrects the oxygen deficit generated by the products of anaerobic metabolism (see chapter 4).

Oxygen Extraction From Venous Blood

As noted in the previous chapter, seals and presumably other diving mammals have large venous sinuses just below the diaphragm (Elsner et al. 1964). During the dive, these reservoirs contain approximately 20 percent of the total blood volume of the seal. In the elephant seal it has been observed that the arterial oxygen tensions decrease more rapidly than the venous oxygen tensions during the early portions of the dive (Elsner et al. 1964). During the latter half of the dive, the inferior vena cava (the large vein that brings blood from the trunk and lower extremities to the heart) has higher oxygen concentrations than the arterial system. When this occurs, it appears that oxygen begins to be extracted from the venous blood to maintain adequate oxygen supplies for the heart and the brain. Consequently, the reservoirs may be an important oxygen storage site for the diving mammals and may help to account for the long durations of their breath-hold dives. Another reservoir of oxygen for diving mammals may be the spleen. With contraction of the spleen, another source of oxygen-rich red blood cells may become available to the core circulation.

Greater Oxygen Extraction From Venous Blood

The blood of diving mammals is more acidic than that of humans. The reason is a reduced buffering (ability to absorb increased acid) capacity of their blood. As the blood becomes progressively more acidic, as associated with exercise and oxygen-deficient (hypoxic) states, more oxygen is released from the hemoglobin molecule. This is a protective mechanism that helps provide more oxygen to tissues in the presence of **hypoxia,** a condition in which body tissues have less oxygen than is needed for them to function normally. This mechanism, termed the **Bohr effect,** improves the efficiency of oxygen off-loading from the hemoglobin molecule in the red blood cell. As the breath-hold dive continues, the blood becomes progressively more acidic due to buildup of carbon dioxide and lactic acid. This makes it possible for additional oxygen to be extracted from the hemoglobin molecule. In the human breath-hold diver as well as in other hypoxic states, the Bohr effect also occurs, but to a lesser degree. This is attributable to our poorer tolerance for acid production in the blood.

Technology to Aid Oxygen Carrying and Storage in the Blood

From the perspective of equipment, there are essentially no practical technological developments for the diver that improve oxygen carrying and storage in the blood in relation to the size of red blood cells, the venous sinusoids, and blood volume. For the SCUBA diver, these benefits in the diving mammals are nonissues because of the self-contained supply of air. Accommodations, in the form of increased blood volumes and percentages of red blood cells, however, are observed in humans who live at high altitudes.

Information about oxygen carrying and storage in the blood of diving mammals can help prevent medical problems of diving in humans. During diving activities, the blood volume should be maintained at optimal levels through avoidance of dehydration. The first step is to recognize that SCUBA diving leads to dehydration. Thus, measures to avoid dehydration associated with diving activities, as listed in table 6.1, are essential. Second, to avoid sludging of red blood cells, medications such as **aspirin** may be of benefit. Aspirin inhibits **agglutination** (clumping together) of blood platelets. **Plate-**

lets have a major role in blood clotting. Consequently, aspirin reduces the likelihood of blood clotting and sludging. Some authorities recommend that aspirin be incorporated in all decompression sickness treatment protocols, not only for the reasons just mentioned, but also because aspirin acts as an anti-inflammatory agent and reduces the reaction between the nitrogen bubble and the blood vessel lining. In the 1970s, Chryssanthou reported on substances, which he named smooth muscle activating factors, that offered protection from decompression sickness in laboratory animals (Chryssanthou, Teichner, and Antopol 1971). Antagonists to these substances make the animal more susceptible to decompression sickness. Unfortunately, because of lack of interest on the part of other investigators, this potentially beneficial research has not been pursued.

For completeness, hyperbaric oxygen (HBO) therapy must be mentioned in any discussion of techniques to improve the oxygen-carrying capacity of the blood. **Hyperbaric oxygen therapy** is a type of breathing therapy in which the patient is placed in a chamber and breathes pure oxygen at pressures greater than 1 ATA. Usual treatment pressures are at 2 ATA to 2.4 ATA, which is equivalent to the pressure experienced at a 33- to 46-FSW (10- to 14-MSW) depths. For diving problems, the HBO treatment pressures usually start at 2.8 to 3.0 ATA (60 to 66 FSW or 18 to 20 MSW). Hyperbaric oxygen at 2 ATA forces 10 times more oxygen into the plasma (the liquid portion of blood) than breathing room air. These effects are verified by Dalton's and Henry's Laws (see chapter 1). Hyperbaric oxygen

Table 6.1	Measures to Avoid Dehydration Problems in the Sport Diver
Measure	**Comment**
Adequate fluid intake	The clearer the urine appearance, the better the hydration.
Moderate exercise in warm, humid climates	Sweating can be a large source of fluid losses.
Allowing time to acclimatize to warm environments by initially modifying activities	Acclimatizations are initiated after three to four days, but full effects may take several weeks.
Avoiding alcoholic beverages	Alcohol, although a fluid, causes dehydration as it is eliminated from the body.
"Loading up" on water or clear fluids before diving	Diving accelerates insensible fluid loss.
Not diving if symptoms of dehydration are noted	Symptoms include light-headedness, confusion, weakness, parched mouth, little or no urine production, concentrated odorous urine, dry skin, headaches.

	Table 6.2 Approved Uses of Hyperbaric Oxygen Therapy by the Center for Medicare-Medicaid Services (Medicare)	
Condition	**Primary effect of HBO**	**Secondary effect of HBO**
1. Carbon monoxide poisoning	Mass effect (CO washout)	Mitigate reperfusion injury
2. Decompression sickness	Bubble reduction	Mass effect (nitrogen washout)
3. Arterial gas embolism (AGE)	Bubble reduction	Mass effect (nitrogen washout)
4. Gas gangrene	Oxygen penetration of relative barriers (dead tissues, edema)	Bacteriological (inhibit bacterial growth and toxin formation)
5. Acute traumatic peripheral ischemia	Increased oxygen in low-flow states (injured vessels, edema)	Angiogenesis (new blood vessel formation)
6. Crush injuries and suturing of severed limbs	Oxygen penetration of relative barriers (edema)	Edema reduction
7. Progressive necrotizing infections	Oxygen penetration of relative barriers (infected tissue, edema)	Bacteriological; inhibit bacterial growth and toxins
8. Acute peripheral arterial insufficiency	Increased oxygen delivery in low-flow states	Edema reduction
9. Preservation of compromised skin flaps or grafts	Oxygen penetration of relative barriers (edema)	Edema reduction
10. Chronic refractory osteomyecitis (bone infection)	Oxygen penetration of relative barriers (bone and skin tissue)	Angiogenesis
11. Osteoradionecrosis (bone death from radiation)	Oxygen penetration of relative barriers (bone and skin tissue)	Angiogenesis
12. Soft tissue radionecrosis (soft tissue death from radiation)	Oxygen penetration of relative barriers (dead tissue, scar tissue)	Angiogenesis
13. Cyanide poisoning	Mass effect (washout of cyanide)	Mitigate reperfusion injury, as in CO poisoning
14. Actinomyosis (bone infection from a fungus)	Oxygen penetration of relative barriers (infected tissue)	Angiogenesis
15. Diabetic foot wounds	Increased oxygen delivery in low-flow states	Bacteriological

Conditions 2 and 3 (and possibly 1) are those in which HBO is used for divers. The Undersea and Hyperbaric Medical Society (UHMS) has a list used by the FDA (Food and Drug Administration) and many insurance carriers as a guideline for appropriate hyperbaric oxygen (HBO) usage. The UHMS list includes 13 conditions, but the conditions are analogous to those in the above Medicare list.

can be helpful in treating conditions in which low oxygen levels in tissues interfere with healing or function. Fifteen different disease conditions have been approved by the Center for Medicare-Medicaid Services (Medicare) for the use of HBO as listed in table 6.2. Hyperbaric oxygen recompression therapy is the standard of practice for treating decompression sickness and arterial gas embolism (see chapter 15).

For the sport diver, HBO is not a practical consideration for improving durations of breath-hold dives. However, under experimental conditions, breath-holding times are increased after breathing of oxygen on the surface and even more so when oxygen is breathed under increased pressure in a hyperbaric chamber. This is attributed to the additional oxygen that becomes physically dissolved in the plasma. Our studies have failed to demonstrate improved weightlifting or running performances immediately after HBO exposures.

For Further Review

1. How is oxygen transported?
2. How are oxygen storage capacities increased in diving mammals?
3. How do diving mammals' and humans' red blood cells differ?
4. What is the role of myoglobin?
5. How does blood acidity affect oxygen off-loading to tissues?
6. What factors contribute to dehydration in human divers? How are these avoided in diving mammals?

MEETING THE CHALLENGES OF THE COLD WATER ENVIRONMENT

C hapter 1 introduced the enormous thermal chal-lenges of the aquatic environ-ment, which are illustrated in figure 7.1. Heat is lost by three methods: **conduction** or direct transfer; **convection,** or indi-rect transfer as a consequence of moving of the surrounding air or fluid environment; and **radiation,** or warming of a remote object without warm-

Chapter Preview

- Challenges of the cold water environment
- Mechanisms that preserve core temperature in diving mammals
- Heat-conserving mechanisms that complement the diving reflex
- Body shape and its affect on heat conserva-tion
- Role of metabolism in heat production
- Equipment for thermal protection of the human diver

ing of the intervening medium. This latter effect is inconsequential for the human diver. The high specific heat and thermal conductivity of water make it much more challenging to the diver's heat-conserving mechanisms than is air. Diving mammals have adaptations that meet these challenges; vestiges of these adaptations are seen in the human diver. Technology makes it possible for the human diver to meet the thermal challenges of the aquatic environ-ment effectively.

Anatomy and Physiology

For practical purposes, body heat conservation involves two compartments, the core and the periphery. The core includes the structures within the head, neck, and trunk. The periphery includes the extremities (arms and legs) plus the skin of the head, neck, and trunk. Heat conservation mecha-nisms in mammals are directed at preserving the **core temperature** (i.e., the

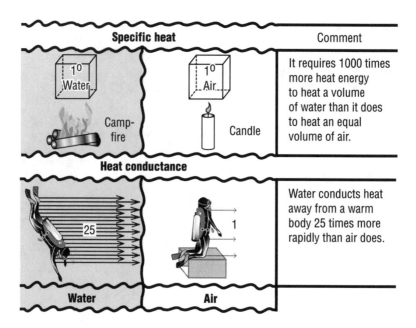

FIGURE 7.1 Thermal challenges of water compared to air. The combined effects make immersion in cold water very challenging for the diver.

temperature of the vital organs in the head and trunk such as the heart, brain, lungs, and liver) at the expense of the periphery. When warm blood flows from the core to the periphery, heat is carried away from the core. If the ambient (the outside, external, surrounding) temperature is cooler than the core temperature, heat is lost to the environment, and the temperature of the blood drops. The periphery radiates heat in the blood from the core to the surrounding water as diagrammed in figure 7.2.

The nervous system regulates the amount of blood that flows to the periphery, but muscle activity and the muscles' oxygen demands also influence the blood flow. With heat conductance 25 times greater than that of air, the water rapidly conducts heat away from the periphery as the warmth of the peripheral tissues tries to warm the surrounding water. The cool blood from the periphery returns to the core, where it is rewarmed at the expense of cooling the core, and then returns to the periphery to further exchange its heat with the surrounding water. The rate at which heat is lost from the immersed human body to the surrounding water is so rapid that the limiting factor is how fast warm blood from the central core can be carried to the skin (Beckman 1963). Diving mammals effectively meet these challenges through adaptations complemented by the adaptations used to meet the cardiovascular and respiratory challenges of the dive.

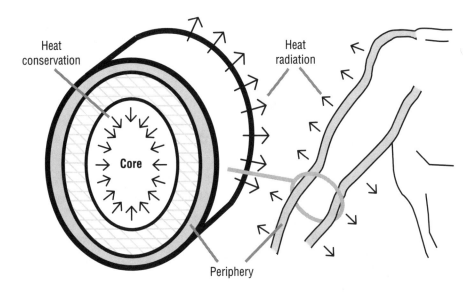

FIGURE 7.2 Heat losses to the environment. The challenge is how to keep the warm core blood from moving to the periphery where it will be cooled by the surrounding cold water.

Much information exists regarding the effects of human immersion in cold water. Breath-hold divers drop their core temperatures 2 to 10 degrees F (1.2 to 7.3 degrees C) during two and one-half hour diving sessions in 80 to 90 degree F (26 to 32 degree C) water (Bond 1966). For human swimmers and divers, this is considered warm water. The average decline in core temperatures of the Ama (commercial diving women) of Japan for a 45-minute session is 3.3 degrees F (1.7 degrees C) during diving in the summer in 77 to 79 degree F (25 to 26 degree C) water and is 3.9 degrees F (2.2 degrees C) during diving in the winter in 50 to 55 degree F (10 to 13 degree C) water (Kang et al. 1963). These changes were noted before the Ama divers began using neoprene wet suits.

Measurable drops in core temperatures occur after humans are removed from severe exposures to cold water (Behnke and Yaglou 1951). This phenomenon is termed **temperature afterdrop** and is attributed to obliteration of the diving reflex and the movement of cold blood from the periphery to the core. We observed that seated divers in neoprene wet suits exposed to 40 degree F (4.4 degree C) water for six hours only had 1 to 2 degree F (0.6 to 1.2 degree C) declines in their core temperatures. The nadir of their temperature drop occurred during rewarming for the reasons just noted. Probes along the extremities demonstrated progressive declines in temperature from the core to the hands, with the hand temperature recordings approaching the temperature of the surrounding water. These observations confirm that the diving reflex is a demonstrable heat-conserving mechanism in humans and is effective in the diver who remains nearly motionless in the water. This has important ramifications for survival after accidental immersions in cold water.

Sudden immersion in cold water has serious consequences. Immersion in 40 degree F (4.4 degree C) water for one hour is estimated to be fatal for 50 percent of victims (see chapter 12). Studies showed that showers in 77 degree F (25 degree C) water increased ventilation because of deeper and more rapid breathing. Respiration cannot be controlled voluntarily during immersion in freezing water (Keatinge and Nadel 1965). However, after repeated exposures the respiratory responses decrease. This is one of several acclimatizations to cold water that occur in human breath-hold divers.

Diving mammals show evidence of cold stresses from diving. During the surface recovery phase of strenuous dives, seals have been observed to shiver on the surface (Scholander, Irving, and Grinnell 1942b). This is thought to be due to return of cold blood from the periphery associated with obliteration of the diving reflex, coupled with the 50 percent reduction in metabolism while the animal is submerged during the dive. Shivering is a heat-generating mechanism that occurs as a response to cooling of the core. However, it is especially counterproductive in water, where more heat is lost by the shivering muscles in the periphery than is generated by the increased metabolism from shivering.

Shunting of Blood As a Heat-Conserving Mechanism

Shunting of blood from the periphery and maintaining it in the core, components of the diving reflex, are important heat-conserving mechanisms for the diving mammal. Through isolation of the core from the periphery, the radiator effect of the extremities is obliterated. The temperature of the extremities and the blood in the extremities approach the temperature of the surrounding water during the period of shunting. Meanwhile the core loses almost no heat to the extremities. During recovery on the surface, the shunting reflex is terminated. What happens to the cooled blood in the extremities during this time? It is returned to the central circulation. Since aerobic metabolism generates almost 20 times more heat (450 vs. 24 kilocalories) than anaerobic metabolism, the diving mammal rewarm the cooled blood without significantly dropping its core temperature.

Cessation of urine production and avoidance of the excretion of urine (at the same temperature as the core) to the ambient water during the dive are other heat-conserving mechanisms observed in diving mammals. They occur secondary to their shunting adaptations. This contrasts with what happens in the human breath-hold and SCUBA diver. Increased urine production in humans occurs because of reflexes associated with immersion (see chapter 6). This factor, plus psychological–physiological effects from the stresses of breath-holding and exposure to cold water, causes involuntary diuresis (excretion of urine into the water). Urination into the water causes substantial heat loss from the core because of the heat lost with the excreted urine.

In the human, vestiges of shunting exist as a heat-conserving mechanism. Our lungs and liver contain more blood when the skin is cold than when it is warm (Glaser, Berridge, and Prior 1950). This is consistent with effects expected from the dive reflex with shifts of fluid from the periphery to the core. However, with activity, in contrast to what happens in diving mammals, shunting is overwhelmed by the metabolic activities of the muscles used to propel the breath-hold diver. One study showed that in cold water, 41 to 59 degrees F (5 to 15 degrees C), core body temperatures actually decreased more during working than during resting (Keatinge 1961). The heat generated by the work activity was insufficient to compensate for the heat loss resulting from the flow of warm blood to the extremities. Blood was required to supply oxygen to the muscles in the extremities that were doing the work. The heat from this blood flow was conducted to the ambient cold water. Subjects with **ectomorphic somatotype** (tall, thin, lean type of body build) cool more rapidly while swimming than while remaining motionless in the water. Divers with **mesomorphic somatotype** (strong, muscular body build) and **endomorphic somatotype** (short, squatty body build) cool less rapidly when motionless in cold water because of the improved insulating properties of their body builds. The builds of diving mammals tend to resemble the endomorphic somatotypes, as shown in figure 7.3.

These observations have applications for human breath-hold divers who dive in cold water as well as for people accidentally immersed in cold water. The deep-diving Ama of Japan minimize their swimming efforts. They descend passively by holding on to a basket weighted with rocks. On the bottom, they harvest food products while pulling themselves along with their hands and using slow, broad sweeping movements of their lower extremities. The male dive tenders then pull them to the surface. In situations of accidental immersion, people should avoid struggling and vigorous swimming movements since these accelerate blood flow in the actively moving extremities, promote loss of heat from the periphery to the surrounding cold water, and hasten the return of cold blood to the core.

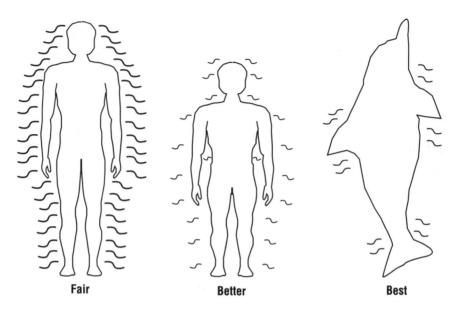

Fair　　　　　　Better　　　　　　Best

**FIGURE
7.3** Body shape and heat conservation.

Body Shape As a Heat-Conserving Adaptation

The more the diving mammal's body shape approaches that of a sphere, the better the preservation of the core temperature as illustrated in table 7.1. The sphere is the most perfect shape for conserving heat. The body's core is analogous to the mass of an object, while the periphery represents the surface area. In contrast to a sphere, a radiator is an object with a large surface area-to-mass ratio and ideal for exchanging heat with the external environment. Whales, seals, dolphins, and other diving mammals have massive cores as compared to the sizes of their appendages (fins and flukes). Furthermore, in contrast to the situation in the human breath-hold diver, the muscles that move the appendages of diving mammals lie primarily in their main body axis. The fins and flukes of diving mammals consist entirely of fibrocartilage, bone, and skin webbing. In contrast to muscle, these tissues have very low oxygen demands, can tolerate long periods without oxygen, and essentially do not increase their oxygen demands between rest and activity.

In the absence of the dive reflex and its shunting component, muscle blood flow may increase 40-fold between rest and activity in humans. In humans who are not obese, it is estimated that 71 percent of the body mass is within one inch (2.5 centimeters) of the surface and that 63 percent of the body surface is covered by the skin of the head, neck, and extremities (Carlson et al. 1958). These numbers contrast sharply with what is observed in diving mammals with their massive main body axes and relatively minimally sized fins and flukes, as noted in table 7.2. The ratio of trunk surface areas is 2.4

Table 7.1	Relative Changes in Surface Areas in Three-Dimensional Shapes With Equal Volumes	
Shape	**Volume (relative)**	**Surface area (relative)**
Sphere	1	3
Cube	1	6
Pyramid	1	12
Prism	1	16.5

Table 7.2	Skin Surface Area (Percentages) in Humans and Porpoises			
Animal		**Trunk (A)**	**Extremities (B)**	**Ratio (A/B)**
Human (burn surface area calculations)		36	54	.67
Porpoises (integrated cross-sectional computations)		86	14	6.1

times greater in porpoises than in humans, whereas extremity surface areas are 3.9 times greater in humans..

Insulation Properties of Subcutaneous Tissues

The insulation property of subcutaneous fat is another factor that offers protection from the cold environment. In humans, this can vary as much as 15-fold (Beckman 1963). In whales, fatty tissues serve two purposes. First, they are storage reservoirs for the body's metabolic needs during migrations from cold feeding waters of the polar environments to the warm equatorial waters for birthing. During these four- to six-month migrations the whales do not feed and instead rely entirely upon their fat stores. Second, the fat tissue functions as an insulator to afford protection from cold polar and deep waters. The insulation layer may also offer protection from the tremendous pressures associated with deep dives.

Insulation in humans varies because of the thickness of the subcutaneous fat tissues and their blood flow. Women have more subcutaneous fat than men. The difference is threefold in the female Ama divers of Japan as compared to their male partners (Hong, Rennie, and Park 1986). Korean women, whether divers or not, were found to have three times the body insulation capacities that American men of comparable fat thickness had (Rennie 1965). **Body insulation capacity** represents the difference between rectal (core) and skin temperatures divided by the rate of heat loss from the skin. A 6 percent increase in total body fat was needed to achieve the same effect in protecting the Korean male from cold water that was naturally present in his female diver counterpart (Rennie 1965).

Another form of insulation is that provided by fur and hair. Not all mammals rely on fat stores and "ideal" body shapes to meet the challenges of cold water. The polar bear exemplifies a mammal that does not rely on these forms of insulation. Although polar bears are extraordinary swimmers, often found in freezing waters as far as 50 miles (80 kilometers) away from land, they are not divers in the same class as diving mammals. The polar bear's fur is its primary protection from cold water. Metabolism of fatty foods is a secondary mechanism for heat generation in this animal. Fur is also the primary form of protection from cold water for the sea otter. In order for sea otters to meet the challenge of cold water, they must constantly groom their fur coats. In contrast to the polar bear and sea otter, the other diving mammals and the human breath-hold diver do not have significant additional protection from cold water because their hair or fur is either nonexistent or covers too little of the total body surface area.

Metabolic Heat Production

Metabolic heat production is another method of meeting the thermal challenges of diving. Regulation of the metabolic rate (energy and heat production from utilizing food) and reduction of shivering thresholds are two factors that accomplish this. In Eskimos, a diet consisting entirely of protein elevates their basic metabolic rate, heat-producing ability, by 20 percent. Rats' swimming durations to exhaustion were significantly better in those animals fed a high-protein diet as compared to those fed a high-carbohydrate diet. The caloric intake of the Ama of Japan was approximately 1,000 kilocalories a day greater than that of their non-diving counterparts (Kang et al. 1965). Their basal metabolic rates were 5 percent higher in the summer and 35 percent higher in the winter than those of similar-sized Japanese women who did not dive. Oxygen consumption paralleled the changes in basal metabolic rates and increased as much as 40 percent during the winter diving months.

DIVING SCENARIO

A COLD WATER RECORD

A purported record for swimming without thermal protection in cold water was reported in a world-class female ultraswimmer. She was able to swim for 25 minutes in 32 degree F (0 degree C) Antarctic waters. Factors that contributed to this remarkable feat included superb conditioning, which allowed her to sustain an extremely high level of metabolic activity during the swim; a wrestling-inspired weight training program; her female sex; and her body shape. At five feet six inches (1.7 meters) and 180 pounds (81.6 kilograms), her body mass index was 29. The normal level for the index, based on a height–weight ratio, is 21 to 24.

Swimmers conditioned to cold water are able to increase their metabolic rates without shivering (Carlson et al. 1958). Channel swimmers have surprisingly small decrements in core temperatures during swims in 61 to 64 degree F (16 to 18 degree C) water. This has been attributed to their conditioning, which allowed them to sustain metabolic rates two to three times greater than in the Ama divers of Japan (Kang et al. 1965).

The endomorphic somatotype is better suited for this type of swimming activity, as shown in figure 7.3. Thermal comfort during diving in cold water, with similar thermal protective gear, is better tolerated in the breath-hold diver than the SCUBA diver. Breath-hold diving seems to be as well tolerated with respect to water temperature comfort as SCUBA diving in water temperatures 50 degrees F (3.3 degrees C) or warmer. This is attributable to the increased metabolic activity required to breath-hold dive with energy expended for ascents, descents, and swimming on the surface.

Reduction of the shivering threshold is another important heat-conserving mechanism. Shivering is a reflex-like action arising from small, rapid contractions of muscles. Although shivering increases the body's heat production five- to sevenfold as a consequence of the effects of the muscle contractions, its requirements for oxygen and metabolites outweigh its beneficial effects. Consequently, during immersion in cold water, the result of shivering is a greater loss of heat than without shivering. The reason is that tremendous heat losses occur when peripheral vasoconstriction is terminated in order to provide a blood supply to the muscles involved in shivering. The diving women of Korea were able to remain in 82 degree F (28 degree C) water for three hours without shivering despite a decline in their core temperature of 1.8 degrees F (1.0 degree C) (Rennie 1965). Their non-diving counterparts with similar body builds and comparable fat thicknesses were unable to tolerate this exposure to cold water without shivering.

SCUBA divers who repetitively dive in cold water develop acclimatizations to improve their tolerances for this challenge (Skreslet and Aarefjord 1968). Research identified three stages in the acclimatization process. The first, the unacclimatized stage, was characterized by an increase in metabolism during the cold water exposure through muscle activity and shivering. During the second stage, while core temperatures declined, metabolic activity did not compensate for heat losses. The reason appears to be **habituation** (unresponsiveness after continuing exposures to the cold water stimulus) of the brain. The acclimatized state, which took about 45 days to achieve, was characterized by a constant core temperature while increases in metabolic activity were negligible. This probably occurred because of heat conservation caused by the lowering of shivering thresholds and the reduction in heat transfer from the core to the periphery. In less than three weeks after the cold water diving activities stopped, the acclimatizations disappeared.

Countercurrent Heat Exchange

Another method by which heat is conserved is countercurrent heat exchange. It is based on a thermodynamic principle stating that if two fluid streams are adjacent to each other but are of different temperatures, heat will transfer from the warmer to the cooler stream. If fluid-filled tubes such as arteries and veins, which flow in opposite directions, lie side by side, heat transfers from the warm conduit to the cold one as diagrammed in figure 7.4. Thus,

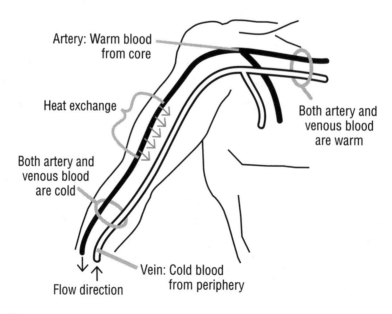

Artery: Warm blood from core

Heat exchange

Both artery and venous blood are warm

Both artery and venous blood are cold

Vein: Cold blood from periphery

Flow direction

FIGURE 7.4   Countercurrent heat exchange.

as warm arterial blood is pumped away from the core, its heat is exchanged with the cold venous blood returning from the core. The arterial blood that now flows to the extremities is cold, so little heat is lost to the surrounding water from the arterial blood. Meanwhile, the heat-exchanged warm venous blood is returned to the core. The slower the flow, the more effective the heat exchange.

With shunting from the diving reflex and nearly total obliteration of blood flow to the periphery, countercurrent heat exchange may not be an important consideration for heat conservation in diving mammals. However, as the duration of the dive approaches its end, shunting from the diving reflex becomes less efficient. Metabolites from anaerobic metabolism begin to return to the core via the cold venous blood from the periphery. The metabolites signal the diving mammal to surface. Initially the blood flow is slow as the shunting response begins to lose its effectiveness. At this time, countercurrent heat exchange is likely to be very efficient in the diving mammal, since the slower the flow the more efficient the heat exchange. This mechanism may prevent cooling in the diving mammal during ascent and before aerobic metabolism (which is about 20 times more efficient than anaerobic metabolism) can be resumed with breathing air on the surface.

Technology to Meet the Challenge of Diving in Cold Water

Exposure suits help the human diver meet the challenges of diving in cold water. It is interesting to note that the female divers of Japan and Korea have begun to use wet suits for their breath-hold diving, food-collecting activities. Alas, the fascinating adjustments seen with "unprotected" exposure to cold water are no longer being observed and men are now doing the majority of the dives (Kang et al. 1983). The choices for thermal protection include a variety of types, qualities, and levels of protection. Modern exposure suits can provide thermal protection for diving even in freezing waters. However, as protection increases, so do the disadvantages. Air-rewarming devices associated with the SCUBA regulator are another piece of thermal equipment. The following section describes the choices divers have for thermal protection gear.

The Dive Skin

The "skin" or Lycra suit is at the "least-protection" end of the spectrum. This suit is made of a thin single-layer nylon or nylonlike material analogous to the material used for making swimming suits for competitive swimmers. At the most, it provides a degree or two of increased warmth during diving in warm waters. Is this minimal amount of protection of any real value? The answer is yes, for several reasons. First, the suit provides protection from exposure to the sun (see chapter 12). While this may not be significant for the SCUBA diver, it is significant for snorkel and breath-hold divers who spend large proportions of their diving time swimming on the surface. Second, the skin suit provides protection from contact with marine animals that can inflict injuries to the human skin, such as jellyfish, fire corals, and barnacles (see chapter 12). Third, it is a useful undergarment between the diver's skin and an overlying wet suit or dry suit. The Lycra suit can be easily rinsed thoroughly with fresh water or even cleaned with soap and water after each series of diving activities to prevent accumulations of organic debris that could act as skin irritants. Finally, the degree or two of thermal protection increases comfort during diving in warm tropical waters.

Hypothermia (abnormally low body temperature) can occur insidiously in warm tropical waters since the water temperature may still be 15 to 20 degrees F (8.4 to 11.2 degrees C) cooler than normal body temperature. The diver may become hypothermic after repetitive SCUBA dives when fatigue and dehydration begin to interfere with the body's own heat-generating and -conserving mechanisms. A degree or two of increased comfort from wearing the dive skin, notwithstanding its other benefits, makes it a worthwhile investment. Rubberizing the dive skin allows the diver to experience the same level of comfort as in water with a degree or two higher temperature.

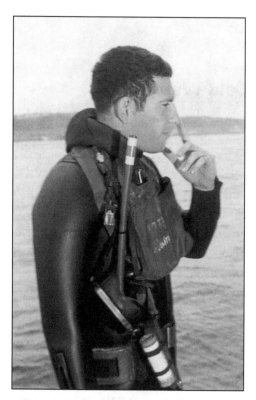

The standard neoprene wet suit affords adequate thermal protection during diving in waters of moderate temperature (48-74 degrees F or 8.9-23 degrees C).

Neoprene Wet Suit

The neoprene **wet suit** is the next level in the hierarchy of thermal protection devices for the diver. Wet suits do for the diver what clothing does for the Eskimo. They create a "tropical" environment around the skin. The principle is simple. Water enters the neoprene cells and is warmed by the diver's body heat. This, of course, requires heat transfer; but once the water is warmed, the suit insulates the diver from the cold surrounding water. The water trapped in the foam cells greatly reduces conductive and convective heat losses. The neoprene is of two types, closed foam and open foam. The open-foam suit is less efficient at conserving heat since water can enter and leave the foam cells, thereby allowing some convective as well as conductive heat losses to occur. With closed-foam neoprene wet suits, minute air bubbles act as insulators. Water movement is restricted to the space around the closed cell; thus there is less movement of water, and conductive heat loss is decreased. The closed-foam cell suit can be used as a dry suit with a neoprene neck seal, latex wrist seals, built-in booties, and an inflator valve. Moisture-wicking undergarments such as Lycra suits are worn under the closed foam.

Wet suits come in a variety of options. For diving in tropical waters, suits that are one-eighth inch (three millimeters) thick work well. They provide protection from the sun and marine animals, as the dive skins do, but also provide comfort for diving in water that is a couple of degrees cooler than would be tolerated with the dive skins. Because of their minimal thickness, they do not interfere much with swimming; nor do they require a lot of additional weight to counteract their added buoyancy. In colder waters, thicker wet suits are used. Some divers configure their wet suits to be twice as thick over the trunk as over the extremities. The thicker parts add additional insulation for the body core while the thinner insulation over the extremities permits greater mobility. Some wet suits may cover the upper limbs only to the above-elbow level and the lower limbs only to the above-knee level in keeping with the principle of protecting the core temperature. Hoods, gloves, and booties are also made of neoprene. A properly fitting hood, most functional if attached to a vest or wet suit jacket, protects the back of the neck and ears. These two areas are very vulnerable to chilling symptoms and cause discomfort when they cool. Trident, or three-fingered, gloves are more effective in keeping the hands warm than five-fingered gloves that have a larger surface area for water contact with the fingers.

Wet suits have several disadvantages. First, because of the compression of the bubbles of the wet suit with an increase in pressure (Boyle's Law), they lose their effectiveness as the diver descends. Consequently, where the water may be the coldest, at the deepest depth of the dive, the wet suit is least efficient. Second, a thick neoprene wet suit provides 20 or more pounds (nine or more kilograms) of positive buoyancy. This requires the addition of lead weights to the weight belt or pockets, or both, in the buoyancy compensator. Although the diver may not notice the additional weight with neutral buoyancy conditions while in the water, it can be a substantial cardiovascular stress when coupled with carrying diving equipment to the water's edge for beach dives. If the diver is prone to a cardiac event, such as a heart attack, it will most likely occur at this stage of the dive. Third, neoprene wet suits tend to accumulate debris from the water that is not always completely removed with typical rinsing or showering. The organic debris can become a source of odor and cause skin irritation.

Principles of heat conservation are essential to maximizing comfort during diving in cold water. Movement of the diver's extremities should be minimized. Violent movements increase the amount of cold water flowing in between the wet suit and the diver's skin. The cold water is not only unpleasant; it can also be a major stress for maintaining the core temperature. A custom-fitted wet suit reduces the chances that water will come in contact with the diver's skin. Once out of the water, the wet suit should be removed as soon as possible to prevent chilling. This is necessary because of the cooling effect of the evaporation of water trapped in the wet suit. Depending on quality and extras such as gloves, hoods, pockets, and booties, wet suits cost from $100 to $300. Closed-foam wet/dry suits cost $600 to $800. Custom wet suits may cost twice as much.

The Dry Suit

The third level of thermal protection is the **dry suit.** The heavy canvas hard hat dry suit is not practical for the sport diver. Although it provides excellent protection from the environment and effectively keeps the diver warm, donning and removing this type of suit require a full support crew. This type of equipment is used in long deep dives in which staged decompression is required and the diver needs to maintain thermal comfort. The thermal comfort results from the fact that the suit is dry inside and has been inflated using the excellent insulating properties of air. This creates a local tropical environment, as discussed earlier, around the diver. Wearing thermal underwear provides additional thermal comfort.

Because of improved seals around the neck, wrists, and ankles, the dry suit is being increasingly utilized for diving in cold water. The outer waterproof layer, with a long watertight zipper in the trunk portion for entry into and exit from the suit, keeps the diver dry. Thermal underwear plus air from the diver's SCUBA tank, used to inflate the suit, provides very effective insulation. With the dry suit, sport divers are able to comfortably tolerate SCUBA dives in freezing waters. Like the wet suit, though, the dry suit has disadvantages. First, only standard neoprene protection is provided for the head, hands, and feet. Second, the air used to inflate the suit adds additional positive buoyancy, upwards of 30 pounds (13.6 kilograms), to the diver and reduces the amount of gas in the SCUBA tank. Finally, if a leak occurs, water enters the suit and essentially all thermal protection from the dry suit is lost. This can be catastrophic during diving in near-freezing waters in which the lethal exposure limit is only a few minutes. Dry suits cost $500 to $1,000 or more. The price is based on customization, quality of fit, and the durability of the dry suit material. Other features include high-quality zippers and designs that allow the diver to don and remove the suit without assistance from others. The trilaminate dry suit, the most technologically advanced of the dry suits, costs about $2,000. An additional $300 undergarment is recommended with its use.

Gas Rewarming Devices

Insensible respiratory heat losses can be reduced by rewarmer systems in the mouthpieces of some regulators. The exhaust air is channeled through baffles so that the heat from the expired air warms the inspired air before it reaches the diver's mouth. Rebreather units also reduce respiratory heat losses since the warmed expired air is circulated through the breathing bags and little heat is transferred to the water environment surrounding the breathing bags.

Hot Water Suits

The highest level of thermal protection is afforded by the **hot water suit.** Hot water is pumped to the suit through a hose. The diver is continuously bathed in warm water that slowly leaks out of the suit. The logistics for using this type of equipment are enormous. Hot water heaters, hoses, pumps, and a full support crew are required. Hot water suits allow divers to work in the most challenging of diving environments such as in deep, cold water commercial diving operations. Because of the expenses and support needed to use this equipment, the hot water suit is limited to commercial diving uses.

For Further Review

1. What adaptations help the diving mammal survive in cold water?
2. Why are active movements and shivering counterproductive for heat conservation in cold water?
3. What acclimatizations do human divers make to cold water?
4. How does heat production differ between aerobic and anaerobic metabolism?
5. What advantages do women have for diving in cold water?
6. What is countercurrent heat exchange? What factors influence its effectiveness?
7. What is the physiological basis for temperature afterdrop?
8. What equipment is used to protect the human diver from cold water?

CHAPTER 8

Propulsion in the Aquatic Environment

> **Chapter Preview**
>
> - Adaptations in diving mammals for movement in the aquatic environment
> - Anatomy and physiology of the propulsion system
> - Body shapes and their influence on the ability to move through water
> - Role of subcutaneous fat and heat exchange in increasing the swimming speeds of diving mammals
> - Swimming speeds of diving mammals and humans and the effects of swim fins
> - Swim fin options

Diving mammals are able to propel themselves through the aquatic environment very efficiently. Humans can become good swimmers, but human swimming feats can hardly be compared with those of diving mammals. It is easy to appreciate how the diving mammals' fins and flukes help to propel them through the water. What may not be appreciated is how other factors such as their hydrodynamic shape and subcutaneous fatty tissue, and possibly a heat exchange system, contribute to their speed in the water. While these latter adaptations have only limited applications for human divers, many of the principles are applicable to surface ship and submarine movement.

Anatomy and Physiology

Movement through the water requires a **propulsion** (mechanics of moving an object) system and energy to drive the system. This is achieved through the musculoskeletal system, with the skeleton providing the structural support and lever arms for muscle movement. The skeletal system is divided into two main sections, axial and appendicular.

Axial Skeleton

The axial skeleton includes the bones in the center of the body, namely the spine, rib cage, and pelvis. It provides support and protection for the structures in the core of the body such as the lungs, heart, digestive tract, excretory system, and the internal portions of the reproductive organs. Although the bones of the head and neck are part of the axial skeleton, in divers they function more like an extremity. In contrast to diving mammals, in humans the neck clearly separates the head and the trunk. Also, the surface area-to-mass ratios of these structures more closely approximate those of the upper and lower limbs than they do of the trunk. The flukes of whales and porpoises are boneless extensions of the axial skeleton, somewhat analogous to tails (which have bones) found on other animals. The flexibility and stability of the flukes are achieved by tendons, cartilage, and tough fiber tissue elements.

Appendicular Skeleton

The appendicular skeleton includes the bones that support the extremities. In humans this includes the four extremities, each with 30 bony elements. Whales, porpoises, and seals have analogous bony components in their fore fins, but the bones of their lower extremities have all but disappeared. The hind flippers of seals, counterparts of our lower extremities, consist of very short bones, almost rectangular stubs. If the highly mobile wrist, hand, fingers, and thumb of humans were covered with a webbed glove, it would somewhat resemble the paddle-like structures of diving mammals as depicted in figure 8.1. The structural differences of the fins of diving mammals eliminate the need for appendicular muscles in their fore fins, flippers, and flukes. The muscles that move the fins and flippers mostly lie in the axial skeleton and are connected by tendons to the appendages.

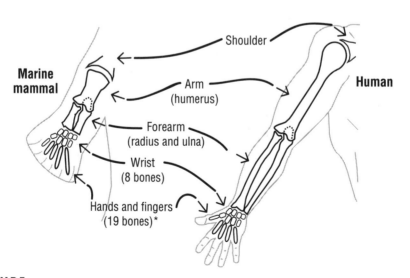

FIGURE 8.1 Comparison of the bony elements of the human upper extremity and the diving mammal's fore fin. * = In humans.

Advantages of Fins and Flippers

The anatomy of the axial and appendicular skeletal systems of diving mammals has advantages for movement as well as for heat and energy conservation in the aquatic environment.

• First, the fins, flukes, and flippers provide a large surface area for contact with water. This is very much like human swimmers' use of hand paddles and swim fins, but with greatly magnified and far more efficient effects. Minimal movements of the fins, flippers, and flukes provide enormous thrust for movement through water that is 775 times as dense as air.

• Second, the heat conservation ramifications are enormous. The heat generated by the muscles to move diving mammals' fins, flippers, and flukes remains in the core. This is different from what happens in humans, where the muscles to provide movement largely lie in the limbs. In diving mammals the joints act as fulcrums. The result is that the muscles in which heat is generated are remote from the fins and flukes where propulsive movements actually occur. Heat generated by muscle contractions for propulsion in the human diver is much more likely than in the diving mammal to be lost to the surrounding water environment.

• Third, the blood circulation required by the fins, flippers, and flukes of diving mammals is minimal. This is the case because these structures are composed of cartilage, bone, fibrous tissue, and skin, which have very

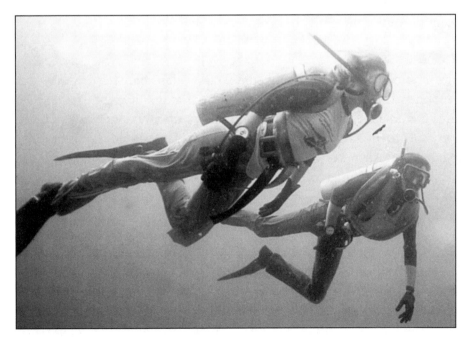

Swim fins meet the propulsive requirements for most diving activities.

low oxygen demands. Also the oxygen demands do not change appreciably between rest and activity. Thus, no significant oxygen deficit is accrued in these structures during the mammals' diving activities.

• Fourth, because of the low metabolic demands of the diving mammals' appendages, the appendages can approach the temperature of the surrounding water and remain at that temperature for long periods without harmful effects.

Joints of the Axial Skeleton

While bones provide support, joints make it possible for movement between the rigid bony segments. The bony structures—primarily vertebrae—in the axial skeletons of diving mammals and humans are similar. The vertebrae are rectangular-shaped bones with archlike structures on their back edges that provide a canal through which the spinal cord passes. The ends of adjacent vertebrae, the articulating surfaces, are nearly flat. Round-shaped pads of fibrous tissue with jelly-like cores, termed intervertebral (between vertebrae) discs, separate one vertebra from another and act as shock absorbers.

The net effect of this anatomy is that only a few degrees of flexion and extension or twisting and bending are possible between two adjacent vertebrae. However, when these few (5 to 10) degrees of motion are multiplied by 24 vertebrae in the human—and by even more in porpoises and whales when the tail segments are included—a substantial amount of motion is possible. This mobility allows almost a 180-degree upward plus downward arc of motion in these diving mammals' flukes.

Shoulder Joints

The shoulder joints of humans and diving mammals have similar bony components. Functionally, however, they are quite different. The shoulder joints of humans allow tremendous mobility, with 360-degree arcs of motion in two planes (front to back and side to side). The shoulder motions of the diving mammals occur in more of a backward–forward direction to move and steer them through the water. The chief method of propulsion for seals and their relatives is through the fore flippers, while in whales and porpoises it is through their flukes.

Muscles of the Axial Skeleton

The propelling of diving mammals, which primarily comes from the muscles in their axial skeletons, is greater than one would expect from any one or two individual muscles acting at a single joint or two linked joints, as with the hamstring muscles that flex both the hip and knee joints. There are several reasons for this power.

Table 8.1	"Paired" Muscles Acting Across the Shoulder Joint	
	Attachments	
Muscle (11 total)	**Anterior (front)**	**Posterior (back)**
Group 1		
Deltoid	✓	✓
Trapezius		✓
Group 2		
Pectoralis major	✓	
Supraspinatus		✓
Infraspinatus		✓
Teres minor		✓
Group 3		
Subscapularis	✓	
Teres major		✓
Latissimus dorsi		✓
Group 4		
Biceps	✓	
Triceps		✓

• First, instead of one or two primary muscles acting across an appendicular joint, many do so for the axial skeleton. In the shoulder joint, for example, at least 11 muscle groups originating in the axial skeleton act to move the joint. They are almost equally divided between attachments on the front and back sides of the chest wall as listed in table 8.1. In contrast, in the neck and trunk there are over 30 muscle groups acting across the axial skeleton, grouped in table 8.2. Although each muscle may have only an individual function or act only across one single joint, such as an interspinalis muscle, each has an enormous additive effect to produce power for the six cardinal motions of the axial skeleton, flexion-extension (forward and backward), lateral bends (to each side), and rotation (twists) to the right and left.

• Second, the muscles of the axial skeleton often have multipenniform attachments as diagrammed in figure 8.2. Typically the fibers of the muscles of the appendicular skeleton are parallel with the longitudinal axis of the muscle action. In multipennate muscles, the fibers converge like the plumes of a feather, as in the deltoid muscle covering the shoulder of the human. This adds additional pulling force by increasing the number of fibers involved in the muscle's action. An analogy for this effect is seen in a "tug-of-war." If

Table 8.2	The Major Muscle Groups in the Axial Skeleton	
Muscle groups	**Number of component muscles (35 total)**	
Transverse costal (rib)	9	
Transverse spinal	6	
Suboccipital (below the skull)	4	
Thorax group	8	
Anterior and lateral abdominal	4	
Posterior abdominal and pelvis	4	

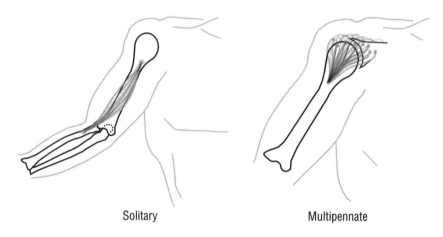

Solitary   Multipennate

FIGURE 8.2   Solitary versus multipennate origins of muscles.

one side pulls on the rope in a straight line while the other side has ropes coming obliquely off the main rope, thereby enabling more than three times the number of people to pull, the obvious winner will be the side pulling in the multipennate arrangement. Because of the overlapping of the origins and insertions of muscles in the axial skeleton, both in humans and in diving mammals, the muscle groups, in many ways, act as multipenniform muscles do.

• Third, the muscles of the axial skeleton are able to function for sustained periods of time at submaximal levels of activity as seen in muscles primarily composed of slow-twitch fibers. In the human, this sustained activity is reflected in the muscles that control our trunk posture. These allow us to sit and stand for prolonged periods of time. The same axial muscles that maintain our trunk control allow whales to do their uninterrupted 6,000- to 10,000-mile (9,600- to 16,000-kilometer) semiannual migrations.

Muscles of the Extremities

The anatomy and mechanics of the muscles of the extremities are somewhat different from those of the axial skeleton. The muscles of the extremities have single—or at the most two or three—discrete muscle origin sites (i.e., attachments to stabilized bony structures). The muscles tend to be long, with well-defined **tendons** that are rope-like connections between the muscles themselves and their insertions, the bone structures to which they attach that are one or more joints beyond the muscle origins. Easily recognized examples include the biceps and triceps muscles in the upper extremities and the quadriceps and hamstring muscle groups in the lower extremities. These anatomical arrangements maximize motions of the joints they cross. They also minimize the circumference of the joints as compared to the greater circumferences of the adjacent muscle bodies, as noted in the differences in circumference of the thigh and the adjacent knee joint. The goal is to provide as much mobility to the extremities as possible, in addition to rapid bursts at near-maximal strength, as seen in muscles with large numbers of **fast-twitch fibers,** muscle fibers that utilize anaerobic metabolism for their actions and thereby are capable of brief, maximal outputs of energy.

Muscle Structure and Contraction

Muscles are composed of smaller and smaller elements as diagrammed in figure 8.3. The elements start with the muscle itself. The muscle comprises groups of fasciculi. The contents of each fasciculus are enclosed in sheaths that are parallel to each other and that all pull in the same direction. Each fascicule is composed of approximately 20 muscle fibers. Muscle fibers are visible with the naked eye. Muscle fibers are, in turn, composed of microscopic structures called myofibrils. Myofibrils contain the contractile elements of the muscles known collectively as sarcomeres.

The myofibrils contain two filaments, **actin** and **myosin,** which are large, elongated protein molecules that are interdigitated and have the ability to slide in and out over each other. The actin and myosin fibers run parallel to the length of the muscle cell and are arranged to overlap at their ends (see figure 8.3). The myosin fibers have hinged crossbridges on them. The crossbridges bind to the actin filaments, pull on them, and cause the overlap to increase. This shortens the sarcomere, and when this summated microscopic overlap is multiplied by the length of a muscle, a contraction is observed. When the muscle is relaxed, the actin and myosin filament overlap is decreased. Relaxation is an active process that requires energy to allow the crossbridges on the actin molecule to elongate. However, energy is required for the contraction process also.

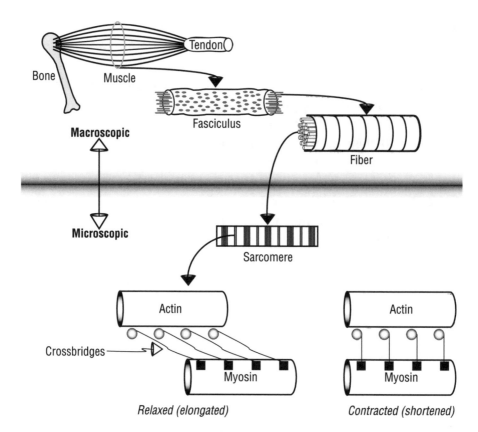

FIGURE
8.3   Muscle contraction mechanism.

The muscles are located in a balanced system. For each muscle or group of muscles that work in one direction **(agonists)**, there is a corresponding group that works in the opposite direction **(antagonists)**. Motor (muscle) control programs that are mediated by the nervous system switch muscles "on" and "off" to produce coordinated movements. The integration of these programs is incredibly precise. If both muscle groups contract equally, there is no movement of the joint on which the muscles act. This type of contraction is termed an **isometric** (no changes in muscle lengths) contraction. If movement occurs, one group of muscles has to relax while the other group contracts. This type of contraction is a dynamic contraction. The coordinated effect allows for myriad activities, from microsurgery to moving mountains and everything else in between.

The ability of muscles to sustain their activity is dependent on two main factors:

• The first factor is the intensity of activity. Muscles that use their energy supplies at a rate equal to or slower than the rate at which they produce energy are functioning aerobically. Those that exceed this level of activity begin functioning anaerobically, building up an oxygen deficit. Muscles contracting at their maximum capacity can do so only for brief periods before the products of anaerobic metabolism interfere with the muscle activity. When this occurs, the muscles cramp (uncontrolled contraction). Proposed reasons for cramping include chemical changes with accumulations of lactic acid, hypoxia (lack of oxygen), inadequate energy supplies, or combinations of these.

• Second, the muscle's ability to function aerobically or anaerobically depends on the relative amounts of fast-twitch and slow-twitch fibers it contains. **Slow-twitch fibers** function aerobically and have the capacity for sustained activity. Myoglobin, found in high concentrations in the muscles of diving mammals, is associated with slow-twitch muscle fibers. Fast-twitch fibers function anaerobically, have the capacity for brief intense work, and build up an oxygen deficit during activity.

Swimming Versus Diving

Muscle activity needed for fast swimming on the surface is quite different from that needed for breath-hold diving. For sustained surface swimming, whether by humans or diving mammals, muscle activity is largely aerobic. Porpoises and whales seem to be more proficient swimmers than seals and sea lions. The swimming speeds of porpoises, at times, appear faster than their muscle masses, fin and fluke movements, and displacement of water would predict. Although porpoises have been observed swimming in the bow wakes of ships moving at 20 to 30 miles per hour (32 to 48 kilometers per hour), a more realistic swimming speed is 16 miles per hour (26 kilometers per hour) in calm water and 14.5 miles per hour (23 kilometers per hour) in rough water (Teague 1968). (Miles per hour rather than knots, which are roughly equal, are used here for convenience.) The 20- to 30-mile-per-hour swimming speeds that have been observed are probably due to these animals' body surfing skills. As boats move through the water, they generate an advancing pressure field—a bow wake. Porpoises apparently use this advancing pressure field to swim, seemingly effortlessly, alongside the fast-moving ships, just as human surfers ride waves into shore.

There are indications that diving mammals minimize swimming movements to increase the durations of their breath-hold dives. Just before starting their descents, they exhale fully (see chapter 5). The changes in buoyancy may be sufficient to allow these animals to descend passively, minimize swimming movements, and thereby conserve oxygen. Even if their buoyancy is only neutralized by the exhalation, which may be the more desirable choice, momentum gained by a few downward swimming movements may be sufficient to allow them to continue their downward descent with minimal energy costs. Correspondingly, when they are ready to ascend, a few upward swimming movements could initiate the momentum to sustain ascent. This would minimize energy expenditures and reduce the chances of depleting oxygen stores and blacking out during ascent.

Buoyancy-controlling and energy-conserving techniques are utilized by human breath-hold divers also. The shallow-water Japanese Ama (Cachido) divers swim to depths of 15 FSW (4.6 MSW) to harvest their foodstuffs on the bottom and then swim back to the surface (Hong et al. 1991). Bottom times average 30 seconds; total dive times, one minute; and surface interval rest and recovery periods, one minute. The deep-diving counterparts (Funado divers) rapidly descend passively with weights to 60 FSW (18 MSW), spend 30 seconds swimming on the bottom harvesting food products, and then are pulled to the surface by their assistants. Descents and ascents take 15 seconds each so that the total underwater time is about a minute. The Funado divers' surface intervals are 60 seconds. Consequently, the energy expenditures of the shallow Japanese Ama divers are greater than those of their deeper-diving counterparts even though the two groups spend approximately equal amounts of time submerged and at rest. These divers through experience have developed the optimal diving patterns for each of their dive profiles (Rahn 1965).

Swimming techniques for surface swimming, without diving gear, and for breath-hold diving among humans are quite different than those of the mammalian breath-hold divers. Human swimming feats can hardly be compared with those of diving mammals. World-class competitive swimmers can sprint for brief intervals from 50 yards/meters to 200 yards/meters at approximately four and one-half miles per hour (7.2 kilometers per hour) and for long distances at three and one-half miles per hour (5.6 kilometers per hour). The range of these swimming speeds is from 22 to 28 percent of porpoises' speeds.

Analyses of upper extremity and lower extremity propulsive efforts in human swimmers show differences between the energy expenditures and efficiencies of these paired appendages. The energy expenditures of the kick, which corresponds to some extent to the fluke movements of porpoises and whales, are two to four times as great as those for the arm stroke, which corresponds to the fore flipper movements of seals (Adrian, Mohan, and Karpovich 1966). Research showed that efficiency of the leg strokes varied from 0.05 to 1.23 percent while that of the arms varied from 0.56 to 6.92 percent, demonstrating that arm strokes are 5- to 10-fold more efficient than the kick. Oxygen consumptions were four times as great for the legs as for the arms in 15-yard (14-meter) swims at 1 yard per second (which equates to swimming 100 yards [91 meters] in 100 seconds). The differences in efficiency and oxygen consumption between the arms and the legs have two explanations:

- First, the propelling movements of the legs are relatively inefficient when compared to those of the arms with their greater mobility.

- Second, the muscles of the hips and lower extremities are among the largest in the body and correspondingly have the highest oxygen demands. Long-distance swimmers apply these prinples to their swimming by emphasizing the arm strokes while reducing kicking to slow efficient movements to maintain stability.

The most efficient swimming rates for underwater swims with fins are 0.7 to 0.9 mile per hour (1.1 to 1.5 kilometers per hour), or about 5 percent of the maximum swimming speeds of porpoises (Donald and Davidson 1954). At greater speeds, efficiencies decline progressively based on oxygen consumption rates. Marked variations are observed with different levels of experience, training, body builds, and water temperatures (Andersen 1960). Swimmers with the lower kick rates and the most nearly neutral buoyancies tend to have the highest swimming efficiencies (Specht et al. 1957). Buoyancy control and energy expenditures are inversely related. One of the most frustrating experiences for human SCUBA divers is the attempt to maintain a constant depth when too positively buoyant. Swimming in the head-down, feet-up position distracts from the dive and rapidly depletes the SCUBA air supply.

Body Shapes and Underwater Swimming Speeds

The shape of an object has an important effect on how well it will move through the water. **Hydrodynamics** is the science that deals with the movement of objects through fluids. The hydrodynamics of the diving mammals help to explain the discrepancies between predicted swimming speeds based on muscle mass and energy consumption and their faster actually observed swimming speeds. The body shapes of diving mammals are blunt, rounded, and balloonlike. Although at first appearance these body shapes might be considered an impediment to moving through the water, in terms of hydrodynamics they represent the epitome of efficiency. The reason is their ability to reduce turbulence and drag. When an object moves through water (as well as other fluids and gases), it creates turbulence. Turbulence represents currents that move at angles different from those of the object moving through the water, as diagrammed in figure 8.4. In contrast, laminar flow refers to the condition in which water flows past an object in parallel planes, thereby avoiding turbulence and resultant drag. Turbulence slows object movements through the water according to the following principles:

- The greater the turbulence, the more drag it places on the object and the more slowly the object moves through the water per unit of propulsive power.
- The faster an object moves through a fluid, the more turbulence it develops.
- The more turbulence an object produces, the less efficient is the use of its propulsive force.

From a hydrodynamics perspective, the body shapes of the diving mammals are ideal for reducing turbulence when moving through the water. Lessons learned from hydrodynamics (and perhaps from studying the diving mammals) have resulted in radical changes in the shapes of submarines. In the past, submarines had knife-like bows (front ends of ships) similar to those of surface ships to "cut" through the water. Now submarines are cigar shaped, with very blunt bows. This shape greatly reduces turbulence while the submarine is underwater, increasing speed as well as reducing noise. Now almost all large ships have large bulbous outcroppings on the bow just below the water line to reduce turbulence when moving through the water.

Other Techniques to Reduce Turbulence and Drag

In diving mammals, subcutaneous fat aids in reducing drag as well as protecting the animal from cold water (see chapter 7). The subcutaneous fatty tissue is of an oily consistency. Its pliability conforms to water turbulence patterns and thereby further reduces drag as the diving mammals move rapidly through the water. This adaptation is not found in the competitive swimmer. However, to improve their swimming speeds, swimmers wear swim caps and shave off their body hair to reduce drag on their bodies while swimming at top speeds. Thin neoprene wet suits frequently used by open-water swimmers not only offer thermal protection, but may also improve performance by reducing drag and increasing buoyancy. Yet maximum swimming speeds of world-class swimmers are only about one-fifth that of the porpoise. Consequently, turbulence and drag effects are much less of an impediment to fast swimming in the swimming human than they are in the mammalian diver.

Heat transfer is an intriguing method of improving the speed of moving through water that has possible applications to diving mammals. Heating a liquid reduces its viscosity, which in turn reduces turbulence when an object moves through the liquid. The reduction in viscosity is due to the increased distance between molecules and the decrease of the cohesive forces

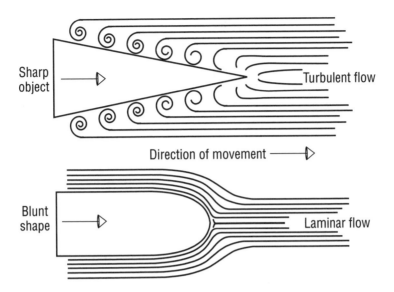

**FIGURE
8.4**   Hydrodynamics: shape versus turbulence.

of internal friction that occur as the temperature of the liquid increases. As mentioned previously, the less turbulent and the more laminar (smooth, flat-like) the flow, the less drag there is on an object moving through the water (see figure 8.4). The skin over the head end of the porpoise is almost bloodless, and the subcutaneous tissue between the skin and the underlying bone is minimal. Laminar flow occurs in this area when the porpoise swims at high speeds because of the blunt, rounded shape of the forward surface of this portion of the diving mammal's body. In contrast, turbulence increases over the diving mammal's body as its shape tapers toward the flukes. This is an area that also has increased **vascularity** (amount of blood vessels) in the subcutaneous tissue. The increased vascularity not only provides a method for dispersion of heat produced by metabolic activity but during swimming at high speeds may also assist in producing a more laminar flow pattern by decreasing turbulence through heat transfer. How much this contributes to the swimming speed of diving mammals has yet to be determined.

Technology to Improve Propulsion in the Aquatic Environment

Swimming fins are used to improve the propulsive ability of human divers in the water. Fins increase the efficiency of moving through the water from 2 to 8 percent (Adrian, Mohan, and Karpovich 1966). This level of efficiency corresponds approximately to that of the arm stroke. Yet swimming with fins is only 20 percent as efficient as walking or running on dry land (Lanphier

1954). Swim fins increase the surface area of the lower extremities. However, there is a limit to the effectiveness to be gained from increasing surface area. This is so because of the power required to move the increased surface area and the decreased mobility that results with increasing fin size. It is interesting to note that the surface area of the porpoise's tail fluke represents less than 5 percent of its total body skin surface area. Consequently, size alone is not the only factor one considers when evaluating the effectiveness of swim fins.

Design, comfort, and mobility are important considerations in deciding which swim fins to use. In the past, progressively larger and more rigid swim fins became popular. These had names such as Jet Fins and Rocket Fins. However, unless the diver had an exceptionally powerful leg kick, they were hard to use because operating them took so much energy. In terms of length, swimming fins vary from short—less than eight-inch (20-centimeter) projections from the ends of the toes—to over three feet (one meter) in length. The longer the fins, the more flexible they tend to be. This latter fin choice is very popular for the breath-hold diver who does spearfishing. The long fins are used presumably for their energy-conserving potential during the dive. A few kicks initiate forward movement, and momentum then continues the diver's progression. This can conserve energy during descent and ascent, especially if the diver is neutrally buoyant. At the other end of the swimming fin spectrum is the Zoomer fin used by competitive swimmers for lower extremity swim training purposes. The fin is short, rigid, and designed for continuous kicking movements. Speed is increased by about 20 percent with the Zoomer fins, given comparable kicking efforts, in relation to speed without the fins.

For SCUBA divers donning gear such as tanks, regulators with dive computers and other monitoring gauges, weight belts, buoyancy compensators, knives, spearguns, game-holding bags, underwater photography equipment, and underwater lights, a fin intermediate in length between the two extremes is most popular. This selection process probably has some empirical basis. Intermediate-length fins are long enough to provide sufficient forward thrust to move the diver through the water, yet they provide enough mobility to allow the diver to constantly change direction and depth.

As with other types of diving equipment, manufacturers have provided many options in fin design for the sport diver. There are options not only for color, fin blade shape, stiffness, and length, but also for features that improve the fins' propulsive ability. Semirigid spines along the edges, and sometimes in the central portions of the fin blades, add stability to the fins while still allowing the majority of the blade to be thin and flexible. A reported disadvantage of this design is that the fins are "too responsive" to foot movements. This makes it difficult for the diver to maintain position in order to stalk marine creatures or do underwater photography. Channels and grooves incorporated into the blade, or at the junction of the foot portion and the blade, or both, are supposed to decrease turbulence at the critical points of the fin, which are at the junction of the rigid foot portion and the mobile blade portion. Force fins with relatively short curved blades and extensions along the blade edges are purported to increase thrust through a water-scooping effect during the upward thrust of the kick. Similar benefits are ascribed to fins with hinge devices or interruptions in their spines at the fin's critical foot-blade portion. The hinges are supposed to help maintain thrust at the endpoints of the upward and downward movements of the kick while reducing turbulence associated with the change of direction of the fin. Split fins are another option. The fin blade is split in two. This tends to cause vortices between the splits that aid in forward thrust and may prevent churning up of silt when the diver is swimming near the bottom.

Another consideration in fin selection is the type of foot portion. The pocket type with a heel strap is the most popular today. Usually the pocket is large enough to allow the diver to wear neoprene booties with protective rubber soles. These booties permit the diver to walk comfortably over rocks, rocks with barnacles, and corals for entry and exit from the water when not wearing fins. Quick-release straps make donning and removal easy, which is especially important when the diver is making surf entries in the presence of waves and surges. Once the foot is inserted and the straps are tightened, the fin is not likely to be accidentally pulled off. If the diver dons fins before entering the water, the extended length of the blade makes walking through the water very challenging, especially if waves and surge are present and the diver is carrying a full complement of gear. In these circumstances, flat-bottomed, relatively rigid fins that are not too long provide definite advantages. Finally, the straps (as well as the back of the heel portion of the foot holder) are the most vulnerable to breakage. While removable straps can be replaced, a tear in a strap that is part of the body of the fin or the shoe-type foot portion will necessitate replacement of the fins.

The incorporated (nonreplaceable) strap or partial-shoe foot holder of the fin also has advantages and disadvantages. It avoids the need to use a bootie, reduces bulkiness, eliminates the need to add extra weights to compensate for the neoprene in the bootie, and makes the fin more streamlined. Usually divers wear a sock or a thin neoprene liner to prevent chafing of the skin with this type of foot holder. The strap and/or partial-shoe foot holder is harder to insert the foot into and is more likely to be pulled off the foot in rough water conditions. This is because the tension of the straps cannot be adjusted to ensure the tightest, most comfortable fit. If the shoe type is used, the opening of the shoe has to be large enough to allow the foot to be inserted, often with some difficulty. However, once the foot is in the fin, it is not held as snuggly as with a pocket and adjustable strap over the heel.

We have found little information about the advantages of one swim fin type over another. One study showed that the preferred swim fin was the one that the subjects had the most previous experience with. Consequently, selection of fins, in contrast to much of the other diving equipment, tends to be a highly individual and experience-based decision. Swimming fins range in price from $30 to over $200.

Underwater propulsion vehicles are another method of assisting divers in moving through the water. Typically, they have a watertight-sealed battery and motor compartment, a teardrop shape (like the contour of a whale), and a propeller enclosed in a cage to prevent injury to the diver. They provide propulsion for 30 to 60 minutes at speeds up to two knots. The duration of the battery charge depends on the speed traveled and whether or not the model includes a light. As with other equipment, these vehicles have advantages and disadvantages. They are very useful for conserving the diver's gas supply while he or she is exploring or searching a large area of the dive site. Also, the power supply is independent of the depth (up to the depth limit of the vehicle, which is about 100 FSW or 30 MSW) as compared to the diver's air supply, which will be used up four times faster at this depth. A major disadvantage is that the underwater propulsion vehicle requires two hands for control. This limits the operator's ability to do activities underwater or take photographs. Since the vehicles are designed to be negatively buoyant, they will sink and may be lost if not held on to continuously. Underwater propulsion vehicles range in price from about $400 to over $1,000.

For Further Review

1. How do the axial and appendicular musculoskeletal structures contribute to movement through the water?

2. What are the similarities and differences between the appendicular musculoskeletal structures of humans and diving mammals?

3. How do muscles contract yet allow smooth coordinated movements?

4. How do adaptations for diving in diving mammals contribute to their swimming ability?

5. How does turbulence interfere with movement in the aquatic environment?

6. How do swim speeds of humans compare with those of the porpoise?

7. How do arm pull, leg kick, and swim fins compare in their efficiency of propulsion?

8. What are the advantages and disadvantages of different types of swim fins?

ORIENTATION IN THE AQUATIC ENVIRONMENT

As amazing as are the previously discussed adaptations of diving mammals to the aquatic environment, without equally remarkable adaptations to orientation, they would not be able to survive. The main adaptations to orientation are observed in two of the five primary senses, their visual and

Chapter Preview

- Aquatic environment's effects on vision and hearing
- Visual and auditory adaptations of mammals in the aquatic environment
- Human divers and how they manage visual challenges while underwater
- Ways in which technology aids navigation in the aquatic environment

hearing systems. This is in contrast to the situation with fish, especially sharks, that rely on highly discriminative lateral-line vibration–pressure sensing and olfactory (sense of smell) systems for major portions of their sensory input in the aquatic environment. These systems, whether vision and hearing or vibration–pressure and smell, make it possible for these animals to navigate, hunt for food, perhaps communicate with each other, and avoid dangers. For the majority of sport divers, sensory input, primarily visual, provides a means to enjoy the beauty and variety of the underwater environment. However, vision also helps with other specific underwater goals such as orientation, food collection, marine biology observations, archeological excavations, equipment inspections, exploration, and hazard avoidance.

Vision in the Underwater Environment

The eyes are the organs of vision. Vision underwater is limited because of water's light transmission properties (about 200 feet [61 meters], maximum distance in the clearest of waters), as well as the amount of turbidity (suspended material) present. Whereas vision with optimal conditions in air is measured in miles, vision in water is usually described in tens of feet (meters).

Diving mammals have adaptations that make it possible for them to use their sense of vision effectively in both environments.

Anatomy and Physiology

The outer surface of the eye is covered with a thin, translucent membrane (the **conjunctiva**) that covers the inner surfaces of the eyelid and is reflected over the front of the eye. This is the portion of the eye that comes into physical contact with the environment, be it air when one is on land or water if one is submerged (without a face mask or goggles). The outer surface of the eyeball contains the **cornea,** which is clear and allows the visual image to be transmitted to the back of the eyeball. In air, about 70 percent of the **refraction** (bending of the light rays in order to form an image on the retina) occurs in the cornea. During submersion, the air–cornea interface becomes a water–cornea interface. Since the cornea's refraction ability is not designed for direct contact with water, objects appear blurred when viewed underwater. The **iris,** the shutter of the eye, lies behind the cornea. The iris gives the eye its color and consists of muscle fibers that have a radial orientation and a round central opening, the **pupil.** As illumination dims, the muscle fibers relax and the pupil enlarges—a process analogous to opening the shutter of a camera. This allows more light to enter the eye. In the presence of bright light, the muscles of the iris contract, thereby constricting the pupil. This reduces the light entering the eye but improves visual acuity since the light rays are more parallel to each other as they pass through the eyeball and focus on the retina.

Behind the pupil lies the lens. About 30 percent of refraction in the human eye occurs in this structure. Whereas the cornea cannot change its refraction, the refractive power of the lens is under physiological control. The lens has the ability to change shape because of its muscular attachments. This allows the eye to accommodate for focusing on objects close up or in the distance. However, this accommodation ability is not sufficient to overcome the **refractive index** (the refractive power of any substance as compared to air) of the water–corneal interface. After reaching the lens, the visual image passes through the eyeball, which is filled with a clear gelatinous liquid called the **vitreous humor.** The image is then received on the **retina,** a nervelike tissue at the back of the eyeball, where it is converted to nerve impulses. The retina has two types of sensory receiving pigments, the **rods and cones.** The cones distinguish color while the rods distinguish black and white images. In dim lighting, the rods are primarily responsible for visual acuity. The nerve impulses are then transmitted by the optic nerve to the brain, where they are processed and interpreted as visual images.

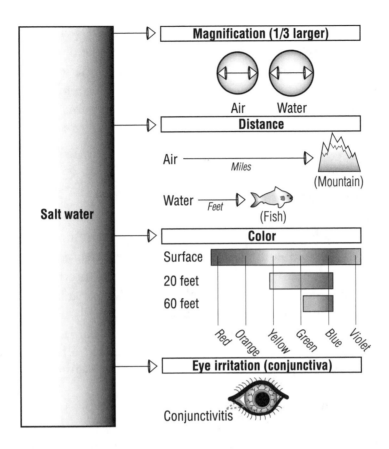

FIGURE 9.1 Effects of immersion in water on vision.

Water has several effects on the interpretation of visual images as seen in figure 9.1. First, the refractive index of water is greater than that of air. Consequently, objects appear about one-third larger or closer up in water than they do in air. Second, with increasing depth, more light is filtered out by the water. There is a selective effect on colors such that red is first lost and then yellow. At the depth of 60 FSW (18 MSW), almost all objects become a monotonous blue-gray color.

Visual Adaptations to the Aquatic Environment

One advantage in vision acuity that diving mammals have over humans is the increased percentage of rods in the retina. This is also observed in animals that are nocturnal or, as in the case of the diving mammals, live in conditions where illumination is dim. The increased proportion of rods helps the animal to discriminate black and white objects in near-dark conditions—the so-called night vision effect. For example, nocturnal predators, such as the great cats, have five times the night vision acuity that humans have.

Porpoises appear to see in or out of the water equally well (Lilly 1961) as a consequence of two known attributes. First, the shape of the lens permits extreme accommodation. This wide range of accommodation helps to compensate for the different refractive indexes of air and water. Second, the iris is a "U"-shaped slit rather than a round opening as in humans. The reaction to different light intensities such as those on the surface and in the water is thought to change the shape of the slit to allow visual acuity both on the surface and underwater.

Technology to Improve Vision in the Aquatic Environment

The main technology to improve visual acuity for the human diver is the face mask and related equipment such as the dive helmet and the swim goggle. This equipment reestablishes the air–cornea interface by creating an airspace between the eye and the glass plate that separates the air from the water. Like most other equipment, these visual aids have desirable as well as undesirable features. In reestablishing the air–cornea interface, they restore visual acuity underwater. Another desirable effect of the face mask and its counterparts is that they protect the eyes from the irritating effects of salt water or chlorine.

Of all the developments that have contributed to the training of competitive swimmers, the swim goggle has to be considered one of the most significant. Before this simple, inexpensive piece of equipment was available, swimming practices were limited to an hour or so because of the irritating effect chlorinated or salt water had on the eyes. Chlorine or salt in the water produces a chemical conjunctivitis that limits swim practices due to pain, tearing, blurring of vision, and seeing halos. Swim goggles protect the eyes from the irritation effects of the chemicals on the conjunctiva and allow for unlimited swim practice times with respect to the eyes.

Without adaptations, swim goggles cannot be used for diving, other than to very shallow depths, because they are not in continuity with the nose or mouth and the pressure therefore cannot be equalized. The Ama diving women of Japan adapted their swim goggles for deep diving by attaching small rubber air-filled bulbs to each eyepiece. With descent and increasing ambient pressure, the bulbs collapsed. This increased the air pressure in the goggles and prevented a pressure differential from building up between the insides of the goggles and the water outside. Thus, "goggle squeezes" were prevented passively; that is, the Ama diver's breath-holding air supply was not used. With this modification, the air-filled, rigid-walled cavities of the goggle were converted to air-filled, flexible-walled cavities that avoided pressure differentials (see chapter 1). For a world record–breaking deep breath-hold dive, a swim goggle filled with fresh water—with lenses designed to

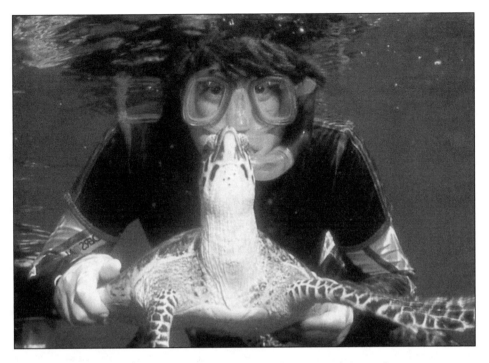

The face mask establishes an airspace between the eye and the underwater environment.

correct for the eye–water refractive index—was used. Since the airspace was obliterated (through the conversion of an air-filled, rigid-walled structure to a fluid-filled, rigid-walled structure), no pressure gradients developed inside the goggles with changes in depth (see chapter 1).

The most undesirable effect of the face mask is that it creates an artificial airspace between the face and the water environment. This airspace is analogous to the natural air-filled, rigid-walled cavities of the body, such as the middle ear spaces and the sinuses, and is therefore subject to barotrauma. This can cause bleeding into the conjunctiva, outward bulging of the eyeballs, and pain (see chapter 13). The larger the face mask, the greater the volume of air needed to equilibrate pressure in the face mask and the greater likelihood of a face mask squeeze.

Face mask squeeze is prevented by exhaling via the nose into the mask. This requires a source of air, either directly from the lungs if the diver is breath-holding, or indirectly from the SCUBA tank or other air source if the diver is breathing compressed gases. Ordinarily face mask clearing does not substantially reduce the air supply in the SCUBA tank because of the small volume of gas required. However, if the face mask leaks due to an inadequate seal, repeated clearing of water from the mask may have a noticeable effect on the air supply.

Some face masks have features designed to facilitate equilibration of pressure in the middle ear spaces as well as clearing of water from the mask. These include the following:

- Indentations in the lower edge of the mask around the nose that make it possible to pinch shut the nostrils for ear-clearing with descent
- Purge valves, also on the lower edge of the mask, designed to drain water from the mask passively by a gravity effect or actively by increasing pressure in the mask through exhalation

Mask straps, purge valves, and the indentations for facilitating ear-clearing tend to be the parts of the face mask that fail most frequently. This occurs because of their thinness and increased handling and movement as compared to other parts of the face mask.

Fogging of the mask can be a great distraction for the diver. It occurs because of condensation of moisture, on the inside of the mask faceplate, from the diver's exhaled air. Fogging is exacerbated by the difference in the temperature between the air inside the mask and the water outside. Defogging agents similar to soaps are very effective in preventing mask fogging, but to be most effective they need to be applied before the inner surface of the glass is wetted. They can cause irritation of the conjunctiva if they come in contact with this part of the eye. Saliva is also used as a defogging agent, but does not seem to be as effective with the new-generation silicon masks as the soap-type defogging agents.

The face mask can cause other challenges for the diver. Because of the differences in the refractive indexes of water and air, peripheral vision is reduced by about one-third while one is wearing a face mask underwater. The diver subconsciously remedies this situation by performing more active neck movements (looking from side to side, up and down, and around) or remaining satisfied to see objects that lie directly ahead. Side and bottom windows, which add bulkiness to the mask, tend to remedy this situation. Water leakage into a mask usually results from wrinkles or folds in the soft, pliable edges of the mask. Hair, a beard or mustache, or the edges of a neoprene hood may interfere with the seal. The pliability of silicon rubber enables divers to make adequate seals over most beards and mustaches. Mask straps that are too tight may cause headaches or uncomfortable pressure buildups on the face where the edges of the mask come in contact with the skin. The inexperienced diver, preoccupied with the other aspects of the dive, may not appreciate that the facial discomfort or headache results from the tightness of the mask straps and will thereby fail to correct the problem. If the straps are too loose, the mask may leak or become too easily dislodged.

As with diving fins, a larger face mask is not necessarily better. The smaller and closer to the eyes the faceplate of the mask is, the better the peripheral vision as noted in figure 9.2. The bulkiness of a large face mask makes it more likely to be accidentally dislodged by surf action or bumping objects. The larger the flat surface of the faceplate, the more it slows the forward swimming speed. As with fins, there are many options available for face masks. Choices include colors, sizes, presence or absence of purge valves and nose-pinching devices, strap design, shape (oval, round, rectangular, with or without side windows, etc.), type of material (silicon, rubber, plastic), glass or plastic faceplate, and airspace volume. The sport diver should try on a variety of masks and select the one that seems to seal the easiest, has the smallest volume, and is the most comfortable. Sport divers on special missions such as archeological explorations may have the opportunity to use full face masks or lightweight helmets with surface-supplied air. Besides providing an uninterrupted supply of surface air, this equipment allows voice communications to and from the diver.

For divers with impaired visual acuity, lenses can be placed inside the face mask to correct the problem. Especially convenient are pressed-fit lenses that adhere to the faceplate when wetted; these are sold in dive shops to correct for loss of near vision. Given the need to read increasingly more sophisticated diving monitors and the dimness of underwater illumination, this small addition to the diving mask becomes a primary safety feature for those with impaired near vision. Face masks range in price from about $25 to over $60 depending on the features and size. Over-the-counter lens inserts cost about $25 while prescription lens inserts, glued into place, may cost $100 or more.

Underwater lights can supplement the visual experiences of diving. A pleasing comment one hears is that photos taken underwater with flash units

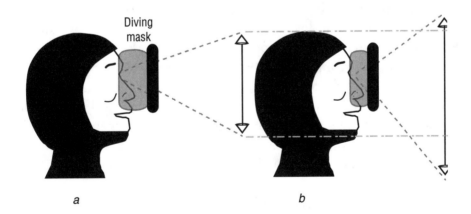

FIGURE 9.2   Peripheral vision and the face mask. *(a)* There is a decrease in peripheral vision due to the refraction index of the water. *(b)* The decrease is mitigated to some extent by moving the faceplate of the face mask closer to the eyes.

are so much more colorful than the scenes actually visualized. The explanation for this is obvious from our previous discussion of the light diminution and color-filtering effects of deeper depths. Dive lights can compensate for these effects. They bring out the myriad colors present in the underwater environment and make night diving a fascinating experience. In contrast to many of our other admonitions about size, the larger and brighter the dive light, the more desirable it is. The size and bulkiness of the light is somewhat offset by its near-neutral buoyancy in water and the greatly improved illumination it provides. Rechargeable batteries are highly recommended, since at full illumination, batteries typically last about 45 minutes. Dive lights, depending on size, battery type, and depth limitations, can vary in price from $25 to over $250.

Vision-Directed Safety Gear

The "dive sausage" and the strobe light are two other pieces of visual equipment that have relevance to the sport diver. Both pertain to dive safety. The dive sausage is a bright orange plastic tube, about six feet (1.8 meters) long and six inches (15 centimeters) wide, that is sealed at one end and open at the other. The dive sausage is stored in a pocket of the buoyancy compensator, tightly rolled up so that it does not take up much space. A diver who becomes separated from the dive group while on the surface unrolls and inflates the sausage, either by placing the mouthpiece of the regulator inside the open end of the tube and filling the tube by pressing the purge valve, or by manually inflating the tube like a balloon. Once inflated, the sausage is held vertically in the water. With its six-foot (1.8-meter) height and bright orange color it can be seen for long distances on the surface of the water. The dive sausage costs $5 or less.

Like the sausage, a blinking strobe light can be seen for long distances on the water. For night dives, the strobe light is very effective as a signaling device for pickups by the dive support boat or as a marker for where the diver is to rendezvous. A compact, waterproof strobe sells for $20 or less. Tubes with **bioluminescence** (light production from living sources) materials will brightly glow in the dark when activated by mixing of the contents, usually done by folding the tube. For night dives, these are attached to tank manifolds and help dive buddies to keep track of each other. These light tubes are nonreusable. They remain effective for about 12 hours and cost several dollars.

Hearing and Related Phenomena in the Underwater Environment

Diving mammals have physical structures related to sound and hearing in water. Sea lions have flaps that close over the external portions of their ear canals when they dive, while seals have no external ear portions at all. The flaps presumably prevent water from entering the ear canals when these animals dive. Porpoises have no ear structures at all. They use an alternative system for sound recognition that we describe further on. The middle ear spaces of the sea lion have several notable differences from those of humans (Odend'hal and Poulter 1966). First, the surface area of the portion of the middle ear bone (the footplate of the stirrup) that helps to conduct sound waves from the eardrum to the inner ear is the same as that of the eardrum itself. In humans the footplate surface area is about 1/20 that of the eardrum. Second, the blood vessels lining the inside of the eardrum and the adjacent middle ear spaces act as sinuses, which fill with blood as the sea lion descends.

These anatomical structures have plausible teleological explanations. The enlarged area of the bony footplate behind the eardrum and the sinuses have possible protective and functional effects:

- First, as a solid object lying behind the eardrum, it may prevent overdistension and perforation of the eardrum with descent.

- Second, the larger area of the footplate may dampen sounds and protect the eardrum from underwater sound trauma (necessary because water transmits sounds five times more rapidly than air does). In contrast, in humans, sounds are multiplied 20-fold because the footplate covers only 1/20 of the eardrum surface.

- Third, the ability to obliterate the middle ear spaces with blood contained in the sinuses offers protection from ear squeezes by eliminating an air-filled, rigid-walled cavity when the venous sinuses fully distend with blood.

- Fourth, as a corollary to this, the large surface area of the bony footplate may be needed in order to transfer the sound energy through the blood-filled venous sinuses to the inner ear.

- Fifth, the venous sinuses, similar to those found below the diaphragm of seals (see chapter 5), may be an additional storage reservoir for oxygen during the breath-hold dive.

An additional hearing-related adaptation that has been described in whales and porpoises aids these mammals in navigation and identification of objects underwater. This adaptation, termed **echo location,** is based on the same physics as **SONAR** (sound navigation and ranging) used for ship navigation, military purposes, scientific studies, and depth determinations. Whales and porpoises emit low-frequency sounds that can travel long distances through the water. After the sound waves strike an object, they are reflected back to the emitting source. When the returned sound waves strike the skin over the porpoises' and whales' skulls, they are transmitted to their brains where they are processed and interpreted. The system in these diving mammals has incredible discriminatory abilities. For example, porpoises can discriminate between edible and inedible fish of equal sizes from distances of many yards (meters) using this echo-location system. In the past there was much interest in the large relative brain weight (weight of the brain in relation to total body weight) of porpoises as compared to humans. Some suggest that the brain size puts these diving mammals on par with humans regarding intelligence. Now, much of the increased size of the porpoise's brain is attributed to elaboration of the echo-location system.

Technology to Improve Navigation in the Aquatic Environment

Many devices are available to help divers improve communications and navigation while on or in the water. These include compasses, sound-emitting systems, handheld sonar units, and the global positioning devices.

Dive Compass

Like the dive knife, the buoyancy compensator, and the sausage tube, the dive compass is an integral part of the diver's safety equipment. While it may not tell divers where they are, the compass can help conserve energy during swimming to and from a dive site. The compass allows divers to navigate on the surface with their heads down and to breathe with a snorkel. This eliminates having to stop and expend extra effort to lift the head out of the water for a visual reference. When in the trough of a swell, the visual references may be temporarily lost, and the compass can be useful in these situations also. Compasses for diving can range in price from $5, for a miniature model that can be attached to the band of a wristwatch, to $60 or more for a model that nests into the cluster containing the dive computer and tank pressure gauge. The compass used for diving should be watertight and fluid filled. A fluid-filled compass avoids pressure differentials that would damage an air-filled compass with changes in depth.

Handheld Sonar and Underwater Sound-Emitting Devices

Handheld sonar units can help locate underwater objects. Because they are bulky and require two hands to operate, their use is totally mission oriented. This means that the sole purpose of the dive using this equipment is to locate an underwater object. Prices for these devices range from $500 to $2,000 or more, depending on their sophistication. An underwater sound-emitting and -transmitting device can be useful for locating a dive buddy, honing in on a counterpart receiver that has been placed on a dive site, or returning to a dive rendezvous point. The system requires two devices. Each has the capability of transmitting and receiving a sound signal. Since water transmits sound so well, the system can be used over long ranges far exceeding the range of underwater vision, even when the visibility underwater is excellent. The principle is simple. The closer the receiving unit is to the in-line position with the transmitting unit, the louder the signal (or with blinking lights, the brighter the signal). The signal diminishes as the receiving unit is rotated away from the in-line position. Prices for this type of equipment begin at about $100.

Global Positioning Device

The global positioning device makes it possible for the dive support craft to precisely navigate to the dive site. Placing the diver directly over the dive site, in contrast to the swim, hunt, and discovery approach to locating the dive target, conserves energy and air supply. At present, however, the device is not available for use by the diver while underwater. Handheld global positioning devices sell for $200 to over $600. The prices depend on how discriminating the device is, as well as its memory and built-in map components. The upper-price, highly discriminating models can locate objects within a radius of 15 feet (4.6 meters) to 20 feet (six meters). The boat fathometer is another device that can help target the dive site. It can precisely identify underwater mounts, walls, or other variations in the bottom contour that will allow the diver to enter the water directly over the intended dive spot.

It is remarkable that the echo-location systems of whales and porpoises have physiological counterparts of all the devices mentioned in the preceding section. The compactness, precision, and versatility of the diving mammals' echo-location systems—with capabilities ranging from that of discriminating fish of similar shapes to making 10,000-mile (16,000-kilometer) migrations—attest to the remarkable workings of these systems.

Dive Watch

The dive watch, although not strictly gear for orientation, is an essential piece of safety equipment. No diver should enter the water without a reliable timekeeping device. It is essential for the diver to be cognizant of the time periods for all portions of the dive. Dive-timer–watch combinations are often integrated into the dive computer. With breath-hold diving, the watch is useful for monitoring durations both underwater and during surface rest periods. A rhythm can be established that allows the diver to do repetitive breath-hold dives over sustained periods of time. More important, the monitoring of bottom times avoids spending too long at depth, which leads to the risk of blacking out during ascents (see chapter 11). In SCUBA diving, the watch is essential for monitoring the inert gas load with respect to bottom times, ascent rates, three-minute rest stops, and surface intervals (see chapter 3).

Dive watches range in price from $25 (probably only appropriate for snorkeling on the surface) to over $1,000. Bezels are a very useful, user-friendly feature for timing diving activities. The more expensive watches have integrated depth gauges with adjustable time and depth limit alarms. Backlighting, preferably automatic versus manual, is another desirable feature, especially for diving at night or where the illumination is poor. Finally, the most expensive, "nondesigner," dive watches contain integrated dive computers with connectors that transfer dive data to computers.

Dive Knife

Finally, for completeness' sake, the dive knife needs to be mentioned. It cannot be classified as orientation gear but is a safety device that should be a part of every diver's equipment. The knife may be lifesaving if it is needed to free a diver from entanglements. Serrated edges make it possible to "saw" through heavy ropes, nylon lines, and strands of kelp, which can be difficult to do with a straight-edged knife, especially if it is not very sharp. Some dive nature preserves, to prevent disturbance of the aquatic environment, do not allow divers to wear sheath knives. In this situation one should carry a folding knife in a buoyancy compensator pocket. The chance of the diver's disturbing the underwater environment by being "plastered" to the bottom because of negative buoyancy is far greater than that from wearing a sheath knife.

An interesting question about the dive knife concerns the best attachment location. A favorite site is on the outside of the leg. This site, which has been glamorized by movies, allows the diver ready access to the knife. However, the leg attachment site interferes with kicking, may cause the sheath to slip down or rotate around the leg, and—more important—can catch the weight belt when it is ditched in an emergency situation. An alternative is to attach a small sheathed dive knife to a D-ring on the buoyancy compensator, where it will be readily accessible by either hand. A second alternative is to attach a larger knife to a thigh pocket in the wet suit or a web belt around the waist. The dive knife should not be attached to a weight belt because if the weight belt is ditched, the knife will no longer be available for an emergency.

Like other pieces of diving gear, the dive knife should be inspected and maintained after each dive period. This includes cleansing, lubrication, and sharpening. Dive knives range in price from $15 to $150. The prices relate to features such as stainless steel or nonferrous metals, rust resistance, size, limited editions with engraved signatures, multiple-use features (hooked, cutting, single- or double-edged, and serrated blades; pry bar and screwdriver tips; and so on), quality of the sheath, fastening devices, storage containers in the handle, and ease and security of the sheathing and sheathing device.

Adaptations: Summary

Although each of the adaptations described in this part of the book are remarkable in themselves, their combined effects make the diving mammals the masters of their environment. The adaptations revolve around three primary effects: (1) improving breath-hold diving times, (2) preventing medical problems of diving, and (3) moving (plus orientation) in the aquatic environment. Adaptations that have major roles for the primary effect often have secondary roles for other benefits, too.

Sustained Breath-Hold Times

The oxygen-conserving reflex makes sustained breath-holding times possible. Its three components are bradycardia, shunting, and energy production by anaerobic metabolism in the skeletal muscles. Supplementary adaptations, which improve the ability to breath-hold as well as prevent medical problems of diving, include (a) oxygen availability from myoglobin, (b) oxygen extraction from venous blood, (c) elevated percentages of red blood cells, (d) diminished sizes of red blood cells, (e) increased tolerance to elevated carbon dioxide and lowered oxygen blood concentrations, (f) negative buoyancy after lung exhalation, (g) improved swimming efficiency, and (h) avoidance of hypothermia.

Preventing Medical Problems of Diving

The respiratory adaptation of diving after exhalation, with associated lung collapse, is the major factor in preventing decompression sickness, air embolism, and nitrogen narcosis in diving mammals. Middle ear barotrauma is avoided by the absence of ear structures, as in the porpoise, and the filling of the middle ear spaces with blood in dilated venous sinuses in seals. Body shape and subcutaneous fat are the primary deterrents to hypothermia; shunting of blood from the extremities, breath-holding, cessation of urine production and excretion, and countercurrent heat exchange are secondary effects that help prevent hypothermia.

Propulsion

The primary adaptations for moving through water and orienting to the aquatic environment are anatomical; these include body shape, muscle anatomy, fin and fluke size and position, and the echo-location center in the brain. Changes in eye structures allow the eyes of porpoises to accommodate for differences in refraction in air and underwater. Echo location provides the orientation and navigation information necessary for whales and seals to survive in the aquatic environment. Secondary changes to improve mobility include turbulence-reducing effects such as subcutaneous fat tissues and heat exchange mechanisms.

Technology As a Substitute for Adaptations

Due to technological achievements, knowledge, and dive planning, human divers can surmount most of the physical, physiological, and medical obstacles of diving. However, in contrast to the diving mammal, which integrates all of these adaptations into a compact, energy-efficient swimming and diving "machine," the human diver encounters negative trade-offs for each technological development. For example, although breathing equipment compensates for the diver's oxygen requirements underwater, it subjects the SCUBA diver to major medical problems and slows swimming speed due to drag. Thermal protection suits shield the human diver from cold water but add bulkiness, reduce mobility, and increase weight (lead weights to counteract the buoyancy of the suit). Masks and other orientation devices slow swimming speed, and many orientation devices interfere with mobility and dexterity because they are handheld. Part III discusses the medical problems of diving, which in many cases are consequences of the technological achievements we have made to become better human divers.

For Further Review

1. What are the important components of the human visual system?
2. How does the aquatic environment affect vision?
3. What structures in diving mammals help them see in the aquatic environment?
4. What are the advantages and possible disadvantages of the face mask?
5. How does the underwater environment affect hearing?
6. What is echo location? How is it used by whales and porpoises?
7. How has technology helped the diver with respect to underwater navigation?
8. Why is the diving watch (or timepiece) an essential piece of diving equipment?

PART III

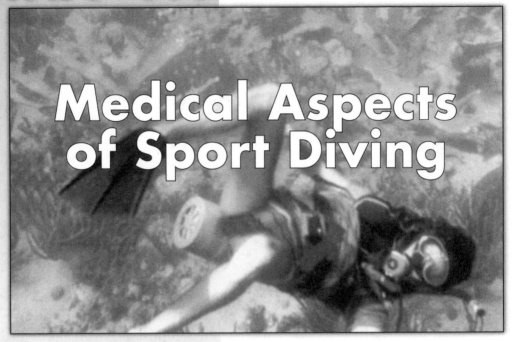

Medical Aspects of Sport Diving

Although the underwater environment is usually safe for the sport diver, medical problems occur at all levels of the dive. This part of the book explores preventive medicine aspects of diving, as well as the medical problems that occur in the diver. Chapter 10 outlines preventive medicine aspects including the conditions that preclude diving, the medical examination for divers, conditions specific to the female diver, and drugs in diving. Chapter 10 also addresses the role of nutrition in diving (not often given much consideration in the sport diver) from a preventive medicine standpoint. Tables in chapter 10 provide a quick reference for conditions that may make the diver susceptible to injury (negative feedback) from the stresses of diving. A reader who needs more information, such as a physician seeking more specific information on an underlying medical condition that may contribute to a medical problem of diving, will find it in appendix B, "Where to Get Help."

Medical problems of diving (MPD) occur when the stresses of diving lead to negative feedback mechanisms that cause injury to the diver. Each of the four phases of the dive—surface, descent, bottom, and ascent—generates stresses that can lead to MPD as listed in table III.1. Five chapters in part III address these problems: chapters 11 and 12—surface; chapter 13—descent; chapter 14—bottom; chapter 15—ascent. This classification not only is logical but also helps a caregiver determine what the MPD is, since a given problem is likely to have had its onset at a particular stage of the dive. From this point, the caregiver can initiate the first-response interventions and decide whether or not the victim needs follow-up medical care. Of course, if there is any question about the need for definitive medical care for an MPD, the decision should always be to seek medical evaluation and care. Chapters 11 through 15, as well as chapter 16, on emergency complications from MPD, present information on the following seven aspects of each MPD:

- Significance
- Causes
- Effects on the body (pathophysiology)
- First-response interventions
- Definitive management
- Prevention
- Return to diving

When appropriate, explanations show why the problems occur and how physiological responses become pathological conditions with the challenges of the dive. The background for much of this information has been presented in parts I and II. Although the chapters in part III include sections on definitive medical care for each MPD, this text is not designed to be a reference for such information. For example, treatment tables for decompression sickness and air embolism are not included. However, we do present the rationale

Table III.1 Medical Problems and Phases of the Dive*			
Surface (chapters 11 and 12)	**Descent (chapter 13)**	**Bottom (chapter 14)**	**Ascent (chapter 15)**
Panic	Ear and sinus squeezes	Nitrogen narcosis	Extra-alveolar air syndromes (including arterial gas embolism**)
Blackout	Thoracic squeeze	Oxygen toxicity	
Environmental problems		Carbon dioxide toxicity	
Injuries from marine animals		Anoxia	Decompression sickness**
		Carbon monoxide poisoning	
		High-pressure nervous system syndrome	

* Complications such as near-drowning, shock, and cardiac arrest may present at any phase of the dive (see chapter 16).
** These two conditions are often linked together as decompression illness.

for selecting the interventions used to treat or prevent each disorder, again referring to information from parts I and II when appropriate. We provide suggestions for answering the important questions of how to prevent future occurrences of the MPD and when to return to diving. Finally, chapters include "Bringing It All Together" sections that present one or more case studies about the MPD, accompanied by comments focusing on the particular medical aspects involved.

MEDICAL PREPARATION FOR DIVING: FITNESS AND NUTRITION

Fitness and nutrition are two components of preparedness for diving. Medical examinations and standards help to ensure that diving is safe for divers of different types and age groups, and also consider differences among male and female divers. Proper nutrition is an important aspect of the safety and enjoyment of diving.

Chapter Preview

- Extent of medical problems of diving
- Medical standards for diving
- Medical examinations for each type of diving
- Medical aspects of women and diving
- Drugs and diving
- Nutrition considerations for the diver

Fitness for Diving

How important is fitness for diving? With an estimated 5 million certified SCUBA divers in the United States and only two or three cases of serious medical problems of diving (MPD) such as decompression illness for every 10,000 SCUBA divers, two conclusions may be drawn about fitness and the related subject of safety in diving: First, diving is an inherently safe sport, and second, diving tends to self-select those who are fit to do the sport. There is validity to both conclusions. Millions of SCUBA dives are done each year; fortunately, serious diving accidents occur very infrequently. Deaths from SCUBA diving accidents have remained level at approximately 100 per year even though the number of SCUBA divers has increased 10-fold over the past three decades. The following facts help to explain these observations:

- Medical problems of diving are either nonfatal or fatal. The number of nonfatal diving accidents far exceeds the number of fatal accidents as shown in figure 10.1.

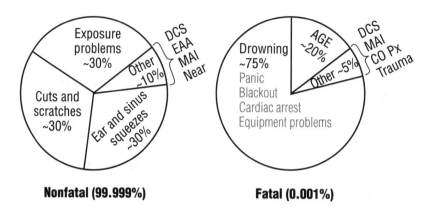

Nonfatal (99.999%)   **Fatal (0.001%)**

FIGURE 10.1   Occurrences of medical problems during diving. AGE = arterial gas embolism; CO Px = carbon monoxide poisoning; DCS = decompression sickness; EAA = extra-alveolar air syndromes; MAI = marine animal injuries; Near = near-drowning; Trauma = traumatic injuries.

- Most nonfatal MPD are minor and appropriately managed by non-physician first-response interventions.

- Only a small percentage of the MPD are a consequence of the actual breathing of compressed gases under increased ambient pressures.

- The most serious MPD occur infrequently, while the most frequent MPD are the least serious.

- Improved training of sport SCUBA divers, including requirements for fitness, contributes to the safety of SCUBA diving.

Medical problems of diving are inherent in each phase of the dive. Problems associated with the surface phase such as panic, blackout, and hypothermia can occur at other phases of the dive. In contrast, arterial gas embolism and decompression sickness (DCS) are associated only with the ascent phase of the dive. Problems such as cardiac arrest, near-drowning or drowning, and shock associated with diving are usually a consequence of one of the other medical problems. The causes of the majority of MPD are usually obvious, such as a puncture wound from a sea urchin spine, an ear squeeze from descent, or symptoms of nitrogen narcosis from diving too deeply. The majority of MPD are treated no differently than their non-diving counterparts. The exceptions are those conditions that arise as a consequence of pressure or the breathing of gas under increased ambient pressure. The treatment of DCS, for example, requires a recompression chamber and supervision by medical personnel familiar with these conditions.

Medical Examinations for Sport Diving

Although a medical examination to begin diving training is not required by the SCUBA diving certification agencies in the United States, each student is required to complete a health questionnaire. If any question referring to a disease condition is answered "yes," a medical examination with medical clearance by a physician is usually required before the prospective student is allowed to begin SCUBA training. While this requirement exemplifies the preventive medicine approach, it also provides the certifying agencies protection from the liability of training a diver who is at risk for a serious MPD. Operators of most sport SCUBA diving charters require that their clients complete a similar health questionnaire and sign a release from liability form before allowing diving under their auspices.

Medical Standards for the Sport Diver

Medical standards for diving is the term used to describe the level of physical and mental health that is necessary for diving. Every type of sport diving requires good physical and mental health. Medical clearance for diving must take into consideration the type of diving that will be done (see table 10.1) as well as the medical condition of the diver. Contraindications to diving are included in figure 10.2 and are based on one or more of the following:

- Safety: the diver's condition poses an unacceptable risk to the diver or the diver's buddies as would be the case with an individual who is morbidly obese.

- Aggravation of a condition: for example, in Raynaud's phenomenon, cold water will cause constriction of blood vessels and loss of circulation to the hands and feet. Aggravation of these conditions may predispose the diver to DCS at these sites.

- Preexisting conditions: for example, a patent foramen ovale in the heart (see chapters 4 and 15) predisposes the diver to DCS.

- Inability to meet performance requirements: this might be observed in a patient with decompensated heart function, which might lead to a heart attack with an exercise challenge.

It is useful to consider the contraindications as absolute, temporary (i.e., will resolve with treatment interventions), or relative. **Absolute contraindications** are those conditions that preclude diving because of their seriousness. Usually in these situations the individual chooses not to dive. Other conditions may impose **temporary contraindications** for diving, such as a ruptured eardrum, pregnancy, or a healing fracture. Once the condition has resolved, diving can be resumed. Finally, there are conditions that impose **relative contraindications** for diving. In these situations sport diving is

Table 10.1	Considerations for the Pre-Dive Examination		
	Types of diving		
Consider-ations	**Breath-hold/ Snorkel diving**	**Recreational SCUBA diving**	**Commercial, technical, and scientific diving**
History	Mainly general health and fitness	Ear, nose, throat, pulmonary, and car-diovascular problems	Diving history; history of diving-related injuries
Physical examination	As appropriate for age (e.g., doctor checkups for school)	General exam plus special attention to ear, nose, and throat; pulmonary; and mental status portions	Examination usually done by undersea and hyperbaric medical physician specialists
Fitness and physical performance	General physical fitness and ability to swim; comfort in the water	Good health; ability to tolerate exercise challenges	High level of fitness consistent with a con-ditioned athlete
Mental status	Ability to under-stand and follow directions	Stable temperament; positive attitude	No evidence of psychopathology
Recom-mended age to start (age)	During childhood (6-7)	After bone maturation (14-15)	Late adolescence (18 or older)

permitted with certain restrictions, for example, in patients who have diabetes or heart disease.

Medical histories provide important information regarding medical fitness for diving. For example, asthma and ear, nose, and throat problems that are well controlled (do not necessitate regular use of medications and do not interfere with physical performance) are not contraindications for SCUBA diving. If there is any risk of pulmonary disease, a chest X-ray is advised. A diver who is older than 40 should have an electrocardiogram with exercise stress testing before beginning diving training. Diabetes, moderate obesity, behavior problems, phobias (especially regarding confined spaces), neu-ropathies, hearing loss, and residuals of severe musculoskeletal injuries are examples of relative contraindications to diving. A history of heart problems is also a relative contraindication to diving. Verification of fitness, stamina, and reasonable cardiac reserve is essential before giving an OK to SCUBA dive in a patient with a history of heart disease. The individual with such a history who is medically okayed to dive should be encouraged to dive in

Cardiovascular disorders

Aneurysms—widened blood vessels that are subject to rupture as in the brain or abdomen

Any cardiovascular problem that requires medication, with function still remaining impaired

Cardiac arrhythmias—irregular heartbeats

Congenital heart problems causing impaired heart function

Congestive heart failure

Hypertension—high blood pressure, moderate to severe

Ischemic—compromised blood flow in the heart muscle; heart disease

Severe deconditioning (temporary)

Pulmonary disorders

Acute (temporary) or chronic lung infections

Asthma requiring medications

Chronic bronchitis

Chronic obstructive pulmonary disease (COPD)

Pulmonary cysts and adhesions

Pulmonary fibrosis (scarring)

Spontaneous pneumothorax—lung collapse (temporary)

Ear, nose, and throat disorders

Acute (temporary) or chronic recurrent middle ear infections, Eustachian tube dysfunction, or both

Chronic sinusitis with or without nasal polyps

Meniere's—inner ear—disease; balance or equilibrium problems

Middle ear surgery

Tympanic membrane rupture (temporary)

Unilateral deafness

Endocrine disorders

Diabetes (relative)

Others with residual impairments even with the use of medications

Hematological disorders

Coagulopathies—blood-clotting problems

Neoplasms—tumors/cancers

Polycythemias—too many red blood cells

Severe anemia (temporary)   *(continued)*

FIGURE 10.2 Medical conditions that are contraindications for diving. This listing is to be used as a guideline, as hundreds of other conditions impose limitations on diving. Usually the problem is so obvious that diving is not even a consideration as an activity for the patient.

Musculoskeletal disorders

Amputations (relative)

Crippling arthritis (relative)

Dysbaric osteonecrosis—bone cell death

Healing fractures (temporary)

Herniated disc (temporary/relative)

Severe traumas/soft tissue injuries (temporary/relative)

Neurological disorders

Alzheimer's—premature senility—disease (relative)

Brain and spinal cord demyelinating disorders such as multiple sclerosis or degenerative diseases (relative)

Cerebrovascular accidents—strokes, with residuals

Epilepsy—seizures

Neuromuscular disorders (relative)

Peripheral neuropathy—nerve malfunction—or peripheral nerve injury (relative)

Severely impaired visual acuity (relative)

Psychiatric disorders

Attention deficit disorder (relative)

Exaggerated fear of open water, sharks, decreased illumination, and so on

Mental illness requiring major tranquilizers, other psychotropic (mind altering) agents, or both

Severe confinement anxiety

Miscellaneous

Age (relative)

Artificial joints (relative)

Colostomy, ileostomy (relative)

Major surgeries (temporary)

Malnutrition (temporary)

Obesity (relative)

Pregnancy (temporary)

FIGURE 10.2   *(continued)*

areas that minimize exertional stresses—for example, should dive off a boat in warm, clear, calm waters.

If the prospective diver is motivated and if complications have not developed from the problems considered to be relative contraindications, sport SCUBA diving is OK. The diver should be aware of ways to avoid injury or complications from the relative contraindication, diving safety practices, and his or her limitations. In such situations a dive buddy who is competent and aware of the diver's relative contraindication(s) should be utilized.

SCUBA Diving for Youngsters   Age should also be a consideration when one is making decisions about sport SCUBA diving. Kids younger than their early teens probably should not SCUBA dive for the following reasons:

- Most diving equipment is designed for larger-sized individuals. Improperly sized diving equipment can slip on the diver and become a safety hazard.

- There is the potential for damage to growth centers of the bones due to gas bubbling in the venous sinusoids with their sluggish blood flow. This would be a preferential environment for gas bubbles to form, coalesce, and enlarge.

- Maturity and judgment in decision making should be at a level that is equivalent to allowing a teenager to drive an automobile.

Nonetheless, youngsters do SCUBA dive. Children who dive should adhere to a dive plan including depth limitations and diving under optimal conditions, with adult supervision.

SCUBA Diving for Older Divers   The decision whether or not older individuals should dive is based on physiological age rather than chronological age. There are no specified upper age limits for SCUBA diving. Because of age-related changes such as decreased muscle strength, joint mobility, stamina, and cardiovascular reserve, older sport divers should dive conservatively; that is, they should avoid "pushing" the dive computer or dive tables to their safe limits and should dive under the conditions recommended for the sport diver with a heart condition. To date, no modifications for diving tables or dive computers have been made that specifically consider age. However, some computers offer personal adjustment modes that reflect how conservative the diver wants to be with respect to the inert gas load (see chapter 3).

Medical Examinations
for Scientific and Deep Technical Diving

Medical examinations for scientific and deep technical divers should be as comprehensive as for commercial divers and should be performed by a physician with special training in underwater medicine. Typically, medical examinations are done before people start these types of diving activities, and on a regular basis, at least every five years, thereafter. As the diver gets older, the examinations need to be done more frequently. For example, the U.S. Navy requires biannual medical examinations for its members between the ages of 50 and 60 and annual examinations after that. In addition to the usual information obtained with a complete medical examination, the periodic medical examination should include the following special health- and dive-related information:

- Changes in health status including medications
- Illnesses or injuries that have occurred since the previous diving exam, that is, the interval history
- Level of conditioning
- Diving activities since the previous medical examination

For scientific, deep technical, and commercial divers, it is also recommended that chest X-rays, blood chemistries, blood counts, audiograms, pulmonary function tests, and possibly X-rays of the major joints be obtained. This latter consideration is especially applicable to divers who make repetitive long, deep, or decompression stop-requiring dives. These types of activities are associated with localized areas of bone cell death, termed **osteonecrosis** ("osteo" = bone; "necrosis" = death). If a large enough area of bone death occurs adjacent to joints, the bone may collapse, leading to arthritis symptoms of the joint. If osteonecrosis is observed, diving is generally not recommended.

Female Divers

Does the female diver require different medical and diving considerations than the male diver? The greater ability of females to tolerate cold water and perhaps thoracic squeeze in record-setting deep breath-hold dives was discussed in part II (see chapters 5 and 7). This suggests anatomical and physiological differences between males and females that have relevance to diving. Other factors specific to females may also have importance to diving. These include menstruation, use of oral **contraceptive agents** (medications that prevent pregnancy) and hormonal replacement therapy, and pregnancy.

Anatomical and Physiological Differences

About one-third of SCUBA divers are females, and the ratio among diving instructors is about the same. Physiological, anatomical, and psychological differences do exist between the sexes and could become important in the underwater environment. The female body contains more fat tissue and less muscle. Theoretically this puts female divers at higher risks for DCS, since nitrogen is lipid (fat) soluble. At the same time, more fat gives some theoretical advantage in cold water since fat serves as insulation. Generally, women have less physical work capacity and stamina. Theoretically, this could make a difference in life-or-death

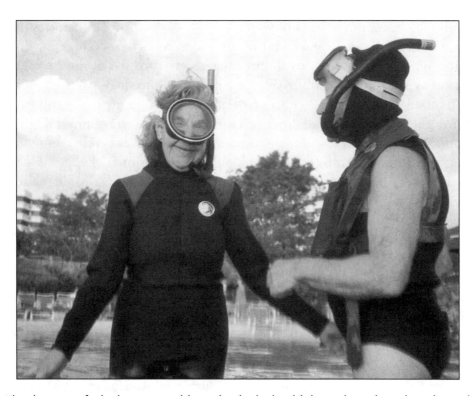

The decision of whether or not older individuals should dive is based on physiological factors rather than chronological age.

situations such as swimming against strong currents or extricating oneself from entanglements.

Even though one-third of divers are female, the ratio of female-to-male deaths in diving is 1 to 10. This may be explained by diving habits rather than anatomical or physiological differences from males. Females tend to select less dangerous or hazardous situations than men. Nonetheless, with appropriate training, female divers can reach the same level of performance as male divers. In some respects they have inherent advantages, such as better tolerance to cold water; and because of their smaller size, women can use their gas supplies more efficiently.

Menstruation and Diving   Two aspects of menstruation deserve discussion in this context: (1) psychophysiological considerations and (2) menstrual blood as an attraction for sharks. Premenstrual and menstrual periods are associated with specific changes in the physiological status of women. These changes may or may not have psychological components. They can produce a range of symptoms that affect physical performance and psychological responses. The female diver must decide whether she wants to dive during these times. However, the change of environment (psychological diversion), the buoyancy effects of water, fluid mobilization (to help resolve fluid retention), and the relaxation provided by a well-conducted dive outweigh the symptoms (in all but their severest forms) of the **premenstrual syndrome** (a combination of emotional, physical, psychological, and mood disturbances that occur after ovulation and normally end with the onset of the menstrual flow) and menstruation. From a physiological point of view, blood loss during menses is almost never severe enough to cause significant **hemodynamic** (blood flow alterations) changes. However, females may be at increased risk for developing DCS. Inside tenders for hyperbaric oxygen (HBO) treatments and treatment of DCS appear to have higher rates of DCS than male tenders. Nevertheless, the information is inconclusive as to whether or not female divers are more prone to DCS than male divers from actual diving activities.

There is no evidence that menstruation increases the likelihood of shark attacks in the female diver. Female divers appear to experience a much lower incidence of shark attacks than male divers, possibly because **hemolyzed** (broken down) red blood cells from menstruation may act as a shark deterrent.

Use of Oral Contraceptive Agents and Hormonal Re-placement Therapy in Diving   Oral contraceptives have side effects. A significant one is the propensity for blood clotting. This causes increased risks for **deep vein thrombosis** (clots), **pulmonary embolism** (venous clots carried to the lungs), cerebrovascular accident (stroke), and **myocardial infarction** (heart attack). However, there is no evidence that oral contraceptives increase the risk of DCS or other diving-related problems. Hormonal replacement therapy may reproduce some of the physiological effects of menstruation, but there is a dearth of information on how this subject applies to diving in the post-menopausal female.

Pregnancy   SCUBA diving is not recommended during pregnancy because of the unknown effects of increased partial pressures of nitrogen on the fetus and the increased propensity for nitrogen deposition in the fetal–maternal lipid tissues. These factors may make the fetus more susceptible to the harmful effects of bubbling than the pregnant woman herself. In addition, if a pregnant woman requires HBO recompression treatment for DCS, the increased partial pressures of oxygen may have **teratogenic** (causing birth defects) effects on the fetus since breathing high pressures of oxygen is toxic to tissues. For these reasons, SCUBA diving is not recommended for pregnant women. Snorkel diving is permissible as long as the woman feels comfortable in the water and in the thermal protection suit if she is using one.

Drugs and Diving

The effects of drugs may be altered under pressure such that side effects acceptable on land in a resting person become unacceptable in the underwater environment with elevated pressure and increased physical activity. Drugs are associated with divers in four ways:

- Treatment of concurrent diseases
- Prevention of MPD
- Treatment of MPD
- Use for "recreational" purposes

When a diver is on a prescription drug, several questions must be answered. First, why does the patient require the medication? Second, are there any known contraindications of the drug for diving? Third, what side effects of the drug could contribute to or worsen an MPD? For example, drugs with sedative side effects will likely make the diver more susceptible to nitrogen narcosis. Drugs with stimulant (excitatory) effects may lower the threshold for oxygen toxicity or panic. Heart and blood pressure medications may predispose the diver to **arrhythmias** (irregular heart rhythms) when the stresses of exercise, pressure, and water temperature are coupled with the drug's effects. One can make appropriate decisions about whether drugs are absolute or relative contraindications to diving based on their categories of action, as listed in table 10.2.

Table 10.2	Drugs That May Interfere With or Should Be Avoided During Diving	
Drug/ Substance	**General mechanisms of action**	**Side effects/Possible problems in diving**
Antihistamines/ Motion sickness remedies	Block histamine (chemicals released in the body that cause allergic reactions) receptors	• Sedation, drowsiness • Impaired cognitive and psychomotor performance
Tranquilizers/ Sedatives	Cause central nervous system (CNS) depression, sedation	• Sedation, drowsiness • Impaired cognitive and psychomotor performance
Antihypertensive drugs	Decrease blood pressure; mechanisms different for different classes	• Decreased ejection of blood from the heart • Decreased cardiac output • Impaired stamina • Increased risk of decompression sickness

(continued)

Drug/Substance	General mechanisms of action	Side effects/Possible problems in diving
Beta-blockers	Block beta-receptors (receptors that stimulate heart action)	• Bradycardia (slowing of heart rate) • Decreased cardiac output • Bronchoconstriction—narrowing of breathing tubes
Angiotensin-converting enzyme (ACE) inhibitors	Block conversion of enzyme that increases blood pressure, used especially for diabetes	• Dry cough • Loss of taste • Rash
Calcium channel blockers	Block calcium channel flow in heart tissues	• Orthostatic (positional) low blood pressure • Dizziness • Syncope (fainting)
Insulin and oral hypoglycemics	Decrease blood glucose level	• Hypoglycemia (low blood sugar) • Altered levels of consciousness • Weakness
Decongestants	Produce local vasoconstriction (reduction in size of blood vessels)	• Rebound phenomena • When the substance wears off or after repeated use, may lead to greater nasal congestion and more difficulty with ear and sinus clearing
Caffeine	Inhibits phosphodiesterase—an enzyme that lessens the listed side effects	• Tachycardia and increased blood pressure • Cardiac arrhythmias • Diuretic (urine producing) action • Dehydration
Amphetamines	Stimulate CNS by releasing biogenic amines (chemicals) from storage sites in the nerve terminals	• Behavioral changes, including erratic diving and increased risk taking • Increased risk of accidents • Panic • Oxygen toxicity • Seizures
Cocaine	Stimulates CNS, blocks neuronal uptake of norepinephrine (a substance in the body that constricts blood vessels and speeds the heart rate)	• Hypermetabolic state • Fatigue • Mental depression • Acidosis • Inability to respond promptly to life-threatening emergencies • Cardiac toxicity, sudden cardiac death • Disturbance of normal heart rhythm • Nasal irritation • Erosion of nasal cartilage • Increased likelihood of an oxygen seizure

Drug/ Substance	General mechanisms of action	Side effects/Possible problems in diving
Opiates	Stimulate opioid receptors within CNS	• Respiratory depression • Altered mood • Impaired psychomotor performance
Tobacco/ Nicotine	Stimulates nicotinic receptors	**Acute effects** • Increases in blood pressure and heart rate • Coronary vasoconstriction • Bronchoconstriction • Decreased oxygen-carrying capacity of the blood • Interference with physical performance **Chronic effects** • Chronic obstructive pulmonary disease • Bronchospasm • Air trapping • Risk of pulmonary barotrauma • Nasal congestion • Sinus and middle ear barotraumas
Alcohol	Acts as CNS depressant	• CNS depression • Interference with mental and physical performance • Increased risk of vomiting • Reduction in blood glucose levels • Weakness and confusion • Blood vessel dilation • Interference with maintenance of body temperature • Diuretic (urine producing) action • Dehydration
Marijuana/ Cannabis		• Impaired cognitive and psychomotor performance • Problems with attention and coordination • Tachycardia (increased heart rate) and increased oxygen consumption • Reduction of cold tolerance and breath-holding capability • Euphoria (feelings of well-being) • General discomfort • Unexplainable apprehension, anxiety, and a desire to terminate a dive prematurely

Some medications have benefits for divers. Divers frequently use drugs to prevent or manage ear squeezes, seasickness, and muscle soreness. Because the use of such drugs is so widespread, experience alone suggests that they have few

BRINGING IT ALL TOGETHER

A 55-year-old male who exercises regularly wants to continue SCUBA diving. He has a history of chronic atrial fibrillation (irregular heartbeat) and was recently placed on Coumadin, a medication that decreases the clotting ability of blood. He seeks an OK from his physician to continue diving. A workup showed that the diver was healthy in all other respects. A graded exercise echocardiogram revealed exercise tolerance consistent with a male half this man's age and no signs of heart dysfunction as the level of exercise increased. Should the diver be allowed to dive?

Answer: The diver needs to consider the benefits and risks of diving. The echocardiogram indicates that the chronic atrial fibrillation condition should not be an absolute contraindication for SCUBA diving. The question is whether the anticoagulant would impose unacceptable risks of bleeding from possible hazards of the dive. From this man's previous diving experiences and safety record, such risks seemed minimal. From a statistical perspective, the chances of serious bleeding from an automobile accident would be far greater than from an injury during diving. From a diving medical perspective, the diver is OK to SCUBA dive.

if any significant side effects for the sport diver. Aspirin is another medication frequently used by divers (see chapters 3, 6, and 15). Anti-inflammatory drugs may reduce the number of treatments needed to manage DCS. If any substance could be considered a wonder drug for divers, it would be oxygen, even though technically oxygen is a respiratory gas rather than a drug. It is the first-line treatment for arterial gas embolism, DCS, carbon monoxide poisoning, and near-drowning. When oxygen is used in nitrox mixes, it reduces the likelihood that DCS will occur (see chapter 2). Finally, oxygen, as used with pressurization in a hyperbaric chamber, is the definitive treatment for DCS as well as the other conditions for which HBO therapy is used (see chapter 6).

Tobacco, alcohol, amphetamines, cocaine, opiates and marijuana, and a number of designer drugs are considered "recreational" drugs. Some are legal; others are illegal. In the context of diving, these substances can be considered to have either "downer" (depression) or "upper" (stimulant) effects. Alcohol acts as a depressant. A very serious consequence of alcohol use is impairment of judgment. Use of alcohol is associated with 50 percent of drowning deaths (including those of SCUBA divers). Tobacco, another legal recreational drug, has stimulant effects from its nicotine. Inhalation of smoke from cigarettes paralyzes the **cilia** (hairlike projections) in the respiratory tract, which in turn interferes with the movement of mucus. This interferes with equilibrating pressure in the middle ear spaces and can lead to ear squeezes. Although divers may claim to dive with impunity while using recreational drugs, use of these drugs by divers is ill advised.

Nutrition Considerations in Diving

The subject of **nutrition** (the science of food values and diet recommendations) and diving is one that usually receives little attention. Divers tend to be physically fit, and sound nutrition is one component of this overall state. In addition, people with nutrition problems tend to be discouraged from participation in diving. At one extreme are people who are morbidly obese, in whom fitting of equipment and buoyancy management can be especially challenging. At the other extreme are persons who are malnourished with nutritional problems usually caused by some other serious condition such as cancer, **malabsorption** (inability of the gut to ingest food) syndromes, or emotional disorders. The seriousness of these conditions with associated weakness, fatigability, and poor exercise reserve makes diving an unlikely recreational activity. Nonetheless, there are nutrition considerations for the diver that can contribute to the safety and enjoyment of this activity.

Anatomy and Physiology

The digestive system is composed of a long muscular tube, the gastrointestinal tract, and a set of accessory organs as diagrammed in figure 10.3. The gastrointestinal tract extends from the mouth to the anus (end of rectum) and is approximately 30 feet (9.1 meters) long. It consists of the oral (mouth) cavity, pharynx (throat), esophagus, stomach, small intestine, large intestine, rectum, and anal canal. The accessory organs include the tongue, teeth, salivary glands, pancreas, liver, and gallbladder. The primary function of the digestive system is to digest and absorb food to provide the body with nutrients, water, and electrolytes.

Digestion and absorption start with eating, that is, chewing food into small pieces, moistening food with salivary secretions, and swallowing, as summarized in table 10.3. Saliva contains **enzymes** that begin to digest carbohydrates in the mouth. Foods react with sensors in the mouth as well as providing odors to the nose to give taste sensations. In the stomach, food particles are degraded by digestive enzymes into simpler compounds. Next, nutrients, water, and electrolytes are absorbed by the small intestine and transported by the circulation to tissues for metabolism and storage. The large intestine absorbs water from the material that was not digested and provides a conduit for its evacuation from the body.

Nutrition and Energy Requirements

Daily energy requirements are based on the basal metabolic rate (BMR) plus the energy required for physical activity (see table 10.4). The BMR is the amount of energy that the body needs at rest to maintain life. It is usually

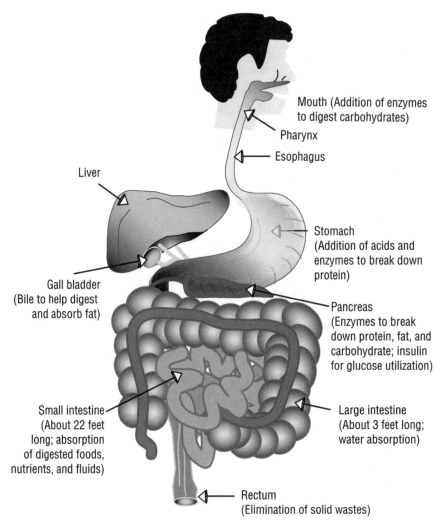

Mouth (Addition of enzymes
to digest carbohydrates)

Pharynx

Esophagus

Liver

Stomach
(Addition of acids and
enzymes to break down
protein)

Gall bladder
(Bile to help digest
and absorb fat)

Pancreas
(Enzymes to break
down protein, fat, and
carbohydrate; insulin
for glucose utilization)

Small intestine
(About 22 feet
long; absorption
of digested foods,
nutrients, and fluids)

Large intestine
(About 3 feet long;
water absorption)

Rectum
(Elimination of solid wastes)

**FIGURE
10.3** Digestive system.

calculated with reference to sleep. The energy of activity is the amount of energy that is necessary to support the physical activity of the person. Energy arises from metabolism of the food we eat. Calorie is the term used to indicate the heat produced by metabolism of food. In the context of nutrition, the term is referred to in 1,000-calorie (kilocalorie) units.

In an average adult, the energy needed for activity accounts for approximately one-third of the total energy expenditures. Energy expenditures with activity increase with the weight of the individual. They greatly increase with strenuous activity. For example, the activities of a sedentary lifestyle for a 150-pound (68-kilogram) male may be 75 kilocalories an hour, or 1,800 kilocalories in 24 hours. For the same-sized individual who is doing moderate activity, the energy expenditure may increase to 100 kilocalories

Table 10.3	Digestion and Absorption of Food and Fluids		
Type	**Enzyme (site)**	**Sites of absorption**	**End products**
Water	–	Stomach and remainder of gut including large bowel	
Carbohydrates	Amylases (mouth, small bowel)	Stomach and small bowel	Monosaccharides (simple sugars)
Proteins	Pepsin, trypsin, chymotrypsin (stomach, small bowel)	Small bowel	Dipeptides (combinations of two amino acids); amino acids
Lipids (fats)	Lipases, esterases (small bowel)	Small bowel	Monoglycerides (single fat chains); free fatty acids
Alcohol	Dehydrogenases (liver)	Stomach and small bowel	

an hour, or 2,400) kilocalories in 24 hours. Energy expenditure is further increased with work in hot, cold, high-altitude, and high ambient pressure environments.

Energy Expenditure With Diving

Diving, like other physical activity, is associated with increased energy needs. Energy expenditure during diving is dependent on the level of activity, the diving depth, and the water temperature. Energy requirements may increase by 30 percent in deep dives, that is, dives over 1,000 FSW (305 MSW).

Sport diving is typically associated with lower energy requirements than comparable activity on land. Energy expenditures for sport diving are estimated to be 5 to 6 2/3 kilocalories per minute for a 150-pound (68-kilogram) man. This means that the average diver may expend 150 to 200 kilocalories in addition to basal metabolic requirements for each 30 minutes of diving time. Since the loss of one pound (0.5 kilogram) of weight is equivalent to 3,600 kilocalories, the exercise from

Table 10.4	Estimated Energy Expenditures With Activities	
Activity		**(Kcal/hr)**
Resting (sitting or sleeping)		60-100
Restful, easy swimming		300-350
SCUBA diving		300-400
Breath-hold diving		500-700
Basketball		800
Fast running		1,000

Examples of expenditures are for an average-sized male.
Note: To lose one pound (0.5 kg) of weight requires a decrease in caloric intake or an increase in activity of 3,600 kcal.

typical diving activities is not expected to cause any noticeable weight loss.

However, when sport divers make three to four dives a day, spend surface intervals doing activities such as swimming and running, and dive into cold, deep waters, energy expenditures increase markedly. The increased energy expenditures from diving in cold water were discussed in chapter 7. Ordinarily, the diver meets the increased energy demands through utilization of fat and other metabolic stores (e.g., glucagons, a form of sugar, in the liver). A person with diabetes, however, may not be able to make the energy conversions due to the lack of insulin and may become hypoglycemic (low blood sugar). The consequences could be disastrous if experienced during a dive because symptoms of **hypoglycemia** include weakness, chilling, confusion, and loss of consciousness. In the water these symptoms could be life threatening. If hypoglycemia is not recognized as the cause of the symptoms, the diver may be inappropriately treated for other possible alterations of mental status in the water, such as DCS, DCI, and near drowning.

Nutrition Recommendations for the Diver

The diver, like everyone else, should have a well-balanced diet with appropriately increased caloric intake according to the planned diving activity. If strenuous diving activities are anticipated, the diver should start building up carbohydrate stores three to six days prior to beginning the dives by "loading up" on complex carbohydrates. In this situation, approximately one-half to two-thirds of the caloric intake should be from complex carbohydrates (pasta, fruits, vegetables, and whole grains along with proteins from low-fat sources). The day before diving, the diver should eat a little less and avoid high-fat foods because they are more difficult than other foods to digest and may contribute to motion sickness.

On the day of the dive, the diver should avoid unusual foods and should eat a small breakfast, rich in complex carbohydrates, at least two hours before the dive. This will provide energy for the dive while leaving the stomach relatively empty during the dive. With an empty stomach, **gastroesophageal reflux** (food moving retrograde from the stomach back into the esophagus) will be minimized. Postural changes (head-down or horizontal positions), air swallowing, and hydrostatic effects on air in the stomach can contribute to gastroesophageal reflux during a dive. It is appropriate to eat snacks rich in carbohydrates during short surface intervals to provide energy for subsequent dives. During longer rest periods between dives, people should eat meals as already described.

Diving tour operators in exotic locations make great efforts to "wine and dine" their clients. Not only is there a temptation to overindulge; there are strong incentives to get one's money's worth from the trip. To avoid nutrition problems, the diver should be mindful of current nutrition recommendations, including recommended daily caloric intake based on lean body weight and the food pyramid for suggested daily food intake as diagrammed in figure 10.4. Approximately 50 percent of caloric intake should be from carbohydrates, 30 percent from fats, and 20 percent from proteins.

Effects of Diving on the Gastrointestinal Tract

Increased hydrostatic pressures depress gastric secretions, increase motility of the gut, and interfere with digestive processes. That is why timing of food consumption is so important before a dive. The general rule is that the diver should avoid having a full stomach before the dive. A full stomach is a predisposition for two possible problems. In gastroesophageal reflux, as discussed earlier, the stomach contents regurgitate (reflux) into the esophagus. Ordinarily, partially digested food contents in the stomach are delivered by the stomach's muscles into the small intestine for further digestion. Since elevated hydrostatic pressure may impair motility function of the gut and the head-down position may result in retrograde movement of the stomach's contents, reflux may occur during submersion. If it does, stomach acid contents reflux into the esophagus, occasionally reaching the throat where

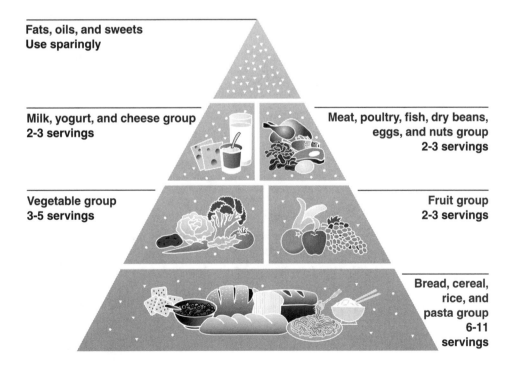

FIGURE 10.4 Food guide pyramid. Daily intakes: carbohydrates 50%, fats 30%, protein 20%.

the division of the trachea and esophagus occurs. The acid contents of the refluxed stomach fluid cause inflammation and damage to the esophagus. If the regurgitated food enters the lungs, it can cause a life-threatening inflammatory response in the lungs.

A second potential problem is barotrauma to the stomach and intestines from gas expansion during ascent. The stomach and large intestine ordinarily contain about one quart (one liter) or more of entrapped gas. Since the intestines are air-filled, flexible-walled cavities, the effects of changes in pressure are usually not noticeable (Boyle's Law—see chapter 1). If large amounts of air are swallowed during diving, it may be necessary during ascent to expel gas by belching or passing it through the rectum. An excess amount of gas in the stomach or intestine during ascent will distend the bowel. Possible consequences are painful cramping sensations, vomiting, and light-headedness (vasovagal effects of gastric distension—see chapter 11). Another consequence from expansion of gas in the gut during ascent is rupture.

Consequently, divers should avoid eating large amounts of gas-producing (legume and cruciferous) foods before diving. During descent and while the diver is on the bottom, the symptoms may be relieved by the compression effects of increased hydrostatic pressure on the air-filled, flexible-walled gut structures (see chapter 1). However, during ascent, re-expansion of the gas will lead to reappearance of the overdistension symptoms. The effect could be compounded by the continued production of gas from the food in the gut so that there would be an even larger volume of gas to expand during ascent. The expanded stomach contents could impinge on the lung volume, interfere with ventilation, and lead to panic. Air swallowing is another source of gas in the gut and may compound the gas formation from the other sources. Accordingly, activities that cause air swallowing, such as gum chewing, should be avoided during diving.

Nutrition in Exotic Areas

Diving is often associated with traveling to exotic places, eating strange foods, and encountering foods that may not have been prepared properly. For example, salads containing vegetables that were not properly washed or were washed with contaminated water may contain germs that cause diarrhea. In most dive areas, for the same reason, tap water should be eschewed and replaced by bottled drinking water. Some tropical seafood dishes may be hazardous to eat because of infection with viruses. For example, eating raw shellfish is a known cause of hepatitis A, a disease that causes liver damage. Some fish may be toxic for humans. For example, one can incur scromboid poisoning from eating tainted fish of the tuna family, ciguartera poisoning from fish that have eaten toxic algae, and puffer (Fugu) fish poisoning from improper preparation.

BRINGING IT ALL TOGETHER

A 50-year-old obese male, about 60 pounds (27 kilograms) overweight, decided to resume SCUBA diving. He was fitted with a wet suit to accommodate his size and arranged to do a recertification dive from a large inflatable boat. With 25 pounds (11 kilograms) of weights he was unable to descend. With 40 pounds (18 kilograms) of weight, he became neutrally buoyant and completed a brief dive without incident. However, he was unable to climb aboard the inflatable boat over the air-filled pontoons even after ditching all his gear. Finally, with three divers pulling him into the boat and two divers pushing him upward from the water, he was brought aboard the boat. What recommendations should be offered to the diver?

Answer: This scenario illustrates some of the problems an overweight SCUBA diver encounters. If the diver remains strongly motivated to dive, then weight reduction is essential. Another approach is to recommend that the person dive only in controlled situations in which a wet suit is not necessary, less weights are required, and a ladder (or ramp or shoreline) can be used to exit the water.

For Further Review

1. Why are different medical exams recommended for divers of different ages and types of diving?

2. What are the advantages of classifying contraindications to diving as absolute, relative, and temporary?

3. What are some of the medical considerations unique to female divers?

4. What are some guidelines for people who want to dive but who require medications?

5. What risks does the use of illegal drugs, alcohol, and cigarettes pose for the diver?

6. Why is nutrition usually not a concern for the sport diver?

7. How should a diver's food choices be modified before diving?

8. What nutrition challenges occur with diving in exotic locations?

PSYCHOLOGICAL AND PHYSIOLOGICAL PROBLEMS OF THE SURFACE

Four types of medical problems of diving (MPD) may arise while the diver is on or near the surface: panic, blackout, exposure, and marine animal injury. This chapter deals with the first of these two, which have psychological and physiological components. The other two are more closely associated with the environment of the diver. The MPD that occur on the surface, unlike almost all of the other

Chapter Preview

- Importance of panic in diving
- Psychological and physiological basis of panic
- Management of the diver with panic
- Significance of blackout in diving
- Physiological aspects of diver blackout
- Classification of the no-panic syndromes in divers

MPD, can also occur at other stages of the dive. In terms of sheer numbers, these problems plus ear squeezes, a descent problem, account for all but a very miniscule percentage of the MPD.

Panic in Divers

Panic arises when stresses, which usually evoke physiological responses and positive feedback, overwhelm the diver and cause negative feedback and pathological responses. On land, the manifestations of panic may primarily be psychological; that is, they affect the person's mental processes. In the water and during diving, the stresses affect the body's functions also. Often the cause of panic, as in most **anxiety** (an unpleasant emotional state with its psychological and physiological responses to an unidentifiable danger or fear) states, is not obvious to the victim, but may be easily recognized by an observer such as the diver's buddy.

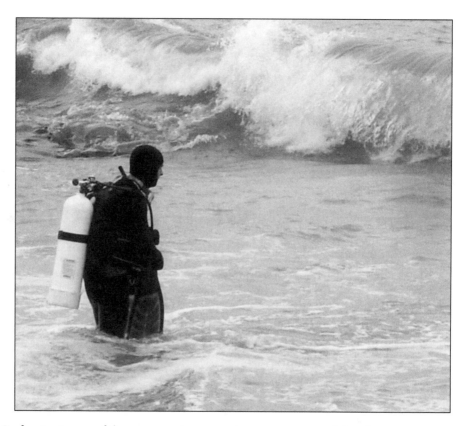

Surf entry is one of the most panic-generating components of the dive.

Significance

Panic is probably the leading cause of death in the sport SCUBA diver. This observation is based on the finding that over half the deaths in SCUBA divers reveal no equipment-related problems or attempts on the part of the diver to correct stresses such as negative buoyancy or entanglements. Undoubtedly, panic is the unidentified cause. Elements of panic without the diver's losing control or experiencing harmful consequences may accompany many diving activities. These events inevitably remain unreported. Sometimes they are recounted by the diver as an "interesting experience" or a "near miss" of a disaster. As figure 11.1 shows, panic is the most serious of the frequent problems divers have and the most frequent of the serious problems. This alone makes panic one of the most important MPD, if not the most important.

Causes

There is no specific cause of panic. Any situation that requires extra effort or is strange from the viewpoint of the diver can lead to panic. Some of the frequent causes of panic are listed in figure 11.2. Most stresses are resolved without conscious effort. Panic occurs when a new stress, be it physical or

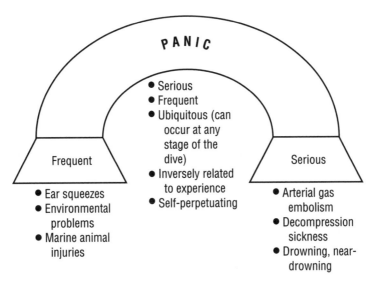

FIGURE 11.1   Panic bridges the gap between frequent and serious MPD.

Aspiration of water
Being pulled away from shore by a rip tide
Being thrown about, having equipment dislodged in the surf zone, or both
Disorientation: losing sight of dive boat due to swells or while diving inside a sunken ship
Entanglements: kelp, lines, equipment
Exhaustion: failure to make headway against a current
Losing sight of one's dive buddy
Negative buoyancy: inability to ascend
Regulator leak or failure, running out of air
Sighting a shark or other large marine animal
Vomiting while breathing with the regulator

FIGURE 11.2   Causes of panic.

psychological, is superimposed on the other stresses with which the diver is already coping. Failure to resolve the new stress adequately during the stage of resistance can result in panic. Panic is not confined to diving activities; it is an example of the **generalized alarm reaction,** biological stress–general adaptation syndrome with its three stages—alarm, resistance, and exhaustion. Manifestations may be seen when people experience severe asthmatic attacks or hyperventilation syndromes, when people with **claustrophobia** (morbid fear of confined or closed-in places) are placed in confining spaces, and when frightened children are confronted with an injection, as well as in many other situations.

Effects on the Body (Pathophysiology)

The unifying factor in all these situations is that once the panic–stress reaction is initiated, the alarm and resistance stages will continue to affect the person even if the inciting event is no longer present. Thus, a self-perpetuating mechanism, which may be referred to as a **vicious circle,** is established. In water-related causes of panic, the mechanisms are analogous, but there are differences as noted in figure 11.3. First, the three components of the stress response—alarm, resistance, and exhaustion—may occur so rapidly in the aquatic environment that the person may not be able to correct the problem during the stage of resistance. Second, in the water the probable consequence of the exhaustion stage is drowning, whereas on land it may merely be collapse and unwillingness to continue the stage of resistance.

Panic in the water leads to a series of predictable responses. Fatigue rapidly develops because of the increased energy demands associated with struggling during the resistance stage. Ventilation may become inefficient due to rapid, shallow breathing. Air may merely move in and out of the larger airways

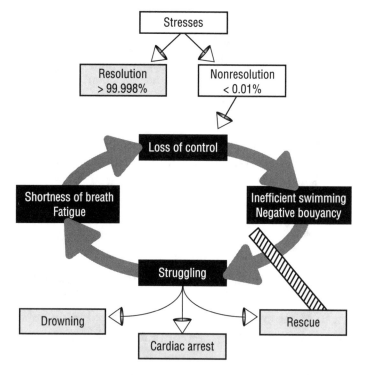

FIGURE 11.3 Panic syndrome.

DIVING SCENARIO

OXYGEN AND THE BRAIN

The brain must be continuously supplied with oxygen in order to maintain consciousness. It is possible to hold one's breath for a minute or two, but during the breathhold time, oxygen carried in the blood is continuously supplied to the brain with each heartbeat. A single missed heartbeat or a moment's interruption of the oxygen supply to the brain can lead to unconsciousness. In the choke hold, for example, consciousness is lost almost instantaneously with constriction of the carotid arteries and interruption of blood flow to the brain.

and not reach the alveoli where gas exchanges in the lungs occur. The consequences are low oxygen levels in the blood, elevated blood carbon dioxide levels, and shortness of breath (air hunger). All this contributes to the person's feeling of panic. With reduced amounts of air in the lungs, buoyancy is decreased. Swimming movements may become inefficient due to fatigue and loss of form. These factors rapidly cause exhaustion and further contribute to the panic. During exercising (struggling) at maximum capacity, exhaustion occurs in only a few seconds even in the well-conditioned individual. If the process continues, one of three things happens in the exhaustion stage:

- The person may become so exhausted that the regulator is released from the mouth; or, if the person is on the surface, the head will not emerge from the water enough to take a breath of air. Aspiration of one mouthful of water at this time may lead to unconsciousness.

- The extreme energy output during the resistance stage of the stress reaction may lead to cardiac arrest, especially in someone who is poorly conditioned or has heart disease.

- The vicious circle of the panic syndrome is interrupted with the person's recovery.

Findings of the panic syndrome include sympathetic nervous system activation (the alarm stage) and the fight or flight response (the resistance stage). Observations in the panic-stricken diver include rapid, shallow breathing; dilated pupils; a terror-stricken facial appearance; paleness of the face; and inefficient swimming movements. The person may struggle to climb out of the water as a drowning man grasps at a straw. At this point, control is lost, actions are irrational, and the person would not be expected to initiate simple corrective procedures such as inflating a buoyancy compensator, releasing a weight belt, or cutting free of entanglements.

First-Response Interventions

Since time is so crucial in managing the panic syndrome and preventing complications such as drowning and cardiac arrest, the first responses are of paramount importance. The vicious circle of the panic syndrome must be interrupted at the earliest possible moment. Merely thinking that something is wrong during the dive, the pre-alarm stage, is sufficient reason to curtail activities, rest, and reevaluate the situation. The following interventions can interrupt the vicious circle of the panic syndrome:

• Correct or eliminate the cause: This may be as simple as pulling the person through the surf zone. Examples of other simple measures include freeing a tank valve from entanglement in kelp, re-placing a face mask, switching from breathing with a snorkel to breathing with a regulator, or drifting with a current rather than swimming against it.

• Improve the breathing pattern: The person should breathe deeply and slowly, inhaling to the fullest extent possible (one should absolutely *not* breath-hold if ascending).

• Improve buoyancy: Ways to improve buoyancy are to inflate the buoyancy compensator, release the game collection bag, drop the weight belt.

• Rest: If on the surface and the water is calm, the person should back float with the head out of the water and breathe the surface air directly.

• Reevaluate the situation: Determine why panic occurred and how it can be prevented; form a plan for safely returning to shore or the dive boat.

• Reassure: Instill confidence in the person that everything is OK and there will be no new problems.

Definitive Management

There is no definitive management for the panic syndrome. If the diver is fortunate enough to interrupt the vicious circle, there usually are no residual effects. However, complications can arise from problems secondary to the panic syndrome, such as aspiration (inhalation) of water, near-drowning, heart muscle injury, muscle–ligamentous strains (from struggling), and lung injury–air embolism as a result of breath-holding during ascent. Except for the latter condition, the definitive management for these complications is no different than for their non-diving counterparts.

Definitive management should also consist of discussion with the diver about the events leading to the panic syndrome, how it was interrupted, and how it can be prevented in future dives. If underlying psychiatric issues exist such as phobias, the diver might be advised to stop diving. Physical conditioning should also be addressed; if it is less than optimal, the recommendation for an exercise program should be given. In summary, if no complications

BRINGING IT ALL TOGETHER

An 18-year-old male diver was doing his first "deep" SCUBA dive. He adjusted his buoyancy on the surface to the point of being neutrally buoyant. He wore a three-eighths-inch (one-centimeter) wet suit. Descent to the 100-FSW (30-MSW) bottom was easily accomplished. On the bottom he felt "heavy," but did not add air to his buoyancy compensator. After a few moments on the bottom, he tried to ascend in the vertical position, but because of his negative buoyancy his fins stirred up a cloud of silt that quickly enveloped him. He inflated his buoyancy compensator with no apparent lifting effect. He struggled even harder (inefficient swimming movements; attempts to climb out of the water as though it were a ladder) to ascend, but only made the situation worse.

Fortunately the diver's partner appreciated the gravity of the situation and released the panic-stricken diver's weight belt. With the improved buoyancy, the diver began to ascend. Although initially out of breath from struggling and overbreathing his regulator, he reached the surface uneventfully.

Comment: This scenario illustrates how fast a panic syndrome can evolve as well as how easy it is to interrupt the syndrome with the proper corrective actions. The main admonition to offer the diver is that of instituting neutral buoyancy for each stage of the dive.

---

occur, definitive management for the panic syndrome should be directed toward providing the diver with an understanding of the panic syndrome and how it can be avoided in future water-related activities.

Prevention

Key to the problem of panic in divers is prevention. The more experienced the diver, the less likely the occurrence of panic. SCUBA diving training agencies realize the importance of panic control and include discussions and training in panic prevention in their certification courses. In-water panic prevention training includes drills to manage a loss of air supply, training in clearing a flooded mask, and harassment (pushing, shoving, tugging on equipment, pulling off equipment, breath-hold underwater swims, conditioning, etc.) drills. The diving industry as a group has done much for panic prevention in divers. Almost all approved diving operations require panic prevention equipment including an octopus (spare) breathing source, a buoyancy compensator integrated with the diver's air supply, a tank pressure gauge, a whistle, and a sausage tube.

Return to Diving

If the panic syndrome is interrupted and no residual injury such as water aspiration or heart injury has occurred, the diver may return to diving as soon as rested. However, the admonitions discussed earlier should be reviewed, and any indicated corrective actions should be taken before resumption of diving.

Blackout and Other No-Panic Syndromes

The **no-panic syndromes** are a diverse collection of MPD. Whereas panic is the most significant problem of the SCUBA diver, blackout is the most significant problem of the breath-hold diver. In about half the cases of drowning, the causes are not clearly identified. The no-panic syndromes are likely the causes of these unrecognized causes of drowning. For the breath-hold diver in particular, the no-panic syndromes are probably the leading cause of death. These syndromes are characterized by the rapid loss of consciousness **(blackout)** in the water without warning, panic, or a struggle for air. This contrasts sharply to presentations of the panic syndromes as discussed previously. The no-panic syndromes are associated primarily with two different diving techniques. They occur in

- breath-hold divers who alter their normal physiological warning signs by hyperventilation, deep diving, or a combination of the two; and
- experienced divers using rebreather diving equipment that alters the concentrations of the **respiratory gases** (oxygen and carbon dioxide).

More than a dozen different conditions can lead to blackout during diving.

Significance

Any condition involving loss of consciousness is serious. Often the consequences ensuing from loss of consciousness are more serious or cause more serious injuries than the loss of consciousness itself. To appreciate the significance of this statement, one only needs to think of the loss of consciousness that leads to an automobile accident or a fall and resultant head injury. In the water, loss of consciousness has very serious consequences. Without immediate rescue and resuscitation, drowning occurs. Without an obvious cause of death, which is characteristic of the no-panic syndromes, the person's demise is usually attributed to drowning. This leads to imprecision in the reporting of statistics for the no-panic syndromes. Specific causes of a no-panic syndrome should be sought for all situations in which consciousness is lost in the water.

Causes

At least 15 different causes of the no-panic syndrome are identifiable. Several of the causes of blackout are discussed more completely in other chapters (see chapters 14 and 15). The causes of the no-panic syndromes can be classified into four categories:

- Hypoxic
- Cardiovascular
- Narcotic
- Miscellaneous causes

Hypoxic Causes of Blackout   When oxygen levels in the brain fall below critical levels, consciousness is lost. The exact levels vary. Factors that cause the variations include the acidity of the blood, the volume of blood flow, the temperature of the blood, and the presence or absence of other factors that can alter the level of consciousness, such as drugs or nitrogen **narcosis** (a condition of deep stupor or unconsciousness produced by a drug, chemical, or gas). The following six conditions represent blackout caused by brain hypoxia.

- Breath-holding blackout. This is the prototype of the no-panic syndromes. It has been termed shallow-water blackout and hyperventilation blackout, but the preferred term is breath-holding blackout. A typical scenario starts with intentional hyperventilation to prolong a diver's breath-hold time. **Hyperventilation** delays the desire to breathe by blowing off carbon dioxide; oxygen stores are not increased. Usually the diver is preoccupied with a goal—an underwater swim for distance, a depth excursion, or an increased breath-hold time. Consciousness is lost before the diver has an irrepressible desire to breathe. Once consciousness is lost, spontaneous breathing movements resume and the diver will drown if prompt interventions are not instituted.

- Distraction blackout. This is a variation of breath-holding blackout. In this situation the diver is near the breath-hold break point but delays surfacing because of distraction resulting from desire to complete an underwater goal, for example, rousting a lobster out of a crevice. The loss of consciousness occurs while the diver is distracted by the goal or during ascent.

- Diffusional blackout. Diffusional blackout is associated with deep breath-hold dives. As the diver descends, the lung volumes decrease in accordance with Boyle's Law. The partial pressures of the gases in the lungs increase correspondingly. For example, a breath-hold dive to 66 FSW (20 MSW or 3 ATA) reduces the lung volume to one-third of its original volume while at the surface. Concomitantly, the partial pressures of the gases in the lungs increase threefold, boosting oxygen diffusion from the lungs to the blood stream by this factor. At pressure, this increases the breath-hold time; however, during ascent, the reverse occurs. When the lung oxygen tensions fall below the blood oxygen tensions, there is reverse diffusion of oxygen from the blood to the lungs. With the fall in blood oxygen levels, consciousness is lost during the ascent.

• Dilutional blackout. This type of blackout occurs because of mechanical failures or technical errors in setting up rebreather diving systems that use carbon dioxide scrubbers (canisters with materials to absorb carbon dioxide). If oxygen is added to the rebreather circuit at rates that are too low, the diver will lose consciousness from hypoxia without any "air hunger" (conscious desire to breathe) since carbon dioxide continues to be absorbed. With use of rebreather equipment that supplies oxygen at a constant rate to the rebreather circuit, the accidental use of air rather than pure oxygen in the SCUBA tank will result in the addition of inadequate amounts of oxygen to the circuit. For example, if oxygen addition to the rebreather circuit is set at one liter (about one quart) a minute and the tank is filled with air (21 percent oxygen) rather than pure oxygen, only about one-fifth the required oxygen will be added to the circuit. The result will be loss of consciousness from low oxygen levels but no perception of air hunger or impending loss of consciousness, since carbon dioxide continues to be absorbed. This problem is avoided in rebreather equipment by oxygen sensors that warn the diver if the desired partial pressure of oxygen is not being maintained.

• Valsalvic blackout. Valsalvic (forceful exhalation against blockage of the airway) blackout is associated with the use of SCUBA gear. In this type of blackout, the diver "skip breathes" in order to conserve the air supply in the tank and extend the time underwater. **Skip breathing** is a technique in which the diver delays breathing until he or she nearly reaches the break point to breathe and then exhales explosively into the regulator mouthpiece before the next inhalation. The exhalation against the resistance of the regulator is a type of **Valsalva maneuver.** This results in increased pressure within the lung cavity and decreased filling of the heart. With decreased filling, there is less outflow for delivering oxygen to the brain. If the blood oxygen level is near the point where consciousness will be lost, this decrease in oxygen delivery from the Valsalva-like effect may be sufficient to cause loss of consciousness.

• Tank blackout. If a tank is stored with air in it and water enters, the inside of the tank rusts. Oxygen in the tank combines in a chemical fashion **(oxidation)** with the metal of the tank. This reduces the amount of oxygen in the SCUBA tank. When the tank is used, the diver breathes a hypoxic (low oxygen percentage) mixture. Carbon dioxide levels remain normal in the diver since this gas is exhaled by the open-circuit regulator. If the inspired gas oxygen partial pressure from the tank is too low, consciousness will be lost as a result of hypoxemia (low oxygen tensions) in the blood.

Cardiovascular (Heart and Blood Vessel) Causes of Blackout   A moment's interruption of blood flow to the brain can lead to blackout. The interruption may be caused by cessation of heart activity or blockage of blood flow to the brain. The following are two types of cardiovascular blackout.

• Cardiogenic blackout. This occurs as a result of heart problems such as irregular rhythms and heart attacks. Stress factors (see chapter 1) associated with diving such as panic, hyperventilation, breath-holding, cold water immersion, shunting, disorientation, and nerve reflexes that slow the heart may lead to heartbeat irregularities, especially in divers with underlying heart conditions. Heart attacks are most likely to occur during the most stressful portions of the dive, the donning of equipment, water entry, and surf passage. With cessation of the pumping action of the heart, blood flow to the brain is interrupted and blackout occurs immediately.

• Carotogenic blackout. The familiar name for this condition is **carotid sinus syndrome.** The **carotid sinus** is a sensory organ in the carotid artery (the major artery supplying blood to the brain) that reacts to pressure. Reflexes from its stimulation cause decreases in blood pressure and heart rate. This decreases the amount of blood ejected from the heart with each beat. If external pressure is applied to the carotid artery, reflexes may be initiated for slowing the heart. Carotid sinus massage is sometimes used by physicians in emergency situations to slow the heart rate when it is too rapid. The carotid sinus syndrome is a condition of increased sensitivity of the carotid sinus resulting in dizziness or syncope from diminished brain blood flow to the brain. It occurs in divers as a consequence of wearing neoprene hoods that cause constriction around the neck. In contrast to the other no-panic syndromes in which consciousness is usually lost abruptly, the carotid sinus syndrome is usually associated with precursor symptoms such as nausea, dizziness, headache, and light-headedness before consciousness is lost. If a diver is unaware of the cause of the symptoms, he or she may progress to loss of consciousness. The problem in such situations is thought to be due to tightness of the hood and the resultant stimulation of the carotid sinus. These symptoms can be observed also with restricting venous return from the brain. This is another problem that could arise if the neck portion of the hood fits too tightly.

Narcotic (Sleep Producing) Causes of Blackout   The side effects of many medications include decreased alertness that may progress to loss of consciousness. Poison gases and nitrogen narcosis may have similar affects. There are four causes of narcotic blackout.

• Carbon monoxide poisoning. Elevated concentrations of carbon monoxide in the breathing gas mixture are another cause of blackout in divers (see chapter 14). Fortunately, this problem is rare. Whenever a diver is found unconscious after breathing a compressed gas, the gas in the SCUBA tank or the surface-supplied air source should be analyzed for dangerous levels of carbon monoxide. Carbon monoxide is 250 times more capable of combining with hemoglobin (protein of the red blood cell that carries 97.5 percent of the oxygen in the blood) than oxygen is. Consequently, low concentrations of carbon monoxide cause serious symptoms. Since there is little interference with carbon dioxide elimination, the symptoms of carbon monoxide poisoning are insidious, as in most of the other causes of blackout.

• Nitrogen narcosis blackout. Nitrogen acts as a narcotic when it is breathed under pressure (see chapter 14). The greater the pressure, the greater the narcotic effect. Euphoria is one of the earliest symptoms. Initially, the diver may have a false sense of confidence and do foolhardy things like descending deeper or deciding that breathing through a regulator is unnecessary. In such instances, the diver may panic and swim to the surface while breath-holding. Upon surfacing, problems would likely be due to the rapid ascent and breath-holding rather than nitrogen narcosis, since ascent immediately corrects nitrogen narcosis. Individual responses to nitrogen narcosis are variable. The symptoms represent a continuum of responses with the endpoint being loss of consciousness if the descent is deep enough.

• Drug-induced blackout. Most drug effects on diving have not been explored. Many drugs have sedative effects, and the influence of pressure and nitrogen narcosis may compound these effects. Other drugs may have reversal effects under increased pressure—for instance, a stimulant may become a depressant. The diver should be wary of using drugs, especially "downers," while diving. In all diving accidents, the diver's medication use should be reviewed, since it could be a contributing cause to the problem.

• Hypothermic blackout. Exposure to cold water rapidly lowers the body's core temperature, especially in the absence of thermal protection (see chapter 12). The discomfort of the cold water is soon replaced by interference with manual dexterity. The progression to stupor and loss of consciousness occurs when core temperatures reach 92 degrees F (33 degrees C). At 88 degrees F (31 degrees C), breathing ceases as a result of inactivation of the breathing centers in the brain.

Miscellaneous Causes of Blackout   Several other conditions can cause blackout during diving. Although uncommon, the following three are listed for the sake of completeness.

• Vasovagal blackout. There are many situations in which the diver could become frightened while in the water (see figure 11.2). Analogously to what happens in situations on land that lead to fainting, reflex stimulation of the vagus nerve could initiate blackout. Although this has not been documented in diving, blackout resulting from similar stimuli could occur in the water. Since there are so many possible causes for blackout in divers, this cause may be overlooked without careful reconstruction of the events leading to the blackout.

• Blackout secondary to head injury. Head injury underwater can occur as a result of falling equipment or rapid ascent under a boat or fixed object. If severe enough, it can cause loss of consciousness (concussion). This cause of blackout qualifies as a no-panic syndrome.

• Other medical problems of diving leading to sudden loss of consciousness. Arterial gas embolism (see chapter 15) and seizures from oxygen toxicity (see chapter 14) can cause rapid losses of consciousness in divers. In these situations, they may qualify as a no-panic syndrome. However, both usually have symptoms that precede the loss of consciousness.

Effects on the Body (Pathophysiology)

The common factor in almost all the no-panic syndromes is loss of consciousness resulting from low oxygen supplies to the brain. The desire to breathe is based on changes in the blood levels of oxygen and carbon dioxide. By far the more potent stimulus is the elevation of carbon dioxide. When carbon dioxide levels increase in the bloodstream as a consequence of metabolism, there is a desire to breathe. Ordinarily this stimulus is not perceptible, and breathing is automatic. The breathing reflex can be overcome by conscious control with breath-holding. However, elevated carbon dioxide levels eventually lead to an irrepressible desire to breathe. This point at which one must breathe is named the **breath-hold break point.**

The stimulus to breathe resulting from low oxygen levels is not as strong as that for elevated carbon dioxide levels. If blood carbon dioxide levels remain normal, the desire to breathe as a result of low oxygen levels in the blood usually is not recognized. This is a potential danger anytime oxygen levels fall below levels at which consciousness is lost while carbon dioxide levels remain normal. This situation is observed in about half of the causes of the no-panic syndromes (dilutional, tank, cardiogenic, carotogenic, carbon monoxide, narcosis, drugs, hypothermic, and vasovagal causes of blackout) previously described.

The most common cause of blackout in breath-hold divers is associated with hyperventilation (voluntarily increasing the depth and rate of breathing). Hyperventilation significantly lowers blood carbon dioxide levels while having almost no measurable effect on increasing oxygen stores (see figure 11.4). As the diver breath-holds, oxygen from the blood is used for metabolic purposes, including maintenance of consciousness. Concomitantly, carbon dioxide

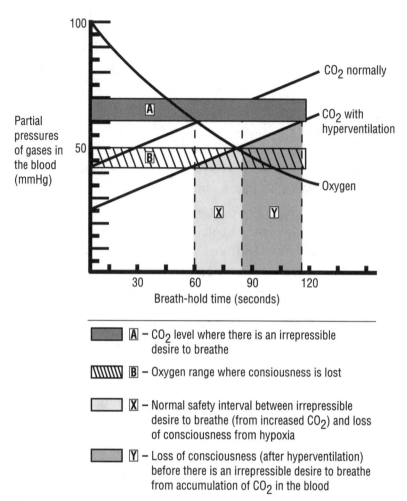

FIGURE
11.4 Blackout associated with breath-holding after hyperventilation.

is produced. With the lower starting point of carbon dioxide secondary to hyperventilation, the signal to breathe is delayed. In the meantime, the blood oxygen levels decrease as oxygen is utilized for metabolism. At a certain point in the breath-hold time, the blood oxygen becomes so low that consciousness is lost. The exact level varies with conditioning and activity. The loss of consciousness occurs before the blood carbon dioxide has reached a level high enough to create an irrepressible desire to breathe. Blackout without warning signs can follow from any of the conditions previously described that lower oxygen supplies to the brain while carbon dioxide levels stay below the level required to initiate breathing.

First-Response Interventions

Since the consequence of loss of consciousness in the water is drowning, the first consideration is rescue. If the person is not breathing, basic life-support measures must be started immediately (see chapter 16). The person should be brought to the shore or the diving boat; resuscitation should not be attempted in the water, where the measures will be less than optimal. However, during the transit to shore it is essential to keep the person's mouth and nose out of the water, since many people who lose consciousness in the water resume breathing spontaneously. As in other situations involving a period of oxygen deprivation to the brain, resuscitation with oxygen should be performed if possible.

Definitive Management

Definitive management for residuals of the no-panic syndromes starts with transportation of the person to a medical center and institution of advanced life-support measures if needed. The cause for the loss of consciousness should be sought to ensure that the most effective treatments are instituted. After assessment at the medical center, specific therapies may be required for treating problems secondary to loss of consciousness, such as antibiotics for infection in the lungs from water aspiration, rewarming for hypothermia, hyperbaric oxygen for carbon monoxide poisoning, and surgery for head injury. Remarkable recoveries are reported after near-drownings. The absence of struggling associated with the no-panic syndromes, plus immersion in water, may initiate the diving reflex (see chapter 4) and maintain oxygen delivery to the brain. Finally, hyperbaric oxygen recompression therapy must not be overlooked for treating decompression illness if the person used compressed gas during the dive and decompression was omitted.

Prevention

Like so many of the other MPD, the no-panic syndromes are largely preventable. Divers need to be made aware of the no-panic syndromes, their causes, and methods of prevention. Breath-hold dives should be timed so that ascent is completed before the breath-hold break point or blackout occurs. Fitness should be maintained to meet the challenges that diving imposes. Diving should not be done under the influence of drugs or alcohol. A dive plan, dive brief, and equipment inspection should precede each dive, especially when closed-circuit SCUBA gear is used. With closed-circuit SCUBA, all safeguards must be followed for setting up and dismantling the equipment. Breath-hold divers should not mix breath-holding with underwater air supplies on the same dive. That is, the breath-hold diver should not breathe from a SCUBA diver's octopus regulator while underwater. In this situation the breath-hold diver may forget to exhale during ascent and rupture the lungs as he or she approaches the surface. Finally, the buddy system must be used throughout the dive. In most instances the diving buddy is the only person who can prevent the disastrous consequences of loss of consciousness in the water.

BRINGING IT ALL TOGETHER

SCENARIO 1: BREATH-HOLDING BLACKOUT

A 16-year-old male competitive swimmer decided to attempt to break his old underwater swim distance record. He heard that hyperventilation would help extend the breath-hold time. Consequently, before starting the swim, he hyperventilated to the point that his fingers and toes were numb. After surpassing his old record, he lost consciousness a few moments later while still swimming. A buddy who was supervising the swim immediately rescued him. The swimmer immediately regained consciousness but continued to cough and retch for a few minutes.

Comment: In this case, numbness, a side effect of hyperventilation, indicated that the swimmer had profoundly lowered his blood carbon dioxide level. Blackout occurred as a consequence of low blood oxygen levels in the brain compounded by the oxygen demands of the underwater swim. Obviously, the breath-hold break point from carbon dioxide had not been reached before consciousness was lost. The coughing and retching were secondary to aspiration (breathing in) of water into the lungs. The reflex for breathing was initiated after consciousness was lost while the swimmer was underwater. Although hyperventilation was inadvisable, the buddy's supervision of the swim and immediate rescue accounted for the absence of serious consequences.

SCENARIO 2: PRESUMPTIVE VALSALVA-ASSOCIATED BLACKOUT

A certified SCUBA diver in his early 30s was diving with two buddies. He had practiced skip breathing on previous dives and told his buddies he wanted to "save" his air supply. The diver became separated from the others and was found dead on the bottom approximately two hours later. There was no evidence of struggling or initiation of self-rescue measures. The diver was still clenching a pry bar and a shell-collecting bag. His weight belt was in place. He had not inflated his buoyancy compensator. An autopsy revealed no apparent cause of death. His heart was OK. The air supply in the tank was free of impurities. The diver's cause of death was listed as drowning while SCUBA diving.

Comment: Examination of the diver's regulator revealed a high resistance to exhalation. This finding coupled with the diver's comment about skip breathing suggests that Valsalvic blackout was the cause of the diver's loss of consciousness and subsequent drowning. Cardiogenic blackout secondary to an arrthymia could be another cause of blackout under these circumstances.

SCENARIO 3: CARDIOGENIC BLACKOUT

A neophyte SCUBA diver in his 50s, poorly conditioned, was trying to make his way through the surf zone in a training dive when he suddenly lost consciousness. Although the diver was quickly rescued and life-support measures were immediately instituted on the beach, he subsequently died. Drowning was listed as the cause of death, although an autopsy revealed advanced disease of the arteries (arteriosclerosis) of his heart.

Comment: The diver's loss of consciousness was likely the result of cardiogenic blackout. The stresses of donning the diving equipment, struggling to pass through the surf zone, and experiencing the relatively cold water probably exceeded the person's reserve exercise capacity and precipitated an abnormal heart rhythm, constriction of a heart artery, or both.

SCENARIO 4: CAROTOGENIC BLACKOUT

A fairly inexperienced 25-year-old man wore a borrowed neoprene wet suit and a tight-fitting hood while SCUBA diving in 25 to 30 FSW (7.6-9.1 MSW) from a shore dive. A few minutes into the dive, he surfaced, complaining that he was uncomfortable, had a headache, and felt light-headed. He decided to terminate the dive and swam on the surface to the beach with his buddy. His symptoms worsened, and he was hardly able to stagger up the beach. The symptoms rapidly ceased after removal of the neoprene hood.

Comment: The diver exhibited a course consistent with a carotid sinus syndrome from a hood that fit too tightly. Fortunately, he realized something was wrong and terminated the dive before losing consciousness.

The no-panic syndromes can interact to make the diver more susceptible to underwater blackout than would otherwise be expected. For example, if a breath-hold diver hyperventilates to extend the diving time and then becomes distracted by some object in the water, loss of consciousness may occur before there is any desire to breathe. Pre-descent hyperventilation plus deep diving may extend the bottom time and lead to diffusional blackout during the ascent. Alcohol and other "downer" drugs lower the tolerance to nitrogen narcosis and make divers more susceptible to the effects of hypothermia. Tank, carotogenic, and cardiogenic blackouts are prone to occur in divers who dive infrequently, are poorly conditioned, or do not maintain and inspect their equipment properly.

Return to Diving

After full recovery from a no-panic syndrome, the diver can usually return to diving activities after a few days' rest. If residuals exist, such as brain injury from oxygen deprivation or lung injury from aspiration, return to diving is not recommended.

For Further Review

1. What similarities exist between the panic and the no-panic syndromes?

2. What differences exist between the panic and the no-panic syndromes?

3. What are the first-response measures for managing the panic syndrome? How do these differ from the first-line responses for managing the no-panic syndromes?

4. How does hyperventilation alter the physiology associated with breathing?

5. What measures should be taken to prevent blackout during diving?

6. Why are deaths secondary to blackout in the water usually listed as drownings?

7. What factors should one consider before allowing a victim of a panic or a no-panic syndrome to return to diving?

8. What panic prevention equipment is available to the diver?

OTHER SURFACE PROBLEMS: EXPOSURE AND MARINE ANIMAL INJURY

Chapter Preview

- Diving-related exposure problems (hypothermia, hyperthermia, sunburn, and external ear canal infections)
- Methods to maintain core temperature
- Significance of sunburn
- Management and prevention of swimmer's ear
- Significance of injuries from marine animals
- Simplified approach to classification and management of injuries from marine animals

From the problems discussed in the previous chapter, we turn to two problems of the surface that are closely related to the diving environment itself. These arise from exposure to the aquatic environment and from injuries caused by marine animals. Like the surface problems discussed in chapter 11, these problems can also occur at other phases of the dive and are not limited to diving activities only. Among the medical problems of diving (MPD), these surface problems are distinctive in two ways. First, they occur more frequently than any of the other diving problems. Second, usually they are so mild or short-lived that they do not materially hamper diving activities. For example, a diver who is cold may terminate the dive early, only to rewarm and resume diving later the same day. The surfer who falls into a bed of sea urchins may pull out as many spines as are easy to remove, leave the remaining ones embedded in soft tissues, and continue the surfing activities. By and large, problems plague not only SCUBA divers but also snorkelers, sun bathers, surface swimmers, surfers, and victims of accidental immersion. Only in the most severe presentations is emergency medical attention needed for these problems.

Exposure Problems

Problems arising from exposure to the underwater environment may seem minor in significance, but in all likelihood they account for more interruptions of diving activities than other types of problems. Exposure problems include hypothermia (decreased body temperature), **hyperthermia** (increased body temperature), sunburn, and infections of the external ear canals (i.e., swimmer's ear). They are ever-present hazards in diving, as well as in many other water-related activities but can effectively be prevented. When they occur—and they do occur frequently as compared to other MPD—their management usually requires simple, commonsense interventions.

Hypothermia

Hypothermia ("hypo" = below; "thermia" = temperature) is a lowering of body temperature. Unless water temperatures are near the core temperature, immersion initiates feedback mechanisms. Initially, these are positive if the water temperature is moderately warm (78-85 degrees F/25-29 degrees C) as the swimmer or diver "adjusts" to the water temperature. This usually occurs through a combination of metabolic heat production (increased activity such as swimming), warming the trapped water in the wet suit if one is being worn, and stabilizing of the skin temperature-sensing structures to the water temperature. **Chilling** denotes the perception of discomfort as the body's heat-conserving mechanisms no longer meet the demands of the cold. When positive feedback mechanisms, primarily metabolic heat production, are exceeded, negative feedback mechanisms lead to progressive lowering of the core temperature. Responses occur in a continuum to the endpoint at which the stimulus to breathe is lost. At this point, metabolic heat production ceases; the core temperature approaches that of the surrounding water.

Significance   Cold water presents a much greater challenge to the body's heat-conserving mechanisms than cold air (see chapters 1 and 7). The additive effects of the specific heat of water and its thermal conductivity make it many times more challenging than air of equal temperature to the body's heat-conserving mechanisms. In fact, the number of hours an individual would survive in air is approximately equal to the number of minutes the same individual would survive in water of the same temperature. Heat can be lost from the immersed diver so rapidly that the limiting factor becomes the rate at which the warm core blood can be transferred to the cold skin and extremity areas.

All divers have probably experienced chilling during diving activities. However, only in the most unusual circumstances is the sport diver unable to terminate the dive before significant hypothermia occurs. In contrast, victims of accidental immersion in cold water, such as in the wreck of the *Titanic*, rapidly cool and die from hypothermia.

Causes   Almost all diving and other water-related activities are conducted in water temperatures less than the core temperature. With minimal activity, the diver is usually comfortable in water warmer than 82 degrees F (28 degrees C). Diving in water with temperatures below this level usually requires thermal protection suits. Diving at deep depths also contributes to hypothermia because of the loss of effectiveness of the wet suit from compression of its air cells, layering of cold water (thermoclines), and insensible heat loss from ventilation at increased pressures.

Effects on the Body (Pathophysiology)   Compared to diving mammals, the unprotected human has only limited abilities to tolerate cold water (see chapter 7). Stocky body build, female sex, and subcutaneous fat tissue provide some natural protection against hypothermia. The first response to immersion in cold water is reduction of blood flow to the periphery in order to preserve the core temperature. The effect is obliterated by shivering and movement. Shivering arises from the rhythmic contraction of muscles in response to cold and is designed to increase heat production. At first inspection, shivering would appear to be helpful for generating body heat to prevent hypothermia, as it increases metabolic heat production five- to sevenfold. However, since it involves the muscles just below the skin surface, shivering actually increases the heat loss during immersion in cold water. The warm core blood is carried to the skin's surface (in order to nourish the shivering muscles) and is rapidly cooled by the cold water in contact with the skin.

In a similar fashion, a diver cools more rapidly when moving the arms and legs since the heat lost through obliteration of the shunting reflex, bringing warm blood to the extremity and exchanging heat with the surrounding water, far exceeds that generated by the increased metabolic activity from exercise. Even with heat generated in association with metabolism from vigorous exercise, the heat production cannot keep up with that lost to the surrounding water. If the heat-conserving mechanisms are maximized, the core temperature may remain near normal while the extremities become painfully cold, numb, and stiff.

Besides the loss of body heat via the specific heat and conduction properties of water, the diver loses considerable body heat via the lungs. This process is termed insensible heat loss. Each breath of air must be warmed to body temperature between the time it enters the mouth and the time it reaches the lungs. Each time the pressure doubles (i.e., with descent), twice as much heat energy is required to warm the same volume of air (Dalton's and Boyle's

Table 12.1	Effects of Progressive Decline in Core Body Temperature	
Temperature in degrees F (degrees C)	**Symptoms**	**Notes**
98.6 (37)	Normal body temperature	
97.0 (36.1)	Temperature noted after 6-hr exposure in near-freezing water in a custom-fitted wet suit in seated divers	Although the core was "warm," the hands and feet were painfully cold
95.0 (35)	Lower limit of "safe" decline noted in conditioned divers	Noted in Japanese diving women without wet suits
94.0 (34.4)	Loss of memory; incoordination	
90.0 (32.2)	Irregular heart rhythms	May lead to death from cardiac arrest
86.0 (30)	Unconsciousness; loss of muscle strength	
Less than 86.0	Death	Depression of heart and breathing activity

Laws). Up to 25 percent of the total metabolic heat produced by the body may be lost via this route.

Progressive lowering of core temperature with colder water or longer duration produces a continuum of symptoms as described in table 12.1. Immersion in near-freezing water often causes involuntary gasps for air. If the person's face is submerged, he or she will inhale water and drowning can occur immediately. This phenomenon explains the nearly instantaneous deaths observed in airplane pilots downed in near-freezing waters during World War II. A one-hour exposure (without benefit of a wet suit) to 40 degree F (4 degree C) water is fatal in 50 percent of cases.

First-Response Interventions and Definitive Management   Struggling and violent movements should be avoided during exposure to cold water. The best chance for survival in cold water exists when one remains as motionless as possible. The person should assume the knee–chest position to conserve heat by making the shape of the body more nearly that of a sphere. The tightly flexed position will also reduce blood flow to the extremities. If several people are present, they should huddle together in the knee–chest position to try to create a small "oasis" of warmer water around themselves through heat conduction and reduction of convective heat losses.

Once the person is removed from the cold water, the wet suit or wet clothing should be removed. Otherwise, further cooling occurs due to evaporative heat losses. Next, the hypothermic diver needs to be rewarmed in one of the following ways:

• External rewarming. If hypothermia is not too severe, rewarming using warm clothes and heated blankets is effective. Even more effective is rewarming by total body immersion in water at 104 degrees F (40 degrees C). Surprisingly, after a person is first placed in the rewarming bath, the core temperature may decline precipitously. This occurs because of the resumption of circulation to the skin and extremities associated with termination of the heat exchange and shunting mechanisms. Consequently, the cold blood in the extremities is returned to the core, and as a result, the body temperature declines. The phenomenon is termed temperature afterdrop. If the person is profoundly hypothermic, to the point that he or she is confused, semiconscious, or unconscious, tourniquets should be placed on the extremities to prevent further core temperature declines from temperature afterdrop associated with rewarming. After the core temperature begins to increase, the tourniquets can be released in a serial fashion to allow the cold blood in the extremities to be returned to the core one limb at a time.

• Core or internal rewarming. Administration of warm fluids into the veins or via a tube into the stomach, or the breathing of warm, humidified air is a very effective rewarming technique. These methods of rewarming require special equipment, as well as setup and monitoring by trained medical personnel. If the diver is conscious, he or she may drink warm fluids such as juices and water. Alcoholic beverages should be avoided. These interfere with heat-conserving mechanisms by increasing blood flow to the periphery and increasing urine production. For these reasons brandy ingestion, a historical treatment for immersion in cold water, is not advised.

Prevention   Prevention is the key to dealing with these problems. Every pre-dive briefing should include information about water temperature and instructions to terminate the dive if chilling occurs. Diver thermal protection exposure suits offer significant protection against hypothermia (see chapter 7). However, the proper thermal protection suit must be selected for the diving conditions. The diver should realize that multiple dives in one day lead to chilling during the later dives. Methods to prevent this, such as using increased thermal protection as the day progresses, reducing the number of dives, or shortening the bottom times, should be utilized.

Return to Diving   Return to diving after minor hypothermia is usually a decision made by the diver when he or she feels comfortable enough to do so. If concurrent conditions such as **Raynaud's phenomenon** (spasm of small arteries supplying blood to the hands and feet) or abnormal heart rhythm patterns exist, the decision to dive needs to be made by a physician trained in hyperbaric and undersea medicine. These conditions are relative contraindications to diving (see chapter 10); but under certain conditions, for example in warm water, diving is permissible.

Hyperthermia and Sunburn

Hyperthermia ("hyper" = above) is an increase of body temperature. Hyperthermia is a much less common problem in diving than hypothermia. Sunburn occurs as a consequence of unprotected exposure to the sun.

Significance   Hyperthermia can cause serious medical problems in divers and swimmers who are performing hard work or strenuous swim activities in very warm waters (over 85 degrees F/29 degrees C). In contrast to positive feedback mechanisms to immersion in cold water, the effects of water that is too warm almost always lead to negative feedback mechanisms and elevation of core temperatures. The reason is that the cooling effects from evaporative losses, a very effective cooling technique in air, are lost during immersion in water. This also occurs on land when one is wearing a dry suit or a wet suit that is still dry before entering the water.

Sunburn may account for more lost days from sport diving than any other MPD. In addition, harmful effects from sun exposure can cause delayed damage to the eyes and the skin in the form of **cataracts** (the opacification of the lens of the eye) and skin cancer, respectively. These effects are accumulative; that is, the more exposure to sunlight, the more likely they are to occur.

Causes   Hyperthermia in diving occurs in three settings:

- During diving preparation, when the diver is expending energy suiting up, getting to the dive site, or working in the hot sun, especially while wearing a thermal protection exposure suit
- In tropical areas when divers are performing high workloads (such as marine archeology projects or military reconnaissance) in the water
- During immersion in hot water such as in therapeutic pools, spas or "hot tubs," or hot springs

Sunburn can occur in a matter of minutes with direct exposure of the skin to sun rays. The rays are most direct between the hours of 10 a.m. and 3 p.m. and during the summer months in the northern hemisphere. During these times of maximum sun exposure, the effects of sunburn occur more rapidly. For the SCUBA diver, sunburn can occur during transit in boats to the diving site and during surface intervals between dives, when the diver is resting and taking advantage of the sunny environment. For the snorkel diver, sunburn may occur while he or she is on the surface, although many people mistakenly think that the water is offering protection.

Effects on the Body (Pathophysiology)   When the water temperature exceeds 85 degrees F (29 degrees C), there is not enough difference in temperature between the skin and the surrounding water for heat to be effectively transferred to the water. Because cooling by evaporative heat loss does not occur during immersion, metabolic activity increases and the diver's core temperature rises. Nausea, headaches, heat seizures, and cardiac arrhythmias are consequences. Death occurs when core temperatures exceed 106 degrees F (41 degrees C). Dehydration increases the risk of hyperthermia by reducing the amount of circulating blood in the body and the normal heat transfer mechanisms from the core to the periphery. Another time the diver is vulnerable to dangerous effects from hyperthermia is while he or she is entering cold water after becoming hyperthermic from suiting up and getting to the dive site. **Coronary occlusion** (heart attack) and dangerous arrhythmias (heart rhythm disturbances) can occur with the shock of the abrupt temperature changes.

The acute effects of sunburn are not usually appreciated until after the exposure, and once present, they can greatly hamper the diver's underwater activities for the remainder of the diving trip. The effects of sunburn on the skin are similar to those of other types of burns. In the mildest forms, first-degree burns, the skin becomes reddened and painful. In the next stage, second degree, blisters form. Skin cell death is associated with third-degree burns. Sunburns are usually first degree but occasionally cause blistering. Any exposure to sunlight that causes sunburn, even in its mildest form, may lead to damage to the skin and delayed effects.

Delayed consequences from sunburn arise from the effects of ultraviolet light on the **DNA** (**deoxyribonucleic acid**; the molecule that encodes genetic information and determines the structure, function, and behavior of the cell) in the **chromosomes** (structures within cells that contain genetic material and have the ability to replicate themselves) of skin cells and the lenses of the eye. Ultraviolet light causes changes in the DNA. With these changes, the messages for replacement of skin cells are altered such that cancerous rather than normal skin cells are produced. Analogous processes occur in the lenses of the eyes to cause cataract formation.

First-Response Interventions and Definitive Management   Management of hyperthermic is threefold: cessation of activity, removal from the hyperthermic environment, and institution of cooling measures. Methods of cooling include spraying the skin with cool water, applying alcohol, covering with wet garments, and other techniques that utilize the cooling effects of evaporation. However, cooling should be gradual, to avoid hypothermia and shock associated with redistribution of fluids in the body. Dehydration may be associated with hyperthermia especially when it occurs with associated sweating. Consequently, fluid administration is indicated. If the person is unconscious, fluid administration by the intravenous route is required. When the diver is conscious and capable of drinking without choking, water and clear juices are the preferred choices for rehydration.

Sunburn is managed by removal from sun exposure. The discomfort associated with first-degree sunburns can be reduced through the use of anesthetic ointments. If blisters occur, they should be cleansed with clean water daily and lightly coated with a burn ointment such as Silvadene. The delayed effects of sunburn, namely skin cancers and cataracts, require the expertise of medical specialists such as dermatologists and ophthalmologists.

Prevention   Methods to prevent hyperthermia in water should seem obvious. If the water temperature is so warm and the diving activities so demanding that hyperthermia is a risk, then durations of dives must be strictly limited. The pre-dive brief should include a review of the symptoms of hyperthermia, namely feeling unpleasantly warm, nausea, headache, and irritability. The diver should respond to the warning symptoms by immediately curtailing the diving activities. Hydration should always be optimized before beginning a dive under these circumstances. Exposure suits, which are recommended for protection from the sun and marine animals, should be as lightweight as possible (e.g., the Lycra diving skin).

Another precaution concerning hyperthermia in divers pertains to the use of a hot tub for relaxation after diving activities. Dive packages often advertise hot tubs as one of the amenities included. Typically the water temperatures in hot tubs are in the 100 to 104 degree F (38-40 degree C) range. Consequently, core temperatures can increase rapidly during immersion. If people in hot tubs are fatigued or sedated by alcohol, they may not appreciate the insidious onset of hyperthermia, or they may become so relaxed that they fall asleep. Serious consequences, from cardiac arrest to drowning, can ensue.

Prevention of injury from the harmful effects of sun exposure can be equally effective. Sunscreens lessen the penetration of harmful ultraviolet rays through the skin. Their effectiveness is listed as an SPF (sun protection factor) based on how long the sunscreen will protect as compared to unprotected exposure. Many sunscreens maintain their effectiveness even after immersion in water. Simply wearing a long-sleeved T-shirt and tights or a Lycra skin is even more effective for preventing sunburn and is highly recommended for the snorkel diver. Zinc oxide ointment will block all sun penetration to the skin and is useful over prominences such as the nose and ears. Its significant disadvantage is that it is wiped off with almost any type of contact. For static situations, such as supervising a dive or lifeguarding, in which exposure to the sun is unavoidable, zinc oxide ointment is effective for protecting these particularly vulnerable areas.

Finally, sun protection equipment should always include sunglasses and a broad-brimmed hat. Although these items are not used during the dive, they offer protection during the trip to and from the dive site and in the dive supervising roles mentioned previously. Sunglasses should be selected based on labels stating that they protect from both ultraviolet A and B radiation.

Return to Diving   The discussion about return to diving after hypothermia is valid also for return to diving after hyperthermia and sunburn episodes. The diver may resume diving when comfortable. Since sunburn is so common and is ordinarily not documented by medical workers as more serious disorders would be, the days lost from diving due to this condition are only estimates but are probably more numerous than for any other single MPD.

Infections of the External Ear Canals

The familiar name for infections of the external canal is **swimmer's ear** since these are so commonly observed in people who swim regularly, as competitive swimmers do.

Significance   Infections of the ear canal, or otitis externa, are important to the diver because they occur frequently. Usually they cause minor problems, such as itching and pain in the ear canal when one is out of the water, but do not curtail aquatic activities. When people dive repetitively in warm, moist environments or polluted waters, the problem is increasingly likely to occur. Its incidence is almost 100 percent in saturation divers (see chapter 2).

Causes   Immersion in water from swimming and diving is an important contributing factor to swimmer's ear because it increases the moisture load to the external ear canals. There is a direct relationship between the incidence of infections of the ear canal and the amount of exposure to aquatic environments. The incidence in swimmers is five times higher than in non-swimmers. Three factors interact to cause otitis externa (see figure 12.1):

• Moisture. The ear canal by virtue of its anatomy is prone to retaining moisture. Moisture retention is proportional to the amount of exposure to the aquatic environment. This is a conditional variable for the development of swimmer's ear. If moisture can be controlled, infections of the ear canal will not develop. Consequently, moisture is the critical variable in

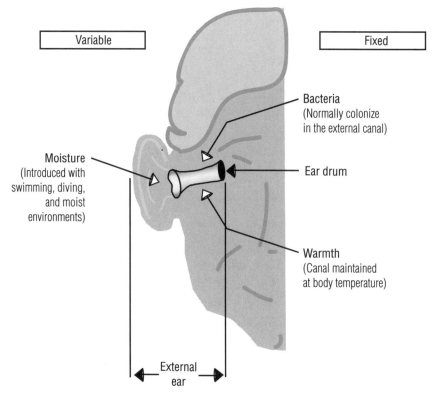

FIGURE
12.1   Factors that interact to cause swimmer's ear.

development of ear infections. It is not possible to keep the ear canals from becoming exposed to moisture during swimming and diving activities. People traveling to moist, high-humidity climates are also prone to developing ear infections because of this increased moisture in the air. Frequently, these factors (diving plus tropical environments) are additive when diving in exotic areas. During saturation dives, the humidity in the habitat or chamber remains at 100 percent. Infections of the ear canal are almost a universal occurrence.

• Temperature. The temperature of the ear canal is very near that of the body core and is ideal for the multiplication of microorganisms. Since the temperature in the inner portion of the ear canal is relatively constant, this variable tends to be independent of exposure or other conditions that lead to otitis externa.

• Microorganisms. Microorganisms normally do not multiply extensively in the inner two-thirds of the ear canal but are present in small numbers in approximately 70 percent of normal individuals. Additional bacteria may be introduced into the ear canal by aquatic activities in conjunction with the moisture that enters the canal.

When moisture is introduced into the canal, the equilibrium is disturbed such that it provides an ideal incubating medium for bacteria multiplication. The multiplying bacteria invade the canal lining, causing symptoms that progress from itching to pain to discharge from the canal.

Effects on the Body (Pathophysiology)   Microorganisms begin to multiply if the canal remains moist. Microorganisms then invade the inner layer of the ear canal, and an infection of the ear canal results. Some individuals are more likely to develop ear infections than others. If the ear canal is excessively long, curved, narrowed, or partially obstructed, water may be trapped within it, making the individual prone to ear infections. Normally the surface layer of the ear canal is slightly acidic, which helps retard the growth of microorganisms. Multiplication of microorganisms, coupled with increased moisture in the ear canal, softens the protective external layer of the ear canal and converts the canal from an acidic to a basic environment.

Signs and symptoms of "swimmer's ear" may develop hours or days after exposure and thus are not always recognized as being associated with an aquatic activity. During the incipient stage, symptoms include itching and pain in the ear canal. The patient may complain that the ear feels wet and full. Tenderness may be noted when the earlobe is pulled, pressure is applied to the canal, or the jaw is rocked from side to side. Pain symptoms are proportional to the degree of canal inflammation but may vary from individual to individual. Occasionally, pus from the ear discharge may cause secondary inflammation around the ear. Debris from a combination of breakdown products of the ear canal wall, bacteria, and earwax may plug the ear canal and decrease hearing.

First-Response Interventions and Definitive Management   Treatment is directed at interrupting the pathophysiology (negative feedback) events just described. First, moisture must be reduced in the ear canal. Ear canal infections are managed with desiccating (drying) agents such as alcohol mixed with acetic (vinegar) acid or boric acid solutions. These solutions can be purchased without a physician's prescription. The acid solutions help convert the ear canal lining back to its normal acid state and also retard bacteria growth. The solutions may also contain **anti-inflammatory agents** to reduce pain, discomfort, and inflammation. If frank pus is observed in the ear canal, then antibiotic solutions may also be placed into the canal. If the skin is reddened around the ear canal, systemic **antibiotics** (medications that kill or stop the growth of microorganisms) may be required. For these latter two conditions, management by a physician is recommended.

Prevention   Infections of the ear canal are prevented or minimized by drying the ear canal after diving and swimming activities. Actively shaking the head with the neck tilted to the side can remove water trapped in the canal. Fanning or using an electric hair dryer (at low temperature settings to prevent burns) directed toward the opening of the ear canal also has drying effects. Use of cotton-tipped applicators to dry the ear canal and remove earwax should be avoided. These can tear the tissues lining the canals and remove protective earwax. Both of these effects make the ear canals more susceptible to invasion by microorganisms. Ear canal hygiene with the use of desiccating agents should be taught to patients who regularly participate in swimming and diving activities.

Return to Diving   As with the other environmental problems, return to diving and swimming is based on the severity of symptoms. When the problem is minor, people usually continue these activities and use eardrops after immersion. For surface swimming, earplugs may be used to prevent water entry to the ear canals. For diving, earplugs must not be used. They may become lodged in the canals with increasing ambient pressure during descent and need to be removed using surgical instruments. The contact pressure effects needed to seal earplugs may also cause irritation of the lining of the ear canals. If more serious symptoms of ear canal infections are present, such as pus draining from the canal or inflammation of the skin around the canal, one should obtain permission from a physician before returning to water-related activities.

Injuries From Marine Animals

Marine animals are among the most fascinating and exotic of creatures. The intended goal of most sport divers is to observe these animals in their natural environments. With only rare exceptions, marine animals are not aggressive. Most of the injuries to humans from marine animals are from passive defense mechanisms that protect the animals in their natural environment. Invariably, injuries to the sport diver occur because of carelessness. If one phrase could summarize the behavior of marine animals, the injuries they cause in humans, and the prevention of such injuries, it would be "Don't tread on me."

Significance

Although over 1,000 species of marine animals can cause injuries to humans, their injury mechanisms are of five types as summarized in table 12.2. This classification simplifies the diagnosis and management of injuries from marine animals. Once the type of injury is determined, the management is obvious. Figure 12.2 lists the basic supplies needed to treat marine animal injuries (for additional supplies, see appendix C). In terms of severity and frequency, most injuries from marine animals are minor cuts, scratches, and irritations

Table 12.2	Injuries From Marine Animals				
Class	**Injury type**	**Examples**	**Pathology**	**Complications**	**Management**
1	Trauma (bite)	Shark, eel	Laceration	Shock	Control bleeding, repair tissue injuries.
2	Sting	Jellyfish, anemones, hydra, corals	Allergic reaction (from poisons contained in nematocysts on the tentacles)	Collapse, respiratory arrest	(1) Inactivate with alcohol or acetic acid. (2) Shave off residual tentacles.
3	Puncture	Sea urchin, stingray, sculpin (fish with spines), cone shell (radicular tooth analogous to a spine)	Puncture wound +/− toxin	Collapse, infection, granuloma formation	(1) Soak in hot (avoid burn) water. (2) Apply tetanus prophylaxis. (3) Be alert to delayed onset of skin infection or joint infection.
4	Poisonous bite	Sea snake, blue-ringed octopus	Envenomation	Respiratory arrest	Provide life support for respiratory arrest, anti-venom.
5	Miscellaneous; indolent wounds, skin rashes	Corals and barnacles, parasites and bacteria	Superficial wounds, rash, infections	Festering wounds, non-healing wounds	Cleanse and scrub wounds to bleeding tissue; leave open to heal by secondary intention; provide antibiotics if needed.

and occur so often that they are among the most frequent MPD. Rarely is an injury from a marine animal serious enough to require medical attention, and only in the rarest of situations is life or limb threatened.

Class 1: Traumatic Injuries

Many marine animals are potentially dangerous because of their size and their ability to bite. Animals in this class include the shark, barracuda, moray eel, and sea lion.

Alcohol solution

Benadryl

Bicarbonate of soda or ammonia
solution

Calamine lotion

Cortisone ointment

Drying powder (talcum powder,
flour, soda)

Gauze compression bandages

Knife

Oral airway (tracheal tube)

Tourniquet

Water-heating device (Sterno can)

**FIGURE
12.2**   Basic supplies for emergency treatment of marine animal wounds.

Causes, Mechanisms, and Presentations   Injuries produced by the animals just mentioned are traumatic; no venoms or poisons are involved. Injury mechanisms are analogous to those caused by bites from their terrestrial counterparts such as dogs and cats. Shark bites are notorious because of media attention. Shark bites to divers have hardly ever been reported. Most shark bites occur in people on the surface, such as surfers or swimmers. Two or more bites on a person are almost never observed; it appears that sharks bite humans mostly when mistaking them for normal food sources, namely seals and sea lions.

First-Response Interventions   Since bite injuries, especially from sharks, can cause massive tissue losses and bleeding, emergency medical care to stop the bleeding and treat shock must be instituted immediately. Emergency control of bleeding with direct compression or pressure over arterial pressure points should be attempted. A tourniquet may be the only method to control bleeding from a severed or badly lacerated limb. Emergency treatment of shock (see chapter 16) includes elevation of the lower extremities to above the heart level and keeping the person warm. Elevation adds blood to the core circulation from the veins in the lower extremities, equivalent to about 10 percent of the total blood volume. One must use discretion when offering fluid to a person in hemorrhagic (blood loss) shock. If not fully alert, the person may aspirate (inhale into the lungs) the fluid and further complicate the shock condition. Additionally, if emergency surgery is required to manage the bite injury, the ingestion of fluids within six hours of anesthesia increases the likelihood of complications from anesthesia.

Definitive Management   Definitive care of bite injuries from diving mammals is analogous to the management of similar types of injuries from other causes. Intravenous fluid administration and antibiotics are started immediately. Tetanus prophylaxis is updated. If the person is in shock, blood is transfused. After primary (vital signs) and secondary (other injury) assessments are completed, the person is taken to the operating room for exploration of the extent of injuries, surgical control of bleeding, removal of dead tissue, and wound closure if possible. Several returns to the operating room may be required and may include skin grafting to close and cover the wounds completely.

Prevention   Most bite injuries and other marine animal injuries can be prevented by adherence to the following admonitions:

- Know your diving area; do not dive in an unfamiliar area without a briefing on the diving conditions and marine animals particular to the area.
- Be aware of the behavior patterns of the marine animals that are potentially dangerous to the diver in the diving area.
- Avoid handling or touching aquatic mammals in their native environments; do not attempt to play with or capture the young animals; respect the animals' territory.
- Do not become attractive bait by swimming with open wounds, dangling fish, or wearing shiny objects that might attract sharks.
- Avoid struggling movements in the water. Sharks may interpret these movements as distress signals and be attracted by them.

Return to Diving   Among human divers there is little experience with bite injuries from aquatic animals. The appropriate time for return to diving would be equivalent to the time the person could resume full exercise activities on land. However, the psychological trauma of the injury in the water environment may dissuade people from returning to swimming and diving activities in the ocean.

Class 2: Sting Injuries
A second group of marine animals inflict their injuries by virtue of stinging apparatuses. Jellyfish, sea anemones, hydras, and some corals are animals in this group.

Causes, Mechanisms, and Presentations   Animals that sting inject toxins into a person by means of nematocysts, microscopic trigger mechanisms embedded in their tentacles or other body parts (see figure 12.3). Although the poison discharged into the wound from a nematocyst may be potent, hundreds of thousands of nematocysts must come in contact with the skin before significant injury occurs. Fatal injuries from the deadly sea wasp jellyfish of Australia indicate that there are always more than 20 feet (six meters) of linear contact between the tentacles and the person's skin.

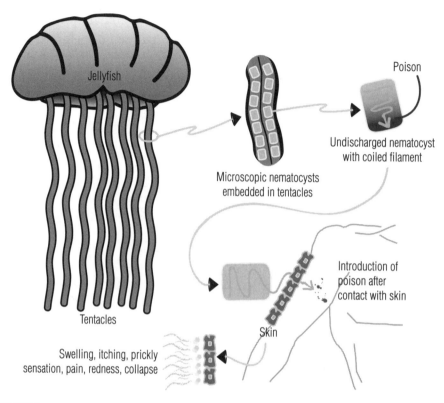

FIGURE 12.3 Stinging mechanism of the jellyfish.

Jellyfish drift or swim slowly by rhythmic contractions of their bodies. The other members of this class are sessile, meaning they are attached to other structures. Usually divers come in contact with the tentacles while swimming or accidentally bumping the other body parts. Symptoms, from the poisons discharged by the nematocysts in order of increasing severity, include the following:

- Prickly, itching sensations
- Welts with burning, excruciating pain
- Headaches and cramps
- Feelings of suffocation and paralysis

In the majority of instances, the symptoms are limited to the first two findings listed above. In sting injuries from the sea wasp, shock and collapse may occur immediately.

First-Response Interventions   Emergency treatment is threefold. First, the nematocysts should be inactivated by rinsing the involved area with alcohol or vinegar. Application of meat tenderizers may be equally effective at this stage.

Usually local residents are able to tell the injured person (or the attendants) what the most effective agent is for the jellyfish in their area. This type of information is useful for presentation in a pre-dive brief.

Second, the residual tentacles should be removed by coalescing them with a drying agent such as flour, baking soda, or diver's talc and then scraping the paste from the skin with a blade. Fresh water, sand, or abrasive cloths should not be used to wash off the tentacles since these agents will stimulate the undischarged nematocysts to release their toxins.

Third, if itching or stinging is associated with the welts, applications of calamine lotion or steroid creams and ingestion of Benadryl usually provide symptomatic relief. If all the tentacles have been removed, hot showers provide temporary relief of the burning and itching symptoms.

Definitive Management   In most cases, emergency treatment is the definitive treatment. If the symptoms progress to headaches and cramps, emergency medical evaluation is recommended. Intravenous steroid administration may be required at this stage. If collapse and shock occur, advanced life-support interventions (see chapter 16) are required.

Prevention   With reasonable precautions, most sting injuries can be prevented. A pre-dive brief should alert the diver to the likelihood of encounters with jellyfish. For example, during certain seasons, jellyfish populations increase. Choppy seas can break the tentacles into fragments so numerous that they literally saturate the diving area. When one is diving in these conditions, a Lycra skin or wet suit offers superb protection against injuries from these animals. It is necessary to take care in removing the dive suit since tentacles may become attached to the outside of the suit and the nematocyst mechanisms remain active whether in the water or not. Wearing gloves prevents sting injuries to the hands. Finally, the maintenance of neutral

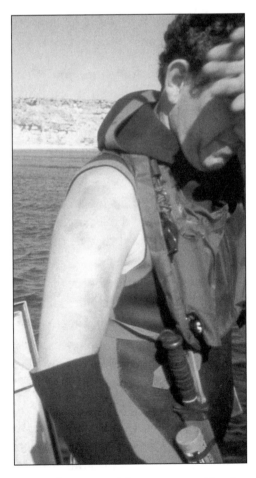

Skin welts can result from contact with a fire coral marine animal.

buoyancy while on the bottom prevents the diver from sinking and accidentally bumping the stinging portions of sessile varieties of these marine animals.

Return to Diving   Divers who have incurred sting injuries may return to diving when they feel OK. In most instances, this is when they are no longer bothered by the itching and stinging sensations. With serious envenomations, as in any other serious medical condition, diving should not be resumed until full recovery has occurred and physical fitness is restored.

Class 3: Puncture Wounds

A variety of marine animals including segmented worms, cone shells, sea urchins, stingrays, and spiny fish (sculpins) have spines or analogous structures. Most of the injuries caused by these animals occur near the shoreline as the person enters the water. Examples of shoreline injuries are stingray injuries and spine injuries from falling into sea urchin beds. Like the stinging animals, these animals are sessile or slow moving. Injuries occur as a consequence of accidental contact, carelessness, or both.

Causes, Mechanisms, and Presentations   Five different varieties of marine animals have mechanisms that can induce puncture-type wounds; all the mechanisms are quite different. Some of the animals have apparatuses to introduce poisons into the wound. In each case, the part of the animal that causes the wound has a protein-type coating (slime) that inflicts severe pain.

• Sea urchins: Surfers or bathers are often injured when they fall onto sea urchin beds and the sea urchins' spines impale the skin, break off, and remain embedded. Divers may be forcefully carried into sea urchin beds by surging seas.

• Stingrays: Injuries occur when bathers run haphazardly into the surf. The sleeping ray reflexively flexes its tail when stepped on and impales its spine into the person, usually at the foot or ankle level.

• Sculpins: Sculpins have spines embedded in their dorsal and pectoral fins. They are very slow moving. Puncture wound injuries to the hands occur when these animals struggle during removal from fishnets or spears. Toxin envenomations often occur with these injuries.

• Cone shells: Cone shells have harpoonlike radicular teeth 1/32 inch (one millimeter) long. They use this device to "spear" food sources. The radicular teeth carry venom into the puncture wound to immobilize the food source. Humans incur injuries when they handle live cone shells and the shells drive their radicular tooth into the hands or fingers.

- Segmented worms. These worms have bristles along the sides of their body segments. When handled without the protection of gloves, the bristles can cause puncture wounds.

Many animals in this group have a venom apparatus associated with their puncture-producing wound devices. In addition to the poisons themselves, the spine injuries usually cause severe pain due to the slime and debris (which coats the puncturing devices) introduced into the wound. As in any puncture wound, infections may develop. Symptoms from marine animal puncture wounds are predominately pain, often excruciating. In the rare instances in which poisons are introduced, such as in sculpin fish puncture wounds, shock, collapse, and respiratory arrest can occur.

Two of the cases in "Bringing It All Together" illustrate how different clinical presentation may be in injuries from sea urchin spines.

First-Response Interventions   Fortunately, the venoms or slime and debris that are impaled into the wound with the injury and cause the excruciating pain are inactivated by heat. Soaking the involved area in water as hot as is tolerable produces dramatic, definitive, and immediate improvement. Two to three hours of soaking may be necessary before the person no longer experiences pain when the injury site is removed from the hot water. Care must be taken not to scald the skin, since the excruciating pain may interfere with temperature interpretation. Analgesics (pain-relieving medications) and antihistamines (allergy-reducing medications) may help to control pain and inflammation.

Spines that are readily accessible should be removed immediately. Those that are not should be removed only if they become symptomatic, but the wound should be observed for the development of a subsequent infection. Embedded sea urchin spines, especially in joints, may become a nidus for granuloma (a type of scar tissue) formation, perhaps requiring surgical removal.

Definitive Management   In most cases, the emergency treatment of immersion in warm water is also the definitive treatment. As in other types of puncture wounds, tetanus prophylaxis must be updated. The person also must be alert to the possibility that infections can occur at the wound site days after the injury (see case studies later in the chapter). In the unusual situations of shock and collapse from these injuries, advanced life-support interventions and steroid administration may be required. An antivenom for stone fish puncture wounds is produced by the Commonwealth Laboratories of Australia.

Prevention   Divers entering water where marine animals of this group are known to reside should be appropriately briefed before commencing diving activities. The pre-dive brief should include information about each animal's appearance, the location of the puncturing devices, the animals' habits, their aggressiveness, and situations in which injuries occur. Wearing gloves and booties helps prevent some of the injuries, but spines from sculpins, sea urchins, and stingrays are likely to penetrate neoprene.

Return to Diving   Most divers resume diving activities after the pain subsides. Medical attention for these injuries is sought only if complications such as delayed onset infection or granuloma formation occurs. When these problems have been resolved with medications, surgery, or both, the diver may resume diving without restrictions.

Class 4: Poisonous Bites

The blue-ringed octopus and the sea snake are included in the class of animals that can inflict poisonous bites. Sea snakes are found in Indo-Pacific waters, while the blue-ringed octopus is found in Australian waters. Injuries to divers from these animals are rare or nonexistent. We include them in this section for completeness and because they are a possible source of injury or death to the diver.

Causes, Mechanisms, and Presentations   Bites from these poisonous marine animals occur when they are mishandled, usually out of the water, for example, in fishing nets or when found washed up on the beach. The sea snake's venom is more toxic than the cobra's, but its mouth and fangs are so small that they cannot bite through a thin wet suit. When bites occur, they are usually on the hands, and envenomation is sufficient to cause symptoms only 25 percent of the time. With significant envenomation, muscle stiffness, passage of red-brown urine (**myoglobinuria**), paralysis, and collapse occur in that order of severity. Symptoms appear two to six hours after the bite. A bite, with envenomation, from the blue-ringed octopus may lead to immediate collapse and death.

First-Response Interventions   People bitten by sea snakes should be immediately placed at rest and transferred to the nearest medical facility. Application of a loose tourniquet to slow venous return proximal to the bite is desirable. The tourniquet should be loosened for 90 seconds every 15 minutes. The person may drink clear fluids. Oxygen is given if the person becomes short of breath. If breathing ceases from paralysis of the respiratory muscles, artificial ventilation should be started.

Definitive Management   Definitive treatment is a continuation of the first-line responses. If the respiratory muscles become paralyzed, the person may need intubation and placement on a ventilator. Intravenous fluids are administered to wash out myoglobin that is released from the muscles by the snake venom. An anti-venom for sea snake bites is available from the Commonwealth Laboratories of Australia.

Return to Diving   Once the person is asymptomatic, he or she may resume diving without restrictions. Muscle stiffness, which is caused by myoglobin

BRINGING IT ALL TOGETHER

CASE STUDY 1

A navy diver was being studied for the effects of immersion in cold water, 40 degree F (4 degree C); he was seated and was wearing a thick neoprene wet suit. During the course of the exposure, the diver became uncomfortable from the cold, but his core temperature dropped only a few tenths of a degree. When rewarmed in a hot water bath, he became confused and started to tremble. His core temperature declined another degree and a half during this time.

Comment: The decline in core temperature was caused by temperature afterdrop. In subsequent immersion studies, tourniquets were placed on the extremities during the initial phases of rewarming and released one at a time to minimize temperature afterdrop.

CASE STUDY 2

A 28-year-old navy diver developed signs and symptoms of swimmer's ear after his first series of diving activities in the tropics. Initially he was managed with a steroid–antibiotic suspension. His symptoms worsened rapidly with complaints that his ear felt wet and full of debris. An alcohol–acetic acid solution was prescribed, and improvement was noted with virtually the first installation of this solution. He said his canal no longer "felt wet." The symptoms cleared completely over the next four days. It is noteworthy that during the following 13 months of his navy tour the diver had no additional episodes but used the alcohol–acetic solution prophylactically after each dive.

Comment: Knowledge of the pathophysiology of swimmer's ear explains why the desiccating, acidifying agent was more effective than the antibiotic–steroid combination. The latter agent, an oil-based suspension, tends to plug the canal rather than clean it of debris. The moist tropical environment plus the diving activities caused the otitis externa. The prophylactic use of the drops prevented recurrences.

CASE STUDY 3

A 28-year-old surfer sustained a stingray injury to the top of his left foot while entering the water. The injury was recognized and managed appropriately with hot water immersion. The surfer's tetanus prophylaxis was current. One week later, after he had run 10 miles (six kilometers), his foot swelled and became red, painful, and warm. He sought medical attention. The diagnosis was delayed onset cellulitis (skin infection) from the stingray puncture wound injury. After antibiotics were started, the condition resolved without incident.

Comment: The stingray puncture wound introduced bacteria into the foot. The stress of the run precipitated the infection even though the run took place a week after the marine animal injury.

(continued)

(continued)

CASE STUDY 4

A 24-year-old diver impaled the tip of his left index finger on a sea urchin spine when he used the hand to push off the bottom. Immediately, excruciating pain occurred at the site of injury. Examination failed to disclose an inflammatory response or gross remnants of the spine in the fingertip. Initially, soaking the hand in cold water as an attempt to lessen the pain worsened the symptoms. After phone consultation with a physician, the diver experienced immediate dramatic relief from soaking the hand in hot water. However, it took a couple of hours of immersion before the patient could remove his hand from the hot water and remain comfortable.

   Comment: This demonstrates how effective soaking in hot water is for relieving pain from a marine animal puncture-type wound. Follow-up medical care in the form of tetanus prophylaxis and observation of a delayed onset infection are recommended.

CASE STUDY 5

A 25-year-old physician who was an inexperienced diver sustained a fairly deep laceration on his leg from the sharp edges of barnacle shells when he entered warm tropical water for a SCUBA dive. After the dive, he placed a disinfectant in the wound and then sealed the edges with Steri-Strips. Twelve hours later, the wound area was red, painful, and draining pus. After conferring with his colleagues, the diver removed the Steri-Strips and vigorously washed out the wound with a surgical scrub brush. The wound was left open and oral antibiotics were started. By the next day the inflammation had subsided, and the patient felt healthy enough to resume diving.

   Comment: The initial wound closure was inadvisable. The quick interventions when infection was noted undoubtedly minimized the infection complication.

---

release and myoglobinuria, usually resolves itself after three or four days. When the respiratory muscles are paralyzed, ventilation support may be required for a prolonged period.

Class 5: Cuts, Scratches, and Lacerations

Cuts, scratches, and lacerations are the most common of all marine animal injuries. They occur from accidental contact with corals, barnacles, and other marine animals that have calcareous (composed of calcium) shells.

Causes, Mechanisms, and Presentations   The causes of cuts, scratches, and lacerations are similar to those described for stings and puncture wounds. Usually these injuries occur when the diver is accidentally impaled into shells while walking through the surf zone, from wave surges, or from negative buoyancy. These types of injuries often seem minor but are usually slow to heal due to the introduction of debris and calcareous material from the shells into the wound.

First-Response Interventions   The most important part of the management of these injuries is washing out the debris—which may be microscopic—

in the wound. Rinsing with fresh water is recommended. One should not attempt to close the wound because doing so may seal in an infection. This is likely to happen when the injury occurs in tropical, high-humidity, warm environments.

Definitive Management   Usually the wound heals with the measures outlined. If not, then formal washout with scraping of the wound base under anesthesia may be required. If the tissues are inflamed around the injury site, antibiotics are administered. Tetanus prophylaxis should be updated.

Prevention   The same measures for preventing sting and puncture wounds are effective in preventing cuts, scratches, and lacerations.

Return to Diving   These injuries are usually so minor that they do not interfere with diving activities if the first interventions are done properly. If infections develop, swimming and diving activities should be stopped until the infection is resolved.

For Further Review

1. What techniques can be used to avoid hypothermia during diving?
2. What are the mechanisms of temperature afterdrop during rewarming?
3. What are the immediate and possible delayed consequences of sunburn for the diver?
4. What factors interact to cause infections of the ear canal (swimmer's ear)?
5. Why is the classification of mechanisms of injury from marine animals useful?
6. What diving equipment helps to protect from marine animal injuries?
7. What is the explanation for pain relief that occurs when one soaks puncture wounds in warm water?
8. How should cuts, scratches, and lacerations from marine animal injuries be managed?

PROBLEMS
ASSOCIATED
WITH DESCENT

Medical problems of diving associated with descent include the ear squeeze, other so-called minor squeezes, and thoracic squeeze. These are examples of direct effects of pressure; gas compression, as described by Boyle's Law, explains why they occur. The

Chapter Preview

- Physics and physiology of barotraumas
- Anatomy of the middle ear spaces
- Causes of ear and sinus squeezes
- Complications that can arise from middle ear barotraumas
- Thoracic squeeze as fact or fiction

ear squeeze is a very frequent problem of the sport diver. Every ascent and descent puts the diver at risk of ear or sinus squeeze. In contrast, thoracic squeeze is very rare, almost nonexistent. Since ear, sinus, suit, mask, and tooth squeeze do not usually cause serious consequences or permanent damage, these may be referred to as "minor squeezes." Thoracic squeeze, which can result in death, is the "major" squeeze.

Minor Squeezes

Even though the human body can withstand marked variations in pressure, the air-filled, rigid-walled cavities such as the middle ear spaces, the sinus cavities, and the lungs, under some circumstances, are susceptible to barotraumas. Also, artificial cavities such as the face mask airspace and air-filled creases in wet suits can lead to barotrauma in the diver. Middle ear and sinus spaces, by virtue of their anatomy, are particularly vulnerable to the effects of pressure change. They probably account for as much **morbidity** (illness) in the diver as the environmental problems do and perhaps more curtailing of diving activities, albeit temporary, than any other medical problem of diving (MPD). The only health problem that the Ama female divers of Japan experienced more frequently than their

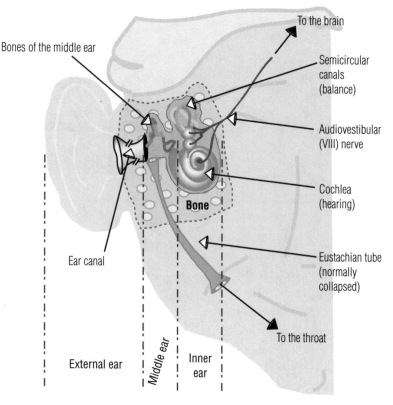

FIGURE 13.1   Anatomy of the middle and inner ear.

non-diving counterparts was chronic inflammation of their middle ear structures.

Causes and Anatomy

The middle ear (figure 13.1) is an air-filled space that is separated from the external ear canal by the eardrum (tympanic membrane). It is connected to the back of the nose–mouth junction (the pharynx) by the Eustachian tube. The Eustachian tube opens during swallowing and allows exchange of air, equalization of pressure, and delivery of oxygen to the middle ear space. The middle ear contains the three smallest bones in the human body. These bones, the hammer, anvil, and stirrup, transmit the sound energy from the eardrum to the inner ear. The four paired sinus cavities are enclosed in the bones of the face. Each has a narrow opening that connects to the nasal passage. Sinus cavities make the skull bones lighter and act as resonating chambers to improve the quality of human speech. Each sinus is lined with a special covering called respiratory **epithelium,** as is the middle ear space. This is similar to the tissues lining the nose and respiratory tree. Respiratory epithelium has a rich blood supply. The diver may create artificial rigid-walled cavities by donning goggles, face mask, and diving suit. A decayed tooth may also allow formation of an air-filled cavity.

The external ear canal must also be considered since impacted cerumen (earwax), **osteomas** (bony masses), diving hoods, or earplugs can generate an artificial air-filled, rigid-walled cavity external to the tympanic membrane. In these cases, even with equalization of pressure in the middle ear spaces, barotrauma results, in the form of a "reverse" or external ear barotrauma. The tympanic membrane is distended outward, and the external auditory canal becomes congested. In this situation, the middle ear cavity is "overpressurized" in relation to the closed cavity between the plug and the tympanic membrane.

Physiology   To avoid barotrauma to the middle ear and sinus cavities during pressure changes, the pressure in these cavities must be equalized continuously with the surrounding pressure. These cavities are all examples of air-filled, rigid-walled cavities (see chapter 1). As the diver descends and the external pressure increases, equalization occurs if the Eustachian tube and sinus ostia (openings) are patent and if the air, at the new ambient pressure, moves either actively or passively into these structures. The air at the new ambient pressure comes from the air tanks when one is SCUBA diving or from the

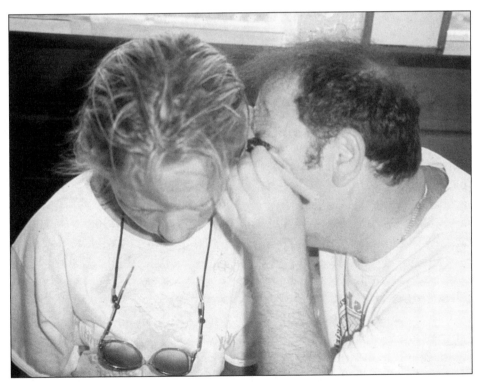

Examination of the ears after a dive frequently shows some evidence of barotrauma to the middle ear structures.

air held in the lungs in breath-hold diving. Because of the pressure–volume relationships, the greatest volume changes per foot of descent occur near the surface. For example, a 15-FSW (4.6-MSW) descent from the surface of the water reduces the volume of a flexible air-filled container by 32 percent. This same 15-foot descent from 85 to 100 FSW (26-30 MSW) reduces the volume by about 3 percent.

Pressure Equalization   Many divers use the Valsalva maneuver (pinching of the nose, with the mouth closed, trying to expel air) to equalize pressure in the middle ear spaces and sinuses. This is an example of an active pressure equalization technique. Experienced divers (and flyers) often equalize pressures passively simply by swallowing, yawning, or protruding the jaw bone. Problems arise when the diver is unable to equalize the pressure between these spaces and the outside environment. Reasons for failure to equalize include the following:

- Inexperience
- Infections causing swelling of the mucous membranes
- Allergies or vasomotor rhinitis (swelling of the passageways of the nose), both of which are aggravated by smoking
- Nasopharyngeal masses such as tonsils, **adenoids** (a mass of tissue in the upper part of the throat, behind the nose, that contains white blood cells and helps with the control of infections), tumors, or scarring from surgery to remove these structures
- Congenital or acquired bony obstruction of these openings

Ear barotrauma during ascent is occasionally caused by occlusion of the Eustachian tube that prevents egress of air from the middle ear cavity. This occurs rarely because the air, at increased pressure in the middle ear and sinus spaces, usually moves out passively with ascent and decrease of the ambient pressure. The use of vasoconstrictors and decongestants may contribute to this problem. If the dive exceeds the drug's period of effectiveness, there may be a rebound phenomenon with increased **congestion** (distension of blood vessels) and a subsequent inability to equalize pressure while ascending.

Effects on the Body (Pathophysiology)

If pressure is not continuously equilibrated in the middle ear spaces and sinuses during descent, pressure differentials develop. The initial positive feedback mechanism of pain, which signals the diver to equalize pressure or halt the descent, quickly changes to a negative (pathology causing) feedback mechanism. This occurs in the form of swelling of the highly vascular epithelial linings of the middle ear and sinus cavities. The swollen vessels reduce the air volume as an attempt to lessen the pressure differential. The eardrum becomes distended inward. A pressure differential less than 3 FSW (1 MSW) is sufficient to cause swelling, fluid leakage, and bleeding of the blood vessels of the eardrum and the middle ear and sinus cavities. Congestion tends to interfere with further pressure equilibration because the swelling narrows the diameter of the Eustachian tube and may even occlude it completely. If the pressure differential is too great, the blood vessels, eardrum, or both, rupture and fill the cavity with blood and water. This converts the cavity into a liquid-filled structure that can now transmit the ambient pressure directly like a "bag of water"(see chapter 1, table 1.3). The clinical findings of ear squeezes are summarized in table 13.1.

In addition to the previously described symptoms, ear squeezes may lead to temporary hearing loss. This is characterized by muting of sounds and is due to fluid accumulations in the middle ear space secondary to barotrauma. With clearing of the fluid, hearing returns to normal. The perforated eardrum can have serious consequences in the water. If cold water comes in contact with the labyrinth (structure that converts balance and hearing sensations to nerve impulses) of the inner ear through the perforation in the ear drum, the diver can lose the sense of equilibrium. Severe **vertigo** (sensation of the room spinning) results. The diver may become disoriented by these symptoms and panic. Usually the disequilibrium symptoms are transitory, disappearing when the water warms to body temperature.

Other medical problems associated with middle ear barotraumas include the following:

• Alternobaric vertigo occurring during ascent: Symptoms of vertigo (room spinning) and disequilibrium suggest that the labyrinth is being stimulated.

Table 13.1	Middle Ear Squeeze Symptoms	
Symptom	**Mechanism**
Pain	Eardrum stretches.
Congestion	Blood vessels swell in response to pressure differential, and fluid leaks through the blood vessel walls into the middle ear spaces.
Bleeding into throat (i.e., blood-tinged sputum)	Pressure differential has become so great that blood vessels rupture and blood flows down the Eustachian tube to the throat.
Bleeding from ear canal	Perforation (hole) in eardrum; now blood flows out of canal as well as into the throat.

The cause of this condition is thought to be unilateral difficulty in equalizing pressures in the middle ear spaces during ascent.

• High-frequency hearing loss and **tinnitus** (ringing in the ear): This problem has been noted to occur with aging and with exposure to loud noises. Pressure trauma, either from ear squeezes or from decompression sickness, may cause minor disturbances in the blood supplies to the labyrinth, which in turn cause hearing loss and tinnitus.

• **Labyrinthitis:** Inflammation secondary to the ear squeeze or infection may spread to the labyrinth. It may take hours or days for the inflammatory process to reach sufficient magnitude to affect the labyrinth. This represents the spreading of the original inflammatory process of the ear squeeze. Since the condition causes abnormal stimulation of the labyrinth, the symptoms are similar to those of alternobaric vertigo.

• **Meningitis:** The perforated eardrum may permit the access of bacteria to the inner ear structures. The infection can ascend to the brain along the pathways of the audiovestibular nerve.

• Reverse ear squeeze: This is observed in inexperienced divers who over-pressurize their middle ear spaces. They think that the pain they are experiencing in their ears with pressure equilibration attempts requires further pressurization of their middle ear spaces.

• Round window rupture: The inner ear structures have two soft tissue windows in their bony walls. These allow the pressure sensations from the middle ear bones to be transmitted to the fluid contents of the inner ear. If one of the membranes ruptures, usually the round window, the effects cause deafness and loss of equilibrium from fluid leaking out of the inner ear space. Surgical repair may be needed to correct the problem.

• Sudden profound deafness: The cause of this serious problem is not known. It has been observed in saturation divers who apparently had had no difficulty clearing their ears during descent. It may represent a variant of decompression sickness (see chapter 15) that affects the inner ear.

The mechanisms of diving suit, goggle, tooth, and mask squeezes are analogous to middle ear and sinus squeezes. However, the rigid-walled, air-filled cavities in these situations are artificially created. When the pressure differential becomes great enough, blood vessels become distended and may even rupture. Signs of red, infected blood vessels in the conjunctivae of the eye and red facial skin are associated with mask and goggle squeezes. Skin welts occur from the suit squeeze. Pain with pressure changes is the symptom associated with tooth squeezes.

First-Response Interventions

The first response to minor squeezes should be to stop the progression of the pathophysiology process. Immediately the descent should be halted. If clearing is not achieved, then the diver should ascend a few feet and attempt clearing again. After clearing is achieved, descent should be resumed at a slower rate. The diver should never attempt to overcome the pain by "swimming though it" during descent. If a squeeze has occurred, decongestant medications and nasal sprays, which can be purchased without prescriptions, can provide symptomatic relief. If serious symptoms such as vertigo are present, the diver should stop and be made to rest. Then immediate arrangements should be made to transfer the patient to a medical facility for further evaluation and treatment.

Definitive Management

Patients with minor squeezes (findings of discomfort, conjestion, muted hearing) need only to be treated with reassurance and cautions against descending at rates faster than they can equilibrate at. Divers with mild and moderate injuries (fluid behind the eardrum) should be treated with oral vasoconstrictors, antihistamines, nasal decongestants, or some combination of these. **Vasoconstrictors** and **antihistamines** (for those who have allergies) help to reduce the swelling and secretion formation, respectively, of the respiratory epithelium. The goal is to maintain patency (opening) of the sinus ostia and Eustachian tubes to permit equalization of pressure and drainage of the secretions. Divers should not use these medications routinely. Repeated use of vasoconstrictors can sensitize the mucous membranes so that they actually swell rather than constrict when the medications are administered. Except in divers with a history of allergies, antihistamines should be avoided because they tend to make secretions more viscous (thick) and interfere with the upper respiratory spaces' own fluid-clearing mechanisms. Antihistamines are notorious for causing drowsiness. Continued requirements for these medications to equalize pressures in the middle ear spaces become a consideration for disqualification from diving.

Rupture of the tympanic membrane should be treated with systemic antibiotics and decongestants. For persistent symptoms, failure of the eardrum to heal, or suspected round window rupture, evaluation and management by an ear, nose, and throat specialist is recommended.

Prevention

Most diving problems related to barotrauma can be prevented if sensible diving practices are followed. Diving should not be attempted without proper instructions. This applies to snorkel divers as well. During the course of instructions the student is expected to gain a fundamental knowledge of barotrauma problems and a facility in equalizing pressures in the middle ear and sinus cavities. If ear, nose, and throat problems are present, the following should be evaluated:

• Condition of the tympanic membrane and its movement with pressure equilibration techniques

• Condition of the external canal with reference to otitis externa, osteomas (bone growths), and cerumen (earwax)

• Position of nasal septum, presence of nasal septal spurring, and hypertrophy of the linings of the turbinates (air channels in the nasal passages)

• Appearance of nasopharynx, especially in the area of Eustachian tube openings

From this information, treatment and clearance for diving can be determined.

Hearing loss must be evaluated also. Its presence, cause, and severity should be established. **Menière's disease** (a serious inner ear disorder), as well as profound unilateral hearing loss, is a contraindication to diving. The risks of diving with profound unilateral hearing loss, especially in view of the propensity for divers to incur ear problems, outweigh the benefits.

Divers avoid the mask squeeze by exhaling via the nose into the mask in order to eliminate the pressure differential developed during descent. With ordinary goggles there is no way to equalize pressures around the eyes; these goggles, therefore, should be used only for surface swimming. One can avoid the suit squeeze by wearing a properly fitting suit and, when using dry suits, divers' insulated underwear. Finally, divers should seek dental attention for decayed teeth before diving.

Return to Diving

With minor ear and sinus squeezes, return to diving is permissible as soon as ear-clearing becomes easy. The medications mentioned may also be used at this stage. Eardrum perforations usually heal in two weeks. People should not dive during this healing period because water may enter the middle ear spaces and cause serious infections. The eardrum should be examined for healing before resumption of diving activities. Profound hearing loss, labyrinthitis (infections of the inner ear structures), and round window rupture must be resolved before resumption of diving can even be considered.

Thoracic Squeeze

Thoracic squeeze is an extremely rare MPD. The question is, does it even warrant a discussion? For several reasons, it does. First, historically this condition was associated with the horrendous condition of total body squeeze. This occurred in hard hat divers when a leak or interruption in their air supply resulted in depressurization of the noncompressible helmet. Because of the enormous pressure differential between the inside of the helmet (surface pressure) and the ambient pressure around the diver's body, the diver's body was forced into the helmet. This was a thoracic squeeze with crushing inward not only of the chest wall but of the entire body. Because of the installation of nonreturn pressure valves at the connection of the air hose to the helmet, it no longer occurs. Second, thoracic squeeze can be associated with breath-hold diving, as a case study later in the chapter confirms. Third, the adaptations that diving mammals have made, as well as the acclimatizations that human divers demonstrate to prevent thoracic squeeze, are fascinating from a comparative physiology perspective (see chapter 5).

Significance

Thoracic squeeze is a MPD that occurs only in the breath-hold diver, and its incidence (number of reported cases with respect to the total population of divers) makes it almost nonexistent. There appears to only be one reported case with pathology reports to confirm that the diagnosis exists. However, the physiology and anatomy of the human lung indicate that this organ is subject to injury consistent with thoracic squeeze. The puzzle is why the condition is not observed more frequently in breath-hold divers, especially those who far exceed their predicted safe breath-hold dive depth limits.

Cause

The cause of thoracic squeeze is believed to be well understood. During descent while breath-holding, the lungs act like air-filled balloons. As descent continues, the volumes of the lungs decrease as described by Boyle's Law. However, once they decrease to their residual volume, the lungs no longer act like air-filled balloons. They act like rigid-walled, air-filled structures analogous to the middle ear spaces. Thus, from a compartment conceptualization perspective, the lungs change from an air-filled, flexible-walled compartment to an air-filled, rigid-walled compartment at the point where they reach their residual volumes (see chapter 1). With further descent, pressure differentials develop between the liquid–solid structures of the body, for example, the blood vessels in the lungs, former air-filled, flexible wall structures, the alveoli, which now act as rigid-walled structures. In an effort to equalize the pressure differential, analogous to what is seen in the ear squeeze, fluid portions of the blood and then blood itself leak into the alveoli. When this occurs, the alveoli no longer exchange gas with the blood vessels surrounding the alveoli, and in effect, the person suffocates from the blood in the alveoli.

Although the cause seems clear, the circumstances leading to this effect may vary. For example, the maximum predicted depth threshold would be the depth that causes the total lung volume to compress beyond the **residual lung volume** (volume of the air in the lungs after full expiration). For an average-sized male who starts his dive with the maximum possible amount of air in his lungs (vital capacity), the threshold would be about 132 FSW (40 MSW). If the diver starts the descent with a lesser amount of air in his lungs, the depth threshold will be correspondingly less (shallower). Conversely, shifting of abdominal contents and dilation of venous sinuses into the lung cavity appear to compensate for the collapsing lungs and allow deeper thresholds to be reached without lung injury (see chapter 5). Hyperinflation of the lungs, another technique that deep breath-hold divers claim to use, may further lower (deepen) the threshold. For whatever reasons, the world record breath-hold dive depths far exceed the divers' predicted thoracic squeeze depth thresholds.

Effects on the Body (Pathophysiology)

Once the **alveolar spaces** (the small air chambers in the pulmonary tissue where gas exchange takes place) begin to fill with fluid and blood, oxygen and carbon dioxide exchange is hampered. If the insult is minimal, the symptoms may go unnoticed. However, if they are more extensive, the person begins to manifest symptoms associated with progressively declining oxygen levels in the blood and body tissues. As discussed in previous chapters, the brain is the organ that is most sensitive to oxygen deprivation. Initial symptoms may be light-headedness and confusion. The heart, in response to low oxygen levels in the blood, beats faster. Shortness of breath from elevated carbon dioxide levels is not noted initially because this gas has about 40 times the diffusion capacity that oxygen has. Therefore, carbon dioxide may still be exchanged with the ambient air while insufficient oxygen is able to enter the bloodstream. This occurs because of the barrier that blood and fluids have created in the alveoli. Consequently, symptoms of low oxygen tensions in the body will be manifested long before those of elevated carbon dioxide levels.

The next stage of progressive oxygen deprivation to the brain is loss of consciousness. Meanwhile, the other most critical organ in the context of oxygen deprivation, the heart, begins to show the effects of hypoxia (low oxygen levels). Although the findings may be variable, irregular heart rhythms are usually the next finding after speeding of the heart rate. As oxygen deprivation worsens, the heart muscles lose their ability to contract. Finally, the heart stops beating. Cardiac arrest from this cause does not respond to **resuscitation** (the restoration to life or consciousness of one apparently dead), and the person dies.

First-Response Interventions

Recovery, resuscitation with oxygen breathing if available, and transport to a medical center as in all other serious MPD are the first-line responses. Recovery may require a swimming rescue if the person loses consciousness while submerged. However, the rescuer should not put him- or herself in jeopardy. Several considerations arise in the decision whether or not to attempt an immediate swimming rescue. First, the sooner the person is rescued, as in any situation of loss of consciousness in the water, the better the chances for recovery. The rescuer or the dive partner cannot be sure what has caused the loss of consciousness, since there are a dozen or more possible causative conditions. Second, if loss of consciousness occurs near the surface, the rescue will be easier than if the person has to be retrieved from the bottom. Third, if the person is sinking and the rescuer is swimming after him or her, the rescuer must make the crucial decision whether or not to continue the descent since the rescuer is at risk for loss of consciousness also (see chapter 11). The events of the rescue may distract the rescuer from recognizing warning signs of air hunger. If the dive partner is unable to retrieve the victim, then it is necessary to summon additional help and perform the retrieval with a diving rescue team. The delay in mobilizing the rescue team will probably make attempts to resuscitate the person futile after the recovery.

Resuscitation in the water should be limited to airway control. If the rescue was rapid, the person may resume breathing spontaneously once on the surface. If the person is not breathing on the surface, cardiopulmonary resuscitation is not recommended while still in the water. He or she should be moved to a platform (boat, pier, etc.) or the shore where resuscitation can be done more efficiently. In addition, the diving reflex or the coolness of the water temperature, or both, may offer protection against the consequences of oxygen deprivation to the brain and heart. Once on the surface, resuscitation with oxygen should be performed if possible. Since oxygen resuscitation equipment is becoming increasingly available on diving boats and at lifeguard stations, this is another advantage of getting the diver out of the water as soon as possible.

Transportation to a medical center should be done expediently. This may require using a boat to bring the person to shore, then transport by ambulance or helicopter. Even if the person appears to be OK soon after the rescue, he or she needs to be evaluated by qualified medical personnel before discharge. While the individual is being transported, vital signs (pulse, breathing rate, and blood pressure) should be monitored, and any changes should be reported to the medical personnel taking over the care. Oxygen breathing needs to be continued during the transit.

BRINGING IT ALL TOGETHER

CASE STUDY 1

A 30-year-old naval officer decided to begin diving training in the navy. He accomplished ear-clearing easily during the training dives to 30 FSW (9.1 MSW). However, he was consistently unable to clear his ears beyond the 50-FSW (15-MSW) depth. This necessitated his withdrawal from diving school.

Comment: The officer's ability to clear his ears at shallow depths, where volume–pressure changes are the greatest for each foot of descent as compared to the deeper depths, is paradoxical. It would seem that factors other than the mechanics of pressure equilibration in the middle ear spaces accounted for his inability to clear his ears at deeper depths. A trial of pressurization in a recompression chamber might help answer the question, but that did not happen for this diver. Ultimately, psychological factors were felt to be a significant contributor to his ear-clearing problem.

CASE STUDY 2

A 27-year-old fit and experienced diver was performing deep breath-hold dives with a buddy at a site where the bottom depth was 80 FSW (24 MSW). He apparently lost consciousness during the final 10 feet (three meters) of his ascent and began to sink. The diving buddy, who was watching from the surface, immediately submerged and retrieved the person at an estimated depth of 40 FSW (12 MSW). Upon being brought to the surface, the diver was not breathing. However, after a few moments of coughing and retching, breathing resumed spontaneously. Gradually the diver regained consciousness as a passing dive boat was being signaled. The diver was taken to a recompression facility about 20 minutes from the dive site. Because of an apparent "full" recovery and no history of breathing compressed gas, the decision was made to not recompress the diver with hyperbaric oxygen.

The loss of consciousness was attributed to blackout and near-drowning. The man was then transferred to a local hospital where he was observed and monitored. For the next hour he felt OK, but his heart rate began to increase. Oxygen breathing via a mask was instituted. Then the diver said he was starting to feel "badly." Complaints included light-headedness, weakness, and confusion. He then became very agitated. Measurements of his blood oxygen levels revealed that they had become dangerously low. For this reason, he was intubated and ventilated with pure oxygen. Nevertheless, his heart rate continued to increase. When it reached 200 beats per minute, he arrested, and all resuscitation efforts were unsuccessful. Subsequently, samples of his lung tissue were sent to two of the preeminent lung pathologists in the United States. Each reported, without collaboration, that the lung pathology was consistent with pulmonary barotrauma (pressure injury) from a thoracic squeeze, and not the findings of near-drowning or air embolism.

This case study poses many questions for discussion:

1. What are some of the possible causes for the diver's loss of consciousness during ascent (see discussion of blackout in chapter 11)?

Answer: Hyperventilation-associated blackout, diffusional blackout, cardiac arrest or arrhythmia, and anoxia.

2. What are some of the reasons the diver began to sink, apparently after losing consciousness near the surface?

Answer: He may have been negatively buoyant to aid the descent. After he lost consciousness, swimming movements to help him reach the surface ceased. In addition, after loss of consciousness the elastic recoil of the lung would lead to passive exhalation and loss of the tidal volume (see chapter 5) and would contribute to negative buoyancy.

3. What happens to a diver's ability to maintain his or her total lung capacity (as much air as the lungs can hold) after losing consciousness?

Answer: With loss of consciousness, the air in the lungs would probably be exhaled passively due to the elastic recoil of the lung tissue.

4. How would the passive loss of air to the residual volume (air left in the lungs after exhaling fully) affect the diver's thoracic squeeze depth threshold?

Answer: It would substantially reduce it. Any further descent would now exceed the thoracic squeeze threshold and likely lead to thoracic squeeze.

5. Why did the diver's heart rate continue to increase even though he was intubated and ventilated with 100 percent oxygen?

Answer: The thoracic squeeze injury interfered with oxygen exchange in the lungs so that insufficient oxygen was being provided to the tissues. To compensate for this the heart rate increased to circulate the blood faster in an attempt to meet the body tissues' oxygen demands.

6. Why did the patient's condition deteriorate several hours after he had regained consciousness and appeared OK for a couple of hours?

Answer: This interval represented the time it took for pressure-induced microscopic bleeding and fluid leakage in the lungs to reach the point of beginning to interfere with ventilation.

7. What signs and symptoms appear as blood oxygen levels progressively decrease? Why may "air hunger" (shortness of breath) not be one of the observations?

Answer: Increased respiratory and heart rates, confusion, restlessness, altered mental status, and loss of consciousness occur with progressive oxygen deprivation to the brain. The altered mental status and loss of consciousness symptoms may mask the "air hunger" symptoms. Also, carbon dioxide diffuses out of the alveolar-capillary boundary of the lungs 40 times better than oxygen diffuses in. Carbon dioxide elevations are primarily responsible for air hunger.

8. Why did the diver develop a thoracic squeeze even though he did not approach his theoretical thoracic squeeze depth threshold (estimated to be 132 FSW or 40 MSW)?

Answer: With loss of consciousness during ascent, he probably lost the tidal volume of air in his lungs. Any descent from this point would reduce his lung volume beyond his residual volume and put him at risk for thoracic squeeze.

9. How might the lung pathology in thoracic squeeze differ from that of arterial gas embolism (see chapter 15), near-drowning, or drowning (see chapter 16)?

Answer: With arterial gas embolism, ruptured alveoli (air sacs) and adjacent blood vessels are expected to be present. With near-drowning and drowning, edema fluid and atelectasis (collapse of the alveoli) are present. In direct confirmatory evidence of near-drowning, drowning is the finding of diatoms (microscopic plants with hard shells) in the alveoli.

Definitive Management

Definitive management is directed toward the patient's needs. If the patient is in satisfactory condition, then all that is required is monitoring of vital signs and observation. The patient may not start deteriorating until several hours after the incident, as oxygen exchange progressively worsens as the patient's own body fluids collect in the lungs. If deterioration occurs, problems need to be addressed expediently. Most are directed toward maintaining blood oxygen levels. This may require intubation and control of breathing with a ventilator. If near-drowning and water aspiration are suspected, antibiotics and steroids should be started. At this stage, close monitoring in an intensive care unit is necessary. Oxygenation of the blood with a heart–lung machine for a sustained period until healing or until further deteriorating in preparation for a lung transplant may be the only way to prevent death.

Prevention

Like all the causes of blackout, thoracic squeeze must be prevented. Prevention is through dive planning and knowledge of why the breath-hold diver is prone to blackout. Breath-hold divers should time their bottom times and start their ascents based on bottom time rather than on the desire to breathe. Deep, record-attempt breath-hold dives, if indeed they should be done at all, need to be closely monitored with standby divers and medical personnel at the scene. Sport breath-hold divers should always use the buddy system and should not perform deep dives in waters where neither diver can comfortably reach the bottom.

Return to Diving

If a diver survives a thoracic squeeze, can diving can be resumed? If the lung insult was minimal, then it is reasonable for the diver to resume diving activities after a suitable length of time. What this time interval is cannot be precisely stated since there are so few reported experiences of thoracic squeeze. Six weeks to three months should be sufficient time for the lungs to heal. However, better criteria are based on X-ray findings and **lung function testing** (diagnostic procedure that measures lung volumes and speed at which air goes in and out of the lung). If these studies are normal, then the breath-hold diver can return to diving after discussion of the preventive measures described previously. If the studies are abnormal, diving activities should not be resumed.

For Further Review

1. What are the factors that predispose the diver to barotrauma of the middle ear?

2. Why should a diver never try to overcome the pain by "swimming through" (keep on descending when unable to clear the ears) an ear squeeze?

3. How do the findings in the ear correlate with the severity of the ear squeeze?

4. How can overzealous use of vasoconstrictors and nasal decongestants be counterproductive in preventing ear squeezes?

5. What complications and additional problems can be associated with ear squeezes?

6. What needs to be considered before resumption of diving after an ear squeeze?

7. How does the three-compartment model help to explain what happens in thoracic squeeze?

8. Why are there questions as to whether or not thoracic squeeze is a concern for breath-hold divers?

BOTTOM PROBLEMS

Six medical problems of diving (MPD) are associated with the bottom phase of the dive. In contrast to descent problems, which result from the direct effects of pressure (see chapter 13), bottom problems better fit into the category of indirect effects of pressure. That is, the longer the duration of the dive, the deeper the dive, or both, the more likely these

Chapter Preview

- Bottom-related problems and why they are prone to occur with closed-circuit SCUBA diving
- Nitrogen narcosis
- Oxygen toxicity
- Carbon dioxide toxicity
- Dangers of hypoxia and anoxia
- Carbon monoxide poisoning and high-pressure nervous system syndromes and how they can affect divers

problems are to occur. Whereas Boyle's Law provides the basis for understanding what happens to the body with descent problems, bottom problems are explained by Dalton's and Henry's Laws (see chapter 1).

In the past, bottom problems were almost exclusively a concern of commercial divers who had equipment that put them at risk for these MPD. Today, with closed-circuit SCUBA equipment available to sport divers, allowing them to remain submerged for sustained periods, dive to deep depths, and avoid carbon dioxide accumulations and oxygen deprivation, bottom problems are a serious concern for this group also (figure 14.1). The efficiency of oxygen utilization from the tanks increases from 5 percent to almost 100 percent. Bottom problems are serious. If corrective actions are not initiated immediately, the diver can lose consciousness while underwater and drown. Because each bottom problem is distinct from the others, the references for this chapter are listed separately by disorders.

Nitrogen Narcosis

Nitrogen narcosis is a clinical condition characterized by **impairment** (a physical or mental condition that reduces the level of function of the involved body part) of mental and neuromuscular performance and changes in mood

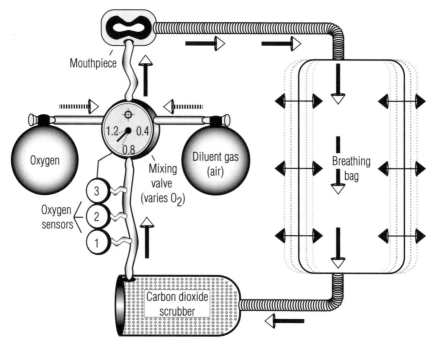

FIGURE 14.1   Schematic of the closed-circuit SCUBA rig.

and behavior due to the increased partial pressures of nitrogen in the breathing medium. Its effects are proportional to the partial pressure of nitrogen in the breathing medium and the duration of the exposure. There are also marked variations in susceptibility to nitrogen narcosis.

Significance

Nitrogen narcosis itself does not cause permanent harm to the body. However, impairment of mental or motor functions underwater can have serious consequences. The great danger of nitrogen narcosis is that the diver will perform irrational, life-endangering acts such as removing the regulator from the mouth or swimming deeper than is safe. For this reason, it is sometimes referred to with the picturesque expression **rapture of the deep.** These acts then put the diver at risk for more serious problems such as panic, arterial gas embolism, blackout, and drowning.

Causes

The cause of nitrogen narcosis is the increased partial pressure of nitrogen in the breathing medium (see chapter 1). This increases the amount of nitrogen dissolved in the body tissues. At some point in the pressure increase, for reasons not understood, nitrogen no longer behaves as an **inert gas** (a gas that forms no chemical combinations with other substances). It begins to affect the human brain similarly to laughing gas and alcohol. The greater the pressure, the more pronounced the effect. When the diver's mental function begins to be affected, the diagnosis of nitrogen narcosis is made. Nitrogen is thought to be forced into the brain tissues in these situations, causing inhibition of brain activity. The rational decision-making and judgment areas of the brain are most affected. Although the effects of nitrogen narcosis lie in the central nervous system, the exact cellular site of action remains a mystery. The following theories have been proposed to explain why nitrogen narcosis occurs:

• Myer-Overton: This theory states that any inert gas will cause an inhibitory effect on the nervous system when enough of the inert gas is forced into the nervous system.

• Quastel-metabolic: According to this theory, high pressures of inert gases interfere with metabolism of the cell. The most sensitive cells are those of the brain. The higher (conscious) centers of the brain are the first to experience this effect.

• Clathrate: Under pressure nitrogen is forced into combination with water and protein molecules to form a clathrate. The clathrate interferes with nerve conduction. The tissues most sensitive to these effects are those of the higher centers of the brain.

• Iceberg: When gases dissolve in water, the water molecules organize into units called "icebergs." It is supposed that each inert gas and anesthetic agent forms its own characteristic iceberg. The iceberg acts on the nervous system similarly to the clathrate.

Effects on the Body (Pathophysiology)

There is a wide range in individual susceptibility to nitrogen narcosis. The diver's fitness, past deep diving experiences, underwater diving, working conditions, and exertion level affect when narcosis will be noted. Many factors influence the diver's susceptibility to nitrogen narcosis (see table 14.1). The first symptoms appear at approximately 130- to 150-FSW (40- to 46-MSW) depths and are similar to those of moderate alcoholic intoxication or the early stages of hypoxia. Whereas one diver may be **narced** (a slang expression for the effects of nitrogen narcosis) at 130 FSW, an experienced diver may be able to function normally at depths of 180 FSW (55 MSW) or more. As the depth increases, all divers show impairment of thought, time perception, judgment, reasoning, memory, and ability to perform mental or motor tasks, as well as increased reaction time. These symptoms represent progressive **inhibition** (restraint of activity) of the higher centers of the brain. They fairly well correspond to a concept labeled the **martini law,** according to which each 50

Table 14.1 Factors That Affect Susceptibility to Nitrogen Narcosis	
Increase[a]	**Decrease[b]**
Alcohol intoxication	Clear visibility
Anxiety	Central nervous system stimulants (not advised for use in diving due to the lack of evidence of their effectiveness, possible dependence, and side effects):
Chilling	
Effects of motion sickness remedies, antihistamines, and sedatives (i.e., "downers")	
	Amphetamines
	Caffeine
Elevated blood carbon dioxide level	
Fatigue	Concentration on a specific mission (e.g., finding a lost object on the bottom)
Individual susceptibility	
Overexertion	Deep sea diving in a "hard hat"
Poor visibility	Experience
Prolonged exposure to depth	Good physical condition
Hypoxia	Warm water

[a] Factors that decrease nervous system function; [b] factors that increase nervous system function, sensory perception, or both.

FSW (15 MSW) of descent has a narcotic effect equal to one martini and the effects are additive. The symptoms in order of progression and severity include the following:

- Mild **euphoria**—a happy state with mild performance impairment that may decrease the ability to work, lessen concentration, interfere with reasoning, and cause short-term memory deficits

- Fixations of ideas, overconfidence, further impairment of mental performance

- Disinterest, disregard for safety (classically, the diver offers his SCUBA regulator to the fish), and uncontrolled laughter

- Intoxication—with severe performance impairment; possible hallucinations

- Total confusion with possibly life-threatening performance impairment

- Stupor and unconsciousness

The onset of narcosis is rapid. Fortunately, recovery is equally rapid. Once the diver ascends to a shallower depth, signs and symptoms of nitrogen narcosis disappear. On the surface some divers may have amnesia, not remembering that they experienced an episode of nitrogen narcosis while underwater.

First-Response Interventions

The immediate management of narcosis is ascent to shallower depths to reduce the partial pressure of nitrogen. The rescuer must try to prevent other more serious problems such as the "narced" diver's removing the regulator or breath-holding during ascent. The rescuer must also be alert to the fact that the person may not want to leave the dreamlike state of nitrogen narcosis and may resist—possibly violently—efforts to ascend.

Definitive Management

For uncomplicated nitrogen narcosis, no definitive treatments are required. However, if nitrogen narcosis has caused problems, such as hypoxia, near-drowning, or unscheduled ascent, immediate measures need to be taken to correct these specific secondary problems.

Prevention

One prevents nitrogen narcosis by not diving too deeply. Divers should adhere to the maximum depth recommendation of 130 FSW (40 MSW) for sport SCUBA diving. In general, substances that depress nervous system function (e.g., **downers,** a slang expression for drugs that depress

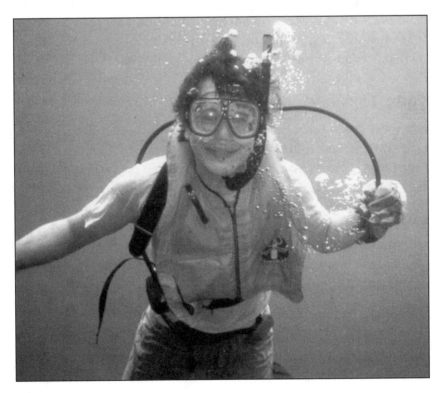

The first symptoms of nitrogen narcosis are similar to those of mild intoxication or the early stages of hypoxia, including impairment of thought and judgment.

the nervous system) lower (make shallower) the threshold depth for nitrogen narcosis. Cold water, alcohol intoxication, elevated blood carbon dioxide levels, fatigue, the effects of motion sickness remedies, sedatives, and longer exposure times increase the diver's susceptibility to nitrogen narcosis. Many of these factors can be avoided or modified with appropriate pre-dive planning and equipment selection. Substances that stimulate nervous system function may increase (make deeper) the threshold depth for nitrogen narcosis.

Because nitrogen narcosis interferes with performance, other gases are substituted for nitrogen when deep diving is required. Helium is the gas most often utilized for this purpose. This permits very deep dives with virtually no inert gas narcosis, but problems do arise from using helium (see discussion of high-pressure nervous system syndrome later in this chapter). Neon, argon, and xenon have also been used as inert gases for diving. Hydrogen has many desirable characteristics as an inert gas, but its explosive qualities make it impractical to use at this time.

Return to Diving

As already noted, by the time the diver reaches the surface, the symptoms of nitrogen narcosis will have cleared. Return to diving is contingent on the diver's feeling OK and the absence of complications that could have occurred with the nitrogen narcosis episode. The diver should be counseled about safe diving practices and methods of avoiding nitrogen narcosis.

Oxygen Toxicity

Exposure to oxygen under increased pressures disrupts function and causes damage to all tissues in the body. As noted in earlier chapters, the brain is the organ that is most sensitive to elevated oxygen pressures. The lungs and the eyes also are more sensitive to oxygen than other body tissues. As with other bottom problems, whether or not oxygen toxicity occurs depends both on the partial pressure of oxygen (depth) and on the duration of exposure. Also, as in nitrogen narcosis, tolerance to elevations of oxygen partial pressures varies from person to person, from day to day in the same person, and with the level of activity.

Significance

Oxygen toxicity is almost a nonexistent problem for the open-circuit SCUBA diver using air since it would require a dive to 300 FSW (91 MSW) for 30 minutes to exceed oxygen toxicity limits. However, diving techniques using nitrox mixtures or pure oxygen put the sport diver at risk for oxygen toxicity (see chapter 2). In addition, should the diver require

BRINGING IT ALL TOGETHER

CASE STUDY 1

A 30-year-old diver with a moderate amount of experience, but no SCUBA dives greater than 100 FSW (30 MSW), was diving under ideal conditions (warm water, no currents, almost 100-foot visibility) along a wall with a group of sport divers. Because of negative buoyancy he gradually drifted down to about 150 FSW (46 MSW). At this point he began swimming after a large fish, away from the wall and toward open water. Fortunately, the diving guide immediately realized something was wrong, descended to the diver, and signaled him to ascend. The diver initially resisted, but after the guide tugged sharply upward a couple of times on the buoyancy compensator straps, the diver seemed to come out of his trance and ascended with the guide holding on to the shoulder strap of the buoyancy compensator. The remainder of the dive was completed uneventfully.

On the surface, when asked to recount his experience, the diver said that as he had drifted downward, he felt warm and glowing all over, a feeling he had not experienced while diving. He thought he had come upon a mermaid and had decided to follow it. He felt the dive guide's tugs on his buoyancy compensator, which apparently brought him back to reality.

1. Had the diver guide not immediately responded to the situation, what could have been the outcome?

Answer: The diver could have rapidly run out of air because of the rapid depletion of air in the SCUBA tank with increasing depth, become more narcotized, or both. Once he realized something was wrong he would probably have bolted for the surface—holding his breath if he had run out of air. If he had lost consciousness during ascent he could have drowned; if he reached the surface, arterial gas embolism could have occurred. Had he continued to sink, he would have become more narcotized and probably would have lost consciousness if his air supply was not used up.

2. What errors in diving did the diver commit?

Answer: The diver failed to appreciate his negative buoyancy. He should have used his depth gauge or dive computer to monitor the depth. He should have stayed with his dive buddy or made sure he did not descend deeper than the dive guide.

3. Why did the dive guide not become "narced" when he descended to rescue the diver?

Answer: The guide likely was experienced enough to tolerate the increased nitrogen partial pressures without narcotic effects at the 150-FSW depth. Further, his focus on rescuing the diver probably afforded an additional degree of protection from nitrogen narcosis.

hyperbaric oxygen recompression therapy for decompression illness, oxygen toxicity is a risk since pure oxygen exposures under pressure are pushed nearly to their limits.

Causes

The cause of oxygen toxicity is an increased "dose" of oxygen in the breathing medium. Four factors contribute to the development of oxygen toxicity: the partial pressure of oxygen, the duration of exposure, the level of activity, and individual susceptibility. Although oxygen toxicity exposure limits exist, they are guidelines only; and at least for navy divers, they have been revised to allow

> ## Diving Physics: The Difference Between Toxicity and Poisoning
>
> **Toxicity,** as in oxygen and carbon dioxide toxicity, results from substances that are normally present in the body but cause damage when present in high concentrations.
>
> Poisoning, as in carbon monoxide poisoning, refers to a disorder that results from the introduction of a substance not normally found in the body. A **poison** is a substance that causes tissue injury or death when taken into the body. However, what defines a poison is also open to question. For example, a medication may cure a disease when taken in correct amounts but damage or kill if taken in excessive amounts.

longer exposures for any particular depth in the ranges used for pure oxygen diving. A standard exposure limit guideline is 2 ATA or 33 FSW (10 MSW) for 30 minutes. With hyperbaric oxygen exposures, these time limits are frequently quadrupled. However, in contrast to the diver, the patient remains at total rest during the treatment and is made comfortable temperature-wise. Consequently, the guidelines predicting the occurrence of oxygen toxicity are less precise than those of other MPD such as blackout conditions and decompression illness.

Effects on the Body (Pathophysiology)

Analogously to the situation with nitrogen narcosis, it is not totally clear why high pressures of oxygen lead to oxygen toxicity. In high concentrations, oxygen appears to inhibit pathways of cellular metabolism in one or more of the following ways:

• Inactivation of sulfur–hydrogen bonds: Many substances vital to cell metabolism contain sulfur and hydrogen links, so-called sulphydryl groups (-SH). Oxygen breaks these links and inactivates the substances. The result is disruption of the normal metabolic pathways and accumulation of intermediate metabolites. These may cause oxygen toxicity.

• Formation of free radicals: Oxygen contributes to the formation of partially reduced oxygen products called **free radicals.** These oxygen products are very active chemically and react with cell membranes and products of **metabolism** (the sum of all the chemical processes taking place in the organism to produce energy). Antioxidants—medications that reduce formation of free radicals—raise the threshold exposure for oxygen toxicity.

• Gamma-aminobutyric acid (GABA): This is a substance in the central nervous system that reduces nerve excitation (firing off of impulses). Increased partial pressures of oxygen reduce the amount of GABA. **Convulsions** then occur because of uncontrolled firing of excitatory nerves. Agents that raise brain levels of GABA protect against convulsions.

• Changes in redox (oxidation and its counterpart, reduction) levels: All metabolic pathways in the body are in electrical equilibrium. Oxygen alters the electrical equilibrium, causing disruption of the metabolic pathways.

• Hormonal modifications: Some **hormones** (naturally occurring substances secreted by specialized cells that affect the metabolism or function of other cells) and steroids cause symptoms of oxygen toxicity to appear at lower thresholds than normal while others prevent symptoms from occurring. For example, high doses of steroids appear to lower the threshold for oxygen seizures.

Central Nervous System Oxygen Toxicity (Paul Bert Effect)   The seizure is the most serious effect of oxygen toxicity. Seizures are associated with short-duration, high partial pressure exposures to oxygen as may occur with diving. Usually the seizure occurs suddenly, but there may be warning symptoms as listed by the mnemonic in figure 14.2. A seizure is a serious enough matter when it occurs on land; but when it occurs in the water, the diver can drown. In those who have a seizure history, convulsions may occur with oxygen exposures much less than the predicted threshold.

Mnemonic: CON-VENTID
CON = convulsion
VENT = ventilation
ID = identification

IDentify the symptoms that precede **CON**vulsion; **VENT**ilate with air to reduce the oxygen partial pressure; (ascend) to prevent a **CON**vulsion.

V	=	Visual disturbances, especially tunnel vision
E	=	Ears: ringing and music sounds in the ears
N	=	Nausea
T	=	Twitching, especially of the lips and hands
I	=	Irritability, anxiety, restlessness
D	=	Dizziness

FIGURE 14.2   Symptoms of oxygen toxicity of the brain.

Pulmonary Oxygen Toxicity (Lorrain Smith Effect)   Pulmonary oxygen toxicity, in contrast to central nervous system oxygen toxicity, is associated with prolonged exposures at lower partial pressures. For example, patients who breathe pure oxygen uninterrupted on the surface for more then 12 hours begin to show signs of pulmonary oxygen toxicity. The alveoli (air sacs) in the lungs begin to leak fluid and collapse (atelectasis). Usually the first symptoms of pulmonary oxygen toxicity are substernal discomfort, cough, and chest tightness that mimic an upper respiratory tract infection. Later, shortness of breath, chest pain, and deficient oxygenation develop in association with decreased vital capacity of the lungs. Ordinarily, pulmonary oxygen toxicity is not associated with diving activities. However, divers are subject to this problem when extended and or repetitive hyperbaric oxygen recompression treatments are given for the most serious presentations of decompression illness (see chapter 15).

Other Effects   Two other manifestations of breathing oxygen at high pressures may have relevance to divers. Oxygen at high pressures can affect vision. This is thought to be due to constriction of the blood vessels in the retina (vision-sensing portion) of the eye, a direct effect of breathing oxygen at increased partial pressures. Decreased visual acuity could interfere with reading dive computer gauges and seeing objects underwater. A second effect is observed in the middle ear spaces. Fluid accumulates in the middle ear spaces, leading to **serous otitis media,** when one breathes pure oxygen under pressure. The condition may be due to oxygen absorption by the lining of the middle ear spaces, causing a reverse ear squeeze or a direct toxic effect with fluid accumulation similar to that seen in the lungs.

First-Response Interventions

Management of oxygen toxicity consists of immediately reducing the partial pressure of oxygen in the breathing medium. This is accomplished in two ways: (1) ascent and (2) switching gas mixtures from pure oxygen to air. In the hyperbaric chamber, this second method is easy to carry out. However, ascent may be the only option for the diver. If a seizure occurs while the person is submerged, he or she should be brought to the surface. Extreme precautions must be followed to avoid rupturing the person's lungs during ascent. This is accomplished by keeping the neck in the extended position. On the surface, attention must focus on airway control and prevention of self-injury, such as chewing on the tongue or banging the head against a hard object. Most oxygen toxicity–related seizures cease immediately upon ascent. After the seizure, the person may be lethargic and require help to get out of the water. All victims of oxygen toxicity seizures require transport to a medical facility and evaluation by a physician.

Definitive Management

By the time the patient is seen by a physician, the seizure usually has ceased. If not, the patient receives **anticonvulsant** medications (medication that prevents or reduces convulsions) intravenously. The presence of other conditions that lower the seizure threshold is investigated. These include concurrent infections, flu syndromes, diving while excessively fatigued, previous history of seizures, and head trauma. These are managed as required. A magnetic resonance imaging study may be done to examine the brain for a seizure focus. If one is found, the patient will likely be placed on anticonvulsant medications.

Prevention

Oxygen toxicity seizures during diving are prevented by pre-dive screening to disqualify those with a history of seizures and by not exceeding the oxygen toxicity depth and time limits during diving with special equipment. The importance of depth limits cannot be overemphasized. As the diver descends, the partial pressures increase proportionally as described by Dalton's Law (see chapter 1). For example, at 66 FSW (20 MSW), the partial pressure of oxygen is three times as great as on the surface. Diving with nitrox mixtures magnifies oxygen partial pressures with increasing depths (see chapter 2). Vitamin E has been given to reduce the incidence of oxygen toxicity seizures for patients receiving repetitive hyperbaric oxygen treatment, but its effectiveness for divers has not been proven. Table 14.2 summarizes factors that can modify the oxygen toxicity threshold.

Return to Diving

Any diver who has had a seizure resulting from oxygen toxicity or some other factor while diving should not return to diving until evaluated and given permission by a physician. If it is ascertained that the seizure was caused by oxygen toxicity and that the oxygen toxicity threshold was exceeded during the dive, return to diving is permissible after the diver has rested for a few days. If the threshold for oxygen toxicity seizures was not exceeded, then a workup for a seizure focus in the brain is necessary. A magnetic resonance imaging study, an electrical brain wave test (electroencephalogram), and examination by a neurologist are the usual procedures. If no reason can be found for the seizure, then return to diving requires the combined decision of a neurologist and a physician with training in undersea and hyperbaric medicine. An oxygen tolerance test in the controlled environment of a hyperbaric chamber might also precede any decision to allow the diver to resume diving. If a reason (abnormal finding in the brain) for the seizure is identified, then the diver is usually disqualified from diving.

Table 14.2	Factors That Affect Oxygen Toxicity	
Increase	**Decrease**
Endogenous (within the body) • Adrenocortical (cortisone-like) hormones • Carbon dioxide • Epinephrine (adrenaline), norepinephrine • Insulin • Thyroid hormones	Endogenous substances (metabolic products produced in the body) • Gamma-aminobutyric acid (GABA) • Glutamine • Glutathione
Exogenous (outside the body) • Amiodarone (for heart arrhythmias) • Amphetamines • Aspirin • Atropine • Bleomycin (for cancer treatment) • Disulfiram (Antabuse—to stop alcohol consumption) • Ibuprofen (Motrin) • Mafenide acetate (Sulfamylon burn ointment)	Exogenous substances • Adrenal cortex blockers • Antioxidants (vitamin E) • Anticonvulsants (seizure prevention medications) • Benzodiazepines (anti-anxiety medications) • Caffeine • Cimetidine (for stomach ulcers) • Lithium • Vitamin C
Special conditions • Exercise • Fever • Hyperthermia • Hyperthyroidism • Stress • Vitamin E deficiency	Special conditions • Adaptation to hyperoxia • Hypothyroidism • Starvation

Carbon Dioxide Toxicity

Carbon dioxide toxicity occurs when the amount of carbon dioxide in the body exceeds physiological levels. The initial responses are positive feedback mechanisms. Elevated carbon dioxide levels are often an indirect signal that oxygen levels in the body are low. When the positive feedback mechanisms for responding to elevations of carbon dioxide are overwhelmed, carbon dioxide may produce unconsciousness and death. In contrast to most of the other bottom problems, which correspond to no-panic syndromes, the symptoms of acute carbon dioxide toxicity are more similar to those associated with the panic syndrome (see chapter 11). This chapter deals with acute, diving-related carbon dioxide toxicity in contrast to effects of chronic exposures such as kidney stones and loss of responsiveness to this gas to stimulate breathing.

BRINGING IT ALL TOGETHER

CASE STUDY 1

A 55-year-old male was diving with a 36 percent oxygen nitrox (nitrox II) mixture. Although he had been SCUBA diving for years, he had just recently been certified in nitrox diving. His diving partner was diving with air. Their goal was to inspect a sunken fishing boat in 120 feet (37 meters) of water. The diver recalled that if he used the same air diving tables his dive partner was using he would have added protection against decompression sickness, which was his biggest concern due to his age and the relatively deep depth of the dive.

After 10 minutes (of a maximum 15 minutes no-decompression time on the air tables) at the 120-FSW depth, the diver began to feel very anxious. When he checked his tank pressure gauge he felt as though he was looking through a gun barrel. In none of his previous SCUBA dives (more than 200) had he experienced anything similar. Even though he had over 750 PSI pressure in his tank, he signaled his partner that he was low on air and started to ascend. During his ascent he began to feel better, and by the time he reached the 15-foot (4.6-meter) rest stop he felt normal. After surfacing and reviewing the events, as well as his nitrox training manual, the diver realized that he violated the maximum oxygen depth limit (110 FSW or 33 MSW) listed for 36 percent oxygen nitrox diving and had experienced preconvulsion symptoms of oxygen toxicity.

Comment: The diver's oxygen toxicity symptoms fortunately did not progress to a seizure. Often the antecedent symptoms are absent, and a seizure is the presenting symptom for oxygen toxicity. As the diver realized after reviewing the events of the dive, he had violated rules of nitrox diving. He did not check the maximum depth limit for 36 percent oxygen nitrox diving, which is 110 FSW, but rather relied on air tables for determining the depth and duration of the dive.

CASE STUDY 2

A 35-year-old female diver who had been diving for several years developed right shoulder pain, after an obvious violation of her dive computer limits, from a long deep dive. The diagnosis of "deserved" decompression sickness (see chapters 3 and 15) was made. During recompression in the hyperbaric chamber the patient became asymptomatic after breathing oxygen for a few minutes at the 60-FSW (18-MSW) depth in the chamber. After 18 minutes into the third oxygen breathing period the patient became tremulous and then began to seize. The attendant inside the chamber removed the oxygen mask so that the patient would breathe air rather than oxygen and protected the patient's head from injury as the pressure in the chamber was brought to the surface level. After a few feet of ascent the seizing stopped.

Although the patient listed no history of seizures when she completed the medical questionnaire before obtaining her SCUBA diving certification, when questioned after her seizure in the chamber she admitted to having had a seizure in the past. This was associated with a head injury from an automobile accident 10 years earlier that had resulted in a concussion (a period of loss of consciousness) and a single seizure after the regaining of consciousness. Anticonvulsants were prescribed, and the patient took the initial supply but then decided not to refill the prescription. She

(continued)

(continued)

had had no seizure problems in the interim 10 years and had forgotten the incident when she filled out her medical questionnaire before starting diving training. The diver was given an electrical brain wave test that showed a small abnormal focus in the movement area of her brain, presumably secondary to the head injury. The next day she was given a second "washout" hyperbaric oxygen treatment after taking a sedative–anticonvulsant medication.

1. What factors contributed to the patient's seizure in the chamber? Why had she not had a seizure during her many previous dives?

Answer: The challenge of breathing hyperbaric oxygen during the treatment for decompression sickness was enough to exceed the patient's seizure threshold. It is unlikely that any of her preceding activities, even while diving, generated oxygen partial pressures that approached those with a hyperbaric oxygen treatment.

2. Should she be given permission to SCUBA dive after this occurrence? If the electrical brain wave test had been normal, would this change the decision?

Answer: Most undersea medical physicians would consider the events in this case study an absolute contraindication for SCUBA diving. If the brain wave test had been normal, a medical OK to dive would be reasonable, since a seizure, without an underlying predisposition, during a hyperbaric treatment is not a contraindication to resume hyperbaric oxygen treatments. In a situation like this diver's, however, a joint decision by an undersea and hyperbaric medical specialist and a neurologist is recommended prior to approval of resumption of SCUBA diving.

3. How reliable is the medical history questionnaire as a prerequisite for SCUBA diving instruction?

Answer: It is a good screening device. However, omissions, either accidental or willful, mean that it is not 100 percent effective as an information source. On the other hand, a complete medical exam with laboratory, imaging, and exercise testing may not detect problems that are willfully omitted from the questionnaire. Furthermore, a comprehensive evaluation with associated studies given without a magnetic resonance study can cost $1,000 or more. A magnetic resonance study costs $1,500 to $2,000.

4. What were the benefits of removing the oxygen breathing mask, having the patient breathe the air in the chamber, and bringing the chamber to the surface for managing a seizure in a hyperbaric chamber?

Answer: These techniques immediately lower the oxygen partial pressure of gas that the patient is breathing. Generally, they are highly effective and the seizure stops within moments of switching to air and starting the ascent.

Significance

For the majority of sport SCUBA diving activities, carbon dioxide toxicity is a nonexistent problem, because carbon dioxide is exhaled into the water with open-circuit SCUBA gear. Even with the most strenuous exercise, carbon dioxide will not accumulate to toxic levels despite the occurrence of extreme shortness of breath and concomitant hyperventilation. With improperly working closed-circuit SCUBA gear, though, carbon dioxide can accumulate to toxic levels. Since the system is closed, if the carbon dioxide scrubber malfunctions, this gas can increase to toxic levels (see chapter 2).

Causes

Carbon dioxide is a physiologically active gas. In the body it arises as an end product of metabolism and moves according to gradients of concentration from the tissues to the blood and then to the lungs, where it is expired. There is an enormous gradient for carbon dioxide to leave the body (see chapter 1). Normally, expired air (5 percent CO_2) contains over 100 times more carbon dioxide than inspired air (0.04 percent CO_2). While increased concentrations of carbon dioxide in inspired air may not be a problem on the surface, they may interfere with the elimination of this gas during diving.

Specific causes of carbon dioxide toxicity include the following:

• No carbon dioxide absorbent: The diver has failed to fill the carbon dioxide canister with Baralyme (the carbon dioxide absorbent) when using closed-circuit SCUBA gear.

• Inactivation of carbon dioxide absorbent: Flooding of the canister, extreme cold, or reversing the air line connections can result in inactivation of or marked decrease in the efficiency of the absorbent.

• Improper filling or setup of the carbon dioxide absorbent canister: The canister must be filled to capacity, the filter screen replaced, and the canister lid sealed properly. Failure to do so will result in ineffective carbon dioxide absorption in the closed-circuit apparatus.

• Working in confined spaces: Breathing the air in a confined space will result in progressive accumulation of carbon dioxide from rebreathing of the expired gas. Working in the head-down position in a deep sea diving rig can also result in carbon dioxide accumulation in the confined space of the diving

---

Diving Physics: Reversing the Carbon Dioxide Gradient With Descent

Q: If foul air on the surface contains 1.5 percent carbon dioxide (partial pressure of 11.4mmHg), what will the percentage and partial pressure be at 100 FSW (30 MSW or 4 ATA)? How does this carbon dioxide tension compare with the normal blood carbon dioxide tension at this depth?

A: *Although the percentages remain unchanged, the partial pressure increases fourfold to 45.6mmHg. Since the CO_2 tension in normal blood is 40mmHg, regardless of the depth, the gradient will be reversed and carbon dioxide will move from the inspired air in the lungs to the blood in response to the gradient.*

suit. As demonstrated by the preceding diving physics problem, if the partial pressure of carbon dioxide is increased due to increased ambient pressure, the likelihood of toxicity is even greater.

Effects on the Body (Pathophysiology)

The body initially responds to elevated carbon dioxide levels with positive feedback mechanisms including **hyperventilation** (an increase in rate and depth of respirations, either voluntary or involuntary) and increased heart rates. These responses are directed at increasing oxygen supplies to tissues, since the body's positive feedback responses to low oxygen are not as obvious as those to elevated carbon dioxide levels. Intermediate responses include **dilation** (widening) of the blood vessels in the brain and increased acidity of the blood. These responses help to ensure an adequate oxygen supply to the critical brain tissues. Endpoint responses that produce negative feedback include nausea, vomiting, feelings of suffocation, confusion, and unconsciousness. Carbon dioxide toxicity symptoms and their causes are listed in table 14.3. Increased physical activity may mask the initial symptoms of carbon dioxide toxicity since the physiological responses are similar. Acclimatizations occur to subacute exposures to elevated carbon dioxide tensions (see chapter 4). An associated presentation of carbon dioxide toxicity is that of burns in the respiratory tract and coughing. This occurs when water comes in contact with the carbon dioxide absorbent. Carbonic acid is produced from this chemical reaction. The fumes are toxic and cause burns when breathed.

First-Response Interventions

Usually the diver, especially if aware of carbon dioxide toxicity from previous diving training, is able to initiate the first-response interventions. The response is threefold: (1) quit the diving activity and exit the elevated carbon dioxide environment, (2) reduce the activity level, and (3) breathe

Table 14.3	Effects of Carbon Dioxide Elevations	
Symptom	**Percent**	**Cause or comment**
Anxiety	>0.5	A feeling something is wrong
Headache	1	Dilation of blood vessels in the brain
Increased respiratory rate	3	Direct effect on receptors; air hunger
Nausea, weakness, discomfort	5	Possibly associated with concomitant hypoxia
Confusion	5-10	Possibly associated with concomitant hypoxia
Loss of consciousness	10	Possibly associated with concomitant hypoxia

air on the surface. If carbon dioxide toxicity develops in the water, aborting the dive usually accomplishes all three purposes.

Definitive Management

Rarely is definitive management required. Usually symptoms resolve immediately with initiation of the first-response interventions. Because of the likelihood of hypoxia associated with carbon dioxide toxicity, if the diver has any residual symptoms, then 100 percent oxygen should be administered and the diver evaluated for hypoxia-related injuries to the heart and brain. The second component of definitive management is to ascertain the cause of the episode. Usually malfunction or improper assembly of the carbon dioxide absorbent system is the cause. If burns have occurred in the mouth and throat, they should be lavaged (rinsed) with fresh water. If shortness of breath or difficulties with breathing are present, observation at a medical facility, monitoring of blood oxygen levels, and breathing of oxygen may be required.

Prevention

Education and training are the best preventive measures for carbon dioxide toxicity. Divers should moderate their activities if hyperventilation is associated with underwater work activities, especially if rebreathing equipment is used. If symptoms persist, the dive should be aborted and the equipment checked for malfunctions. When rebreathing diving equipment is used, all the checks and balances for safe assembly must be strictly followed.

Return to Diving

Once the diver is rested and asymptomatic and the cause of the episode has been determined, the diver may resume diving. If burns in the respiratory tract have occurred, diving should not be resumed until they are resolved.

Hypoxia and Anoxia

Hypoxia and anoxia are the medical terms for low and no oxygen availability, respectively, to tissues. Drowning, of course, is a consequence of anoxia. These two problems occur in all types of diving (see chapter 2). Hypoxia–anoxia problems with breath-hold and closed-circuit SCUBA diving are insidious. Altered levels of consciousness can occur without the usual warning signs and symptoms of hypoxia that are associated with concomitant elevations in carbon dioxide levels. This chapter focuses on equipment-associated causes of hypoxia and anoxia, which are especially a concern with the use of closed-circuit SCUBA equipment.

BRINGING IT ALL TOGETHER

A Navy Special Warfare (SEAL) diver was using closed-circuit pure oxygen gear. After following the guidelines for setting up the equipment and passing the pre-dive equipment checks, the diver began the training exercise. For safety reasons he was connected by a tether line to his dive buddy. A few minutes into the dive he began to experience burning sensations in his mouth, rapid breathing, and coughing. He immediately signaled his buddy to abort the dive and surface with him. After a few minutes of coughing, he was all right except for some minor burn sensations in his mouth. Later a check of the equipment showed that seawater had entered the CO_2 canister but revealed no problems in the equipment itself. The probable explanation for the problem was that water had entered the mouthpiece and had been exhaled into the CO_2 absorbent.

Comment: Although all the checks and balance systems to ensure safety with use of this equipment were followed, a procedural error, such as removing the mouthpiece in the "open" position while in the water, could have allowed water entry into the system and caused this complication associated with of carbon dioxide absorption.

Significance

The interruption of oxygen to the brain for a moment or two causes loss of consciousness. Brain anoxia for more than three or four minutes will result in brain damage (see chapter 1). The body's recognition of hypoxia and anoxia symptoms is paradoxical. If elevated levels of carbon dioxide are associated with the hypoxic–anoxic conditions, **air hunger** (an extremely strong desire to breathe in order to increase exhalation of carbon dioxide) and struggling to restore the oxygen supply occur. If not, the diver may black out without any warning signs or symptoms (see chapter 11).

Causes

Causes of blackout were described in chapter 11. If carbon dioxide levels remain normal while oxygen supplies are deficient, consciousness will be lost without the recognition of hypoxia. This is most likely to occur with closed-circuit SCUBA in which carbon dioxide is reabsorbed while oxygen is added to the system. If the diver fails to add sufficient oxygen to the system, unconsciousness from hypoxia will occur without warning symptoms.

Outright failure of the SCUBA regulator is a rare cause of hypoxia symptoms. More likely, the diver exhausts the air supply in the SCUBA tank. When unable to breathe through the regulator and a dive buddy with an octopus regulator is not nearby, the diver will make an emergency ascent to the surface. If he or she reaches the surface while still conscious and has avoided a gas overexpansion injury to the lungs (see chapter 15), the incident may be disregarded by the diver and he/she will go on with subsequent diving activities as if nothing happened. With loss of consciousness, drowning may result. If the diver holds his/her breath during ascent, arterial gas embolism may occur. A fourth consequence is decompression sickness from too rapid an ascent.

Effects on the Body (Pathophysiology)

The initial symptoms of hypoxia (in the presence of normal CO_2 levels) result in decrements in mental function secondary to oxygen deprivation to the brain. When oxygen availability is abruptly interrupted, loss of consciousness is rapid and may occur without significant warning symptoms. When the oxygen supply decreases slowly, nonspecific signs and symptoms may be noted before consciousness is lost, including the following:

- Impairment in mental function—inability to concentrate, difficulty with cognitive activities, impaired judgment
- Altered level of consciousness—light-headedness, dizziness, giddiness with or without nausea
- Impairment of coordination—impending collapse, altered visual acuity
- Alterations of vital sign(s)—elevated pulse and respiratory rates

Symptoms of hypoxia are not specific and may be confused with other conditions that alter the level of consciousness without air hunger, including nitrogen narcosis, drug effects, head injury, carbon monoxide poisoning, and strokes. However, during diving with closed-circuit SCUBA systems, hypoxia should be the primary consideration with the appearance of any of the signs and symptoms listed.

First-Response Interventions

The essential first-line responses for hypoxia are recognizing the causes and increasing oxygen delivery to the person. If symptoms are mild, breathing of air on the surface is usually sufficient to correct the problem. If the person has apparently drowned and spontaneous breathing is not observed, basic life support must be instituted immediately (see chapter 16).

Definitive Management

If a person who has experienced a hypoxia–anoxia episode does not recover immediately with reestablishment of normal amounts of oxygen in the breathing medium, then further evaluation for brain, heart, and lung injury at a medical facility is required. Elements of near-drowning and possibly decompression illness are likely to be mixed with the hypoxia insult and require additional interventions such as advanced life support, antibiotics, and hyperbaric oxygen recompression treatments.

Prevention

Prevention of hypoxic–anoxic problems requires appropriate training in the use of closed-circuit SCUBA equipment, recognition of the earliest signs and symptoms of these problems, and knowledge of the established methods to manage them. Sensible diving practices to prevent hypoxia–anoxia problems in general, and with closed-circuit SCUBA in particular, include these:

- Swim in pairs: Use the buddy system; for training dives with closed-circuit SCUBA gear, the diving pairs should be tethered with buddy lines.

- Use checkoff lists: Avoid omitting any steps in setting up closed-circuit SCUBA gear; recheck that the oxygen concentrations in the SCUBA tanks correspond to the oxygen concentrations computed in the pre-dive planning conference.

- Follow established protocols: Check oxygen sensors, if this type of equipment is used, at the prescribed intervals.

- Avoid hazardous predicaments: Diving activities should be curtailed if currents are so strong that it is difficult to keep the mouthpiece in place, if obstructions block emergency ascents to the surface, or if visibility is so poor that it is not possible to observe one's dive buddy.

- Have contingency plans for emergencies: Review in the pre-dive brief the emergencies that may possibly be encountered and the recommended methods to manage them.

BRINGING IT ALL TOGETHER

A 34-year-old male was swimming at a depth of 10 feet (three meters) with a pure oxygen rebreather diving rig. A few minutes into the dive, he lost consciousness. He was immediately brought to the surface by his dive buddy (they were swimming with a buddy line because of the hazards associated with using this type of equipment) and regained consciousness immediately without any residual problems. Inspection of the oxygen gas supply revealed that it had been filled with air rather than pure oxygen. Blackout was due to dilutional hypoxia (see chapter 11).

Comment: The gas flow rate from the oxygen cylinder was set for delivering pure oxygen. The amount of available oxygen at this flow rate was only about one-fifth of what it would be with pure oxygen (air contains approximately 20 percent oxygen). This gas flow rate was insufficient to maintain consciousness with the accidental substitution of air. The scrubber removed carbon dioxide from the breathing circuit so that the diver was unaware of any "air hunger" or depletion in the oxygen supply in his breathing circuit.

Return to Diving

If the diver is asymptomatic after an episode of hypoxia–anoxia, he or she may resume diving when feeling rested. Since an oxygen depletion stress was incurred, several days' rest is recommended. If residual problems such as complications of near-drowning are present, these must be resolved before consideration can be given to resuming diving. Then, the recommendation is made based on the criteria for the complications rather than the hypoxia–anoxia incident itself.

Carbon Monoxide Poisoning and High-Pressure Nervous System Syndrome

We briefly discuss carbon monoxide poisoning and high-pressure nervous system syndrome in this chapter for the sake of completeness. Both conditions manifest their symptoms during the bottom phase of the dive. The sport diver is unlikely to encounter either of these conditions because of their rarity and the special conditions in which they occur. The references for this chapter, however, include selected sources on these subjects for further information. Carbon monoxide poisoning has been discussed previously as one of the no-panic syndromes. Its effects as related to durations of exposure and concentrations in the breathing gas are listed in table 14.4. As in the example of carbon dioxide poisoning, the partial pressures of carbon monoxide increase in direct proportion to the depth of the dive. Those responsible for filling SCUBA tanks must ensure that the air in the tank is essentially free of carbon monoxide. Prevention, management, and recommendations for return to diving have been described previously (see chapter 11).

Table 14.4	Carbon Monoxide Exposures and Their Effects	
Parts per million	**Effects**	**Exposure duration**
25	None	Indefinite
100	None	40-hr work week
800	Headache, breathlessness with exertion	1 hr
1,600	Confusion, collapse with exertion	1 hr
3,200	Unconsciousness	1 hr
4,000	Profound coma	1 hr
4,500	Death	Immediately

BRINGING IT ALL TOGETHER

While vacationing in an exotic area, a couple decided to do an off-shore, surf-entry sport dive. They rented equipment from a local dive shop. During the dive, the male diver became light-headed and developed a headache. He attributed his symptoms to the borrowed equipment. After surfacing and explaining his symptoms to his wife, the two decided to end the dive. The light-headedness cleared rapidly, but the diver's headache persisted for several hours. When returning to the dive shop, the couple observed that the air compressor intake hoses were only a few yards away from the gasoline compressor engine in an open area where shifts in wind could cause the exhaust to enter the compressor intake hose. The divers explained their concerns about carbon monoxide poisoning to the dive shop owner. The shop owner took the divers to the local hospital, where they both breathed surface oxygen for an hour. The owner promised them he would extend and move the intake line to a "safe" place and offered them equipment for their next dive free of charge.

Comment: The setting and symptoms indicated that, with a high likelihood, carbon monoxide poisoning was the cause of the problem, although the gas supply in the tanks was not checked for this gas. The carbon monoxide symptoms probably appeared in the male diver because of his larger size and more rapid consumption of the tainted air in the tank. Another explanation is that wind had blown the compressor exhaust into the intake valve of the male diver's tank while it was being filled and that this had not happened while filling the other tank.

The high-pressure nervous system syndrome is a condition associated with deep diving activities. It is thought to be caused by the effects of breathing helium–oxygen mixtures at depths greater than 660 FSW (201 MSW). The initial symptoms are tremors. With further descent, the symptoms can progress to additional nervous system dysfunction, loss of consciousness, and death. The addition of a small amount of nitrogen to the breathing mixture is effective in preventing the syndrome. This small amount of nitrogen does not appear to have a narcotic effect on the diver, even at the great depths where this condition makes its appearance.

For Further Review

1. What are the similarities in the various MPD that occur during the bottom phase of the dive?

2. What are the differences in the MPD that occur during the bottom phase?

3. What bottom phase MPD might be considered panic-producing disorders?

4. What bottom phase MPD might be considered no-panic–producing disorders?

5. Compare and contrast oxygen toxicity of the central nervous system with that of the lungs and identify the importance of each to the sport diver.

6. Why in most circumstances are the bottom MPD associated with special diving equipment?

7. In what situations are special medical interventions needed for management of MPD of the bottom?

8. How does increasing pressure compound the effects of carbon dioxide and carbon monoxide in the breathing mixture?

ASCENT
PROBLEMS

The medical problems of diving (MPD) associated with ascent are usually serious. Every ascent from a compressed gas dive incurs a risk, albeit small, that one of these problems will occur. Whereas many of the MPD previously discussed occur

> **Chapter Preview**
>
> - Extra-alveolar air syndromes and their causes
> - Subcutaneous and mediastinal emphysema, pneumothorax, and arterial gas embolism
> - Significance of decompression sickness
> - Five types of decompression sickness
> - Disordered decompression and bends-proneness factors

more frequently, almost all SCUBA dive planning and monitoring equipment are designed to prevent the ascent problems from happening. The ascent problems are unique to the ascent phase of the dive. Most of the other MPD can occur at other phases, although they are most likely to occur in a particular phase as discussed in earlier chapters. Boyle's, Dalton's, and Henry's Laws help to explain the events that occur with ascent problems (see chapter 1) since they involve components of both direct and indirect effects of pressure. In contrast to almost all the other MPD, the ascent problems generate stresses to the body with which few or no positive feedback mechanisms are associated, that is, the body cannot respond to them in a positive or corrective fashion. If the stresses with the ascent problems precipitate symptoms, they have already reached the negative feedback stage.

The terminology for the MPD ascent problems can be a source of confusion. Arterial gas embolism and decompression sickness are two separate entities. Many prefer to combine the two disorders and refer to both as decompression illness. Earlier in the text we used this term for convenience. There is justification for combining the terms since the pathology of both disorders is based on how bubbles react with tissues during ascent, and the occurrence of air embolism may predispose the diver to decompression sickness. Now it is appropriate to make a distinction between the two conditions, for several reasons:

- Arterial gas embolism and decompression sickness are caused by different challenges of the dive; the dive profiles for the two disorders are usually quite different.
- In the majority of instances their presentations are different.
- The ancillary treatments for arterial gas embolism and decompression sickness, while both require hyperbaric oxygen recompression, may be quite different.
- While arterial gas embolism is associated with two less serious but distinct conditions, decompression sickness may present as a spectrum of problems from nuisances to life-threatening effects.

Accordingly this chapter is divided into two sections. The first section deals with extra-alveolar air syndromes, which include subcutaneous and mediastinal emphysema, pneumothorax, and arterial gas embolism. The second section covers decompression sickness with its limb bends (pain only) and its serious classifications.

Extra-Alveolar Air Syndromes

Extra-alveolar air syndromes are a group of conditions caused by air trapping in the lungs, expansion of the gas volume (Boyle's Law) with ascent to the point of rupturing the alveoli, and escape of gas into body tissues and cavities. Other names for this group of conditions include the air retention syndromes, the pulmonary overdistension syndromes (POPS), air embolism, and burst lung.

Significance

Clinical manifestations and severity of the extra-alveolar air syndromes depend on the location of the free air that escapes the alveoli as shown in figure 15.1. Their presentations vary from very mild conditions that require only observation to life-threatening conditions that require immediate treatment. Arterial gas embolism, the most serious of the extra-alveolar air syndromes, accounts for about 20 percent of the approximately 100 SCUBA diving–related deaths that occur annually in the United States. Although arterial gas embolism happens infrequently, it is considered the most serious SCUBA diving problem since recovery is so highly dependent on immediate hyperbaric oxygen recompression treatment. However, about 50 percent of the presentations resolve completely with the immediate breathing of oxygen on the surface. Arterial gas embolism can occur with an ascent, during breath-holding after breathing of a compressed gas, from depths less than 10 feet (three meters).

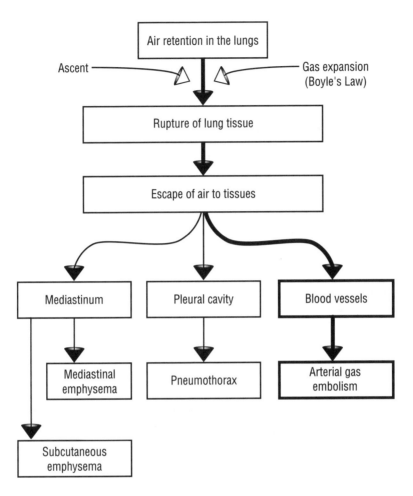

FIGURE 15.1   Genesis of extra-alveolar air syndromes.

Causes

When compressed gas is breathed underwater, the gas enters the lungs at the ambient (i.e., outside) pressure. Should the diver inhale deeply while at depth, breath-hold, and ascend, the air in the lungs expands in volume (Boyle's Law). Once the air in the lungs has expanded to the total lung capacity, further ascent will cause overexpansion and rupture of the alveoli. Gas then escapes. If the air enters the subcutaneous and mediastinal (space between the heart and breastbone) tissue planes, gas bubbles appear in these tissues. If it enters the chest cavity, a **pneumothorax** (lung collapse) occurs. If the overexpansion is great enough in magnitude, blood vessels adjacent to the alveoli also rupture, and air enters the blood vessels, returning to the heart, causing arterial gas embolism.

Breath-holding is not the only reason for extra-alveolar air. Air trapping also occurs in the presence of factors that block air egress from the alveoli, such

Areas of lung collapse (atelectasis)

Asthma

Benign (not cancerous) masses of the lungs or airways

Chronic bronchitis

Chronic obstructive pulmonary disease (emphysema)

Emphysematous (air filled) blebs

Foreign objects (aspirating a piece of a broken or bitten-off mouthpiece of a regulator)

Pleural (lung lining) adhesions

Plugs of mucus

Previous spontaneous pneumothorax

Severe back curvatures (scoliosis)

Tumors of the lungs or airways

Water aspiration and laryngospasm

FIGURE 15.2 Conditions that lead to air trapping in the lungs.

as secretions and bronchiolar constriction resulting from asthma. Another possible cause of extra-alveolar air is the rupture of **emphysematous blebs** (out-pouchings or pockets in the lungs that have weak walls), which may be asymptomatic on the surface and while the person is underwater but rupture due to gas expansion during ascent. Figure 15.2 lists conditions that may predispose to extra-alveolar air syndromes. Cigarette smoking aggravates almost all these conditions. Youthful divers may discount the effects of smoking, claiming that smoking has not affected their diving. However, the effects of smoking on the lungs are accumulative and may take years to manifest themselves.

Effects on the Body (Pathophysiology)

As noted earlier, gas from the ruptured alveoli usually causes one of three problems: mediastinal and subcutaneous emphysema, pneumothorax, and arterial gas embolism.

Mediastinal and Subcutaneous Emphysema   If overexpansion of the lungs and rupture of the alveoli occur near the **hilum** (center where the bronchi begin to branch off) of the lungs or the free air dissects through tissue planes to the hilum, free air may enter the mediastinal space. This condition is termed mediastinal emphysema (air). The air may continue to move upward and come to lie under the skin of the neck and upper chest. In this case the appropriate term is subcutaneous (below the skin) emphysema.

Symptoms of mediastinal and subcutaneous emphysema are usually mild. The diver may experience discomfort or pain under the sternum (breastbone). Air in the **mediastinum** (a potential space between the breastbone and the heart) may go unnoticed except on X-ray examination. Subcutaneous emphysema causes a

> ### *Diving Physics: Elastic Recoil*
>
> Normally the alveoli, which are elastic structures, collapse if a negative pressure is not maintained in the pleural cavity. This phenomenon is termed "elastic recoil." With inhalation, the diaphragm moves downward, which increases the negative pressure. The lungs expand as air is "sucked in" by the pressure differential. With exhalation, the diaphragm and muscles of the chest wall relax. The elastic recoil of the alveoli passively causes air to be forced outward in a fashion similar to the exhaust of air from a balloon when the neck is released.

spongy, cracking sensation in the skin. This may occur high in the neck and cause speech to have a nasal quality. Massive amounts of air here could obstruct the windpipe at the region of the larynx (Adam's apple). The free air in these conditions is not in one continuous mass but diffusely distributed between layers of tissue. Thus, it is not possible to puncture the tissue and suck out the air.

Pneumothorax   If overexpansion of the lung and rupture of the alveoli occur near the periphery (outside margin) of the lung, a pneumothorax may develop. In this situation, free air passes into the **pleural cavity** (the potential space that lies between the pleura [the lining] covering the lungs and the pleura lining the inside of the thoracic cavity). The negative intrathoracic pressure is obliterated, and the lung collapses because of its elastic recoil.

Symptoms of pneumothorax include the sudden appearance of shortness of breath and severe pain in the involved side of the chest. Shock may occur. The diagnosis is usually confirmed by the absence of chest movement on inspection and of breath sounds on auscultation (use of a stethoscope to listen for air movements in the lungs) in the involved side. X-ray examination confirms the diagnosis with the findings of free air in the pleural cavity and collapse of the lung shadow from its normal position adjacent to the chest wall. There are two types of pneumothorax:

• Simple pneumothorax entails a one-time air entry into the pleural cavity. A simple pneumothorax frequently occurs without any significant insult (such as overexpansion) to the lungs. This is termed a spontaneous pneumothorax. Spontaneous pneumothorax may occur during breath-hold diving, with lifting equipment, or even at rest.

• In tension pneumothorax, more air enters the pleural cavity with every breath. This increases pressure in the pleural cavity and causes further collapse of the lung. The pressure may be so great that it causes the collapsed lung and the mediastinal structures to move toward the noncollapsed lung and interfere with its function. A tension pneumothorax is much more serious than a simple pneumothorax. It may cause rapid progression of symptoms leading to collapse and shock. In diving, a simple pneumothorax may become a tension pneumothorax even if additional air does not enter the pleural cavity. If a simple pneumothorax occurs at depth, with ascent air trapped in the pleural cavity, air will expand as ambient pressures decrease. This may produce a tension pneumothorax.

Arterial Gas Embolism   Arterial gas embolism results when air-carrying structures (alveoli and bronchial tubes) rupture explosively from sudden overexpansion. Apparently the recoil also ruptures the blood vessels lying adjacent to these structures. Free air then enters the lung circulation and is carried to the left side of the heart, where it is pumped into the arterial circulation. Once free air enters the bloodstream, the results can be catastrophic, as noted in figure 15.3. The air forms boluses or emboli. The emboli are too large to pass through small blood vessels and thus act as obstructions just as a cork would in a pipe that progressively narrows. The obstructions prevent oxygen and nutrients from reaching tissues. When the emboli block the brain or heart, collapse may occur immediately. The symptoms in the brain and the heart are usually so overwhelming that the symptoms at other sites may be overlooked. Blood tests confirm that multiorgan involvement can occur.

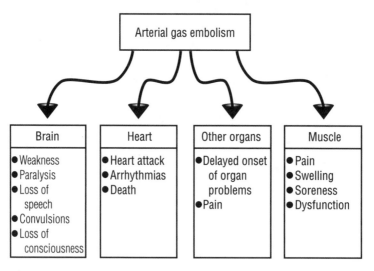

FIGURE 15.3   Presentations of arterial gas embolism.

Whenever a diver breathing compressed gas surfaces and immediately loses consciousness or develops other symptoms associated with a stroke such as weakness, inability to speak, convulsions, or altered level of consciousness, arterial gas embolism is the diagnosis until proven otherwise. Other symptoms associated with arterial gas embolism include the following:

- Tightness in the chest during ascent; coughing and collapsing
- Frothy, bloody secretions from the mouth
- Marbling of the skin; also, a sharply defined area of pallor (paleness) may be noted at the base of the tongue (Liebermeister's sign)
- Heart dysfunction with arrhythmias, pumping problems, or arrest suggestive of emboli to the coronary arteries
- Muscle pain and symptoms from dysfunction of other organs (may be noted a few hours later)

There are no specific laboratory changes diagnostic of arterial gas embolism. Hemoconcentration (increased viscosity of blood) may occur in reaction to the inflammatory response between the blood vessel walls and the air bubbles. This causes fluid to leak from the blood vessels to the tissue spaces. Increased levels of serum creatinine phosphokinase (an enzyme that reflects tissue, especially muscle, damage) correlate with the severity of clinical presentations. Generally X-rays do not detect gas emboli in blood vessels. However, magnetic resonance imaging and **computerized tomography** (a special type of X-ray that makes cross-sectional images of tissues and with the aid of a computer is able to reformat the images to aid in interpretations) scans may detect brain and lung damage and sometimes even demonstrate bubbles blocking blood vessels.

First-Response Interventions

For subcutaneous and mediastinal emphysema, treatment is usually not necessary. Reassurance to the diver that the symptoms are not serious and will resolve without treatment will help relieve anxiety. If there are any signs of difficulty breathing, the diver should inhale 100 percent oxygen and be transported to a medical facility for further evaluation.

Pneumothorax is an emergency that requires immediate medical attention. The diver should breathe pure oxygen while awaiting transfer and en route to a medical facility. Increasing pain and shortness of breath suggest that the pneumothorax is of the tension variety. Those with proper training can decompress the tension pneumothorax in the field with a Claggett needle and a **Heimlich valve** (a valve device that connects to a chest tube or needle).

In the case of an arterial gas embolism, the first-response intervention is the immediate breathing of 100 percent oxygen on the surface. This is so effective that 50 percent of people with arterial gas embolism have complete remission of their symptoms. People who are unconscious should be placed flat on their back. This position facilitates turning the head to the side to prevent aspiration (inhalation of food or fluid into the lungs) if vomiting occurs.

Although one might think that positioning the patient in the head-down position would reduce the bubble load to the brain, because of the decreased density of the bubble compared to the blood this effect probably does not occur. In addition, the head-down position may increase swelling in the brain due to the effect of gravity. Swelling occurs in the brain when it is deprived of oxygen. Because of its confinement within the nondistensible skull, the brain experiences increased pressure with swelling. This further restricts blood flow to the brain by collapsing the thin-walled capillaries and veins (i.e., compartment syndrome). With blockage of venous outflow, arterial inflow is backed up (dam effect). These mechanisms all contribute to brain oxygen deprivation.

If the person is alert, oral fluid administration is recommended to expand blood volume and increase blood flow with concomitant oxygen delivery to the brain. However, too much hydration (fluid overload) can contribute to brain swelling. Swelling of tissues is an inevitable consequence of oxygen deprivation. As noted above, the brain is no exception.

Definitive Management

For subcutaneous and mediastinal emphysema, usually no definitive treatment is required. Observation over a 24-hour period, as a precautionary measure should airway obstruction develop, is recommended. A chest X-ray may show a pneumothorax, emphysematous blebs, or other lung abnormalities. Measurements of oxygen and carbon dioxide tensions and acidity of the blood will ascertain whether or not ventilation is adequate. If not, then some other problem that caused the abnormality must be sought. The subcutaneous and mediastinal air in the tissues is gradually reabsorbed over a period of days.

In the case of pneumothorax, definitive treatment is required immediately. In general, management of a pneumothorax associated with diving is the same as for pneumothoraces from other causes. Following X-rays to verify the diagnosis, a large needle or chest tube is inserted into the collapsed lung cavity and connected to a suction device. If extreme respiratory distress is noted or a chest X-ray cannot be obtained, for example, if the patient is undergoing treatment for decompression sickness in a recompression chamber, the needle or chest tube may be placed based on the findings from the examination. Ruptured alveoli typically stop leaking air within 24 hours of the injury. After 48 hours, the suctioning device is usually removed. If decompression has been omitted or if symptoms of decompression sickness occur, hyperbaric oxygen recompression can be done with the chest tube in place and connected to a Heimlich valve. The treatment for arterial gas embolism is hyperbaric oxygen recompression, which has four effects:

- Reduction in bubble size or actual obliteration of the bubble (forcing the gas in the bubble back into solution in the blood) with elimination of the obstruction
- Oxygenation of hypoxic tissues that resulted from the obstruction, a desirable consequence of the hyperbaric oxygen exposure
- Speedier washout of inert gas from the bubble, which further contributes to the reduction in bubble size or actual dissipation of the bubble
- Attenuation of the inflammatory response that occurs when the nitrogen bubble comes in contact with the lining of the blood vessel (see chapter 3)

If the diver still has signs and symptoms of serious brain involvement at the time of presentation to a recompression chamber, ancillary interventions are necessary. These include steroids; intravenous lidocaine at doses used to treat heart arrhythmias; intravenous fluids; and management of intercurrent problems such as seizures, pneumothorax, hypoxia, and insufficient ventilation. If symptoms improve but do not resolve completely, the initial hyperbaric recompression treatment may be extended, treatments may be repeated, or both. Residual problems, if they exist, require the same type of management that is required for a stroke, such as physical therapy, braces, surgery, and medication to improve function.

Note that it is beyond the scope of this text to include either the algorithms used for decision making regarding arterial gas embolism and decompression sickness or the actual treatment tables. Appendix B includes references to diving manuals such as the *NOAA Diving Manual* and the *U.S. Navy Diving Manual* that contain this information.

If the diver is all right at the time of arrival at the recompression facility or all symptoms clear with treatment(s), one additional "washout" hyperbaric oxygen treatment is recommended 12 to 24 hours later as an additional safety factor.

Prevention

Much can be done to prevent extra-alveolar air syndromes. The diver must never forget to exhale during emergency ascents. Extra-alveolar air syndromes often occur as a consequence of other diving problems such as entanglements, equipment malfunctions, nitrogen narcosis, and panic. There is an inverse relationship between the experience of the diver and the occurrence of these problems. Although divers gain experience through repetitive diving, it is important to note that diver certification programs, proper diving equipment, and pre-dive planning effectively reduce the likelihood that extra-alveolar air syndromes will occur. The pre-dive examination also helps to prevent these problems through detection of predisposing lung conditions (see chapter 10).

Return to Diving

If recovery is complete after an extra-alveolar air event and the cause identified (i.e., the diver panicked and breath-held during ascent), with counseling and retraining the motivated diver may return to diving. The question is, how long is a safe period for recovery? Firm criteria do not exist. For subcutaneous emphysema and mediastinal emphysema it is probably safe to return to diving after a couple of weeks. If a pneumothorax occurs spontaneously, U.S. Navy diving regulations prohibit diving for five years. If it is traumatic, the patient may return to diving after complete lung and chest wall healing, which may take three to six months. For arterial gas embolism, a similar waiting period before return to diving is recommended. In all cases of extra-alveolar air, it is necessary to try to determine the causes and to perform a workup, including plain X-rays, computerized tomography, and pulmonary function studies, before clearing the patient to dive. If neurological (nervous system) residuals exist after an extra-alveolar event, further SCUBA diving is not recommended.

Decompression Sickness

When one is dealing with superlatives about MPD, decompression sickness is the most notorious. Almost everyone has heard of the bends. Whenever a diver has a problem, the first question asked is "Did he get bent?" Even so, decompression sickness occurs only two or three times in every 10,000 ascents from SCUBA dives. Decompression sickness is rightfully labeled a syndrome because of its many presentations, and its signs and symptoms are not always clearly related to the causes. That is, one diver may get bent while the dive buddy with identical dive profiles may show no signs of decompression sickness. Arterial gas embolism and decompression sickness may have many findings in common, which helps to justify using the generic term *decompression illness* for the two conditions. However, they have many characteristics that are different, as noted in table 15.1. Decompression sickness also has been known by many other terms, including aeroembolism (not to be confused with air embolism), compressed air illness, diver's disease, diver's itch, diver's **paralysis** (loss of motor function), dysbarism, silent bends, the chokes, the niggles, and the staggers. Chapter 3 presented much of the information

BRINGING IT ALL TOGETHER

CASE STUDY 1

Several children were playing in a backyard swimming pool. They decided to tie weights to a bucket handle and let the bucket sink, filled with air, so that they could breathe the air in the bucket from the bottom of the pool. After breathing air from the bucket, one of the kids swam to the surface holding his breath. Upon surfacing, he sighed and immediately lost consciousness. Resuscitation efforts by paramedics were futile. The youngster was pronounced dead upon his arrival at the hospital.

Comment: The diagnosis of arterial gas embolism was made. Computations from diving physics show that an ascent from as little as 3 FSW (1 MSW) after full inhalation of air into the lungs will theoretically result in a 10 percent overexpansion of the lungs upon reaching the surface. Compressed gas diving (as in breathing the air in the bucket) and breath-hold diving should not be mixed.

CASE STUDY 2

Upon reaching the 70-FSW (21-MSW) depth, the regulator malfunctioned for a 28-year-old moderately experienced diver. He indicated his predicament by hand signals to his dive buddy, and the dive buddy offered the diver his octopus regulator. Together they ascended at a safe rate, but the diver was having difficulty getting enough air from the octopus regulator. Therefore when he reached the 30-FSW (9.1-MSW) depth, he decided to swim to the surface since he could easily reach this depth when breath-hold diving. Upon surfacing he became confused, weak on the right side of his body, and unable to speak. His predicament was noted immediately by the dive supervisor, who rescued him, brought him aboard the dive boat, and gave him pure oxygen to breathe. After five minutes of breathing oxygen, the diver's symptoms resolved. The diver continued to breathe pure oxygen until the cylinder was empty at about 15 minutes of oxygen breathing time. He was reluctant to seek further medical care since he felt OK except for a little fatigue. He was persuaded by the dive supervisor to report to a hospital that had a hyperbaric oxygen chamber. The diagnosis of decompression illness, resolved with surface oxygen breathing, was made and a "washout" hyperbaric oxygen recompression treatment was given. The diver was advised to have a study for a patent foramen ovale, not dive until cleared by an undersea medical specialist, and have his equipment serviced before resuming diving if given permission to do so.

Comment: The diagnosis of decompression illness was appropriate. The diver could have sustained an arterial gas embolism from breath-holding during the last 30 feet (9.1 meters) of his dive. Alternatively, bubbles from the free gas phase (see chapter 3) could have crossed from the venous side of his bloodstream to the arterial side through a patent foramen ovale. The omission of the 15-foot (4.6-meter) three-minute rest stop during the emergency ascent may have generated enough of a gradient to drive air bubbles across an otherwise silent patent foramen ovale. If a patent foramen ovale study was negative, the diagnosis of arterial gas embolism would have been likely; if positive, then decompression sickness would have been the more likely diagnosis.

Table 15.1 Differentiating Arterial Gas Embolism From Decompression Sickness		
Characteristic	**Decompression sickness (serious presentations)**	**Arterial gas embolism**
Source of symptoms	Spinal cord, joints, brain	Brain, heart
Dive profile	Long, deep	Shallow, short duration
Related problems	Usually absent	Panic, equipment failure
Maximum treatment pressure (ATA)	Usually 2.8 to 3.0	6.0
Surface oxygen effects	Symptoms usually persist	Symptoms clear in 50% of the cases
In-water recompression	Considered in special situations	Not recommended
Diver experience	Substantial	Usually inexperienced

needed to understand what happens when decompression sickness occurs. Here we supplement that discussion by focusing on its clinical aspects.

Significance

Even though decompression sickness occurs infrequently, its prevention is fundamental for all SCUBA and other compressed air diving activities. Essentially almost all elements of dive planning focus on preventing this problem, whether the dive profile, the bottom time, the ascent rate, the rest stop, or the surface interval (see chapter 2). Even though dive computers and dive tables are designed to prevent decompression sickness, its occurrence is not always predictable. For shallow dives, the dive tables seem to be inherently safe. For example, for dives to 60 FSW (18 MSW), modestly exceeding diving table time limits does not correlate well with the advent of decompression sickness. Conversely, this problem is often observed in deep dives (over 130 FSW/40 MSW) even if dive table time limits are not exceeded.

Causes

In 1670 Robert Boyle (of Boyle's Law fame) noted bubbles in the cornea of a viper subjected to decompression. However, it was not until the mid-1800s that decompression from high-pressure environments was associated with joint pain.

The condition was initially called **caisson** (watertight boxes) disease because it was associated with working in these structures during the underwater construction of bridge foundations. Frequently workers experienced joint pains or paralysis that began after they returned to the surface. Caisson disease became known as "the bends" when men working on the Brooklyn Bridge walked with bent-over postures. Their posture simulated the "Grecian bend," a term designating the way fashionable women of the day walked. The bends has persisted as a term for decompression sickness even though the Grecian bend is an image of the past.

Unfortunately for the diver, the lung tissues act like a sieve and the body tissues act like a sponge with regard to the nitrogen (or other inert gases) in the air that is breathed (see chapter 3). Ordinarily all body tissues are in equilibrium with the nitrogen in the air. As the ambient (outside) pressure increases during descent, the "sponge" soaks up (on-gasses) more of the nitrogen. Some body tissues, such as the lungs, blood, and the brain, on-gas the nitrogen very rapidly. Others like bone and tendon come to equilibrium with the nitrogen very slowly. During ascent, the nitrogen that has been forced into the tissues leaves the tissues (off-gasses) as a response to the gradient created by the reduction in ambient pressure. If the ascent is gradual enough or the nitrogen load miniscule enough, the nitrogen leaves the tissues in an orderly fashion. However, if the off-gassing overwhelms the transport in the blood and the release of nitrogen from the lungs, bubbles will form to a much greater extent—as a carbonated beverage will fizz if shaken. Decompression sickness is associated with the formation of bubbles in tissues. The location of the bubble formation determines the presentation; for example, paralysis will occur if the location is the spinal cord, and pain will occur if it is the joint structures.

Four outcomes are associated with ascending from a dive (see chapter 3). The following are the permutations for outcomes of decompression:

- Uneventful: In over 99 percent of ascents from compressed air dives, decompression is uneventful and no symptoms develop in the diver.

- Deserved decompression sickness: Due to overwhelming gradients and omitted decompression, this occurs in one to three of every 10,000 ascents and accounts for about one-half the cases of decompression sickness.

- Undeserved decompression sickness: So labeled in cases in which there have been no apparent violations of decompression procedures; this form accounts for the other half of decompression sickness cases. In turn, about half of these cases are associated with bends-proneness factors, such as a patent foramen ovale, and the other half with disordering events during decompression.

- Nonbubble-related phenomena: These include post-dive complaints from nonbubble-related causes such as trauma, illness, purposes of secondary gain, or psychosomatic factors.

Effects on the Body (Pathophysiology)

The pathophysiology of decompression sickness is an important subject. Large portions of many texts on diving medicine are committed to the topic. The basis for understanding decompression sickness was presented in chapter 3. This section reiterates some of this information while focusing on its clinical aspects, including bubbling effects, noteworthy observations, and classification. Once bubbles form, they may affect tissues in two ways:

- If they are within blood vessels, they may block the circulation to critical tissues such as the brain, heart, lungs, and spinal cord. In this case the condition is referred to as serious or type 2 decompression sickness. The nitrogen bubbles also initiate an inflammatory reaction with the lining of the blood vessel wall. Consequently, even if the bubbles are dissipated by recompression, the inflammatory response may cause irreversible injury to tissues as a type of reperfusion (reestablishment of blood supply) injury. The longer the bubbles are in contact with the blood vessel wall, the more likely it is that permanent damage to the tissues will occur.

- The bubbles may distend pressure-sensitive structures in tissues to cause pain, altered sensations, and skin rashes. Symptoms from bubbles in these areas are termed limb bends, pain-only bends, or minor symptoms, and the condition is classified as type 1 decompression sickness. The mechanisms proposed to cause symptoms are different than for type 2 decompression sickness. It appears that microscopic bubbles form in pressure-sensitive organelles of joint capsules (**Ruffini type 2 corpuscles**) and physically distend the capsules, causing pain in much the same way a stretch injury from a dislocated joint would. A proposed mechanism for the experiencing of abnormal sensations termed **paresthesia** (pins and needles) and **hypesthesia** (decreased sensation) is the presence of microscopic bubbles in the tissues covering nerves. These minor alterations in sensation must be differentiated from the very serious type 2 presentations of paralysis. Microscopic bubbling in the tissue layers just below the skin may account for the skin rash symptoms. In contrast to what happens with type 2 decompression sickness, recompression by itself appears to resolve theses symptoms even if delayed for many hours.

In one-third of the presentations of decompression sickness, findings from both type 1 and type 2 are present.

Nine other observations about decompression sickness and its effects of the body are noteworthy:

1. Batson's plexus of veins: The venous circulation of the spinal cord, especially at the lower thoracic (chest) level, appears particularly susceptible to bubble formation, coalescence, and then enlargement during ascent

because of a plexus (network) of veins, named Batson's, where the circulation is known to be sluggish. This anatomical consideration correlates closely with the high incidence of **paraplegia** (paralysis of the lower half of the body) in type 2 decompression sickness.

2. Catastrophic presentations of decompression sickness in fast tissues: Each tissue has its own nitrogen absorption and release rate (see earlier in this chapter, also chapter 3). The lung has the most rapid rates; one breath at the new ambient pressure will equilibrate the lung tissue with the new partial pressure of nitrogen. The blood is a very rapid tissue also. It takes less than 25 seconds for blood to circulate through the body. Symptoms of type 2 decompression sickness correlate closely with bubble formation in the bloodstream and lungs. The intravascular (within blood vessels) bubbles, if in sufficient amounts, will usually cause catastrophic presentations of decompression sickness.

3. Delayed onset of symptoms: In 10 percent of the cases, the onset of symptoms from decompression sickness may not appear for many hours after a dive is completed. Usually they are of the type 1 variety and are associated with additional off-gassing stresses such as ascending in altitude in an airplane or interfering with off-gassing as a result of falling asleep with a limb in the cramped position.

4. Interference with off-gassing: Impeding the circulation during decompression leads to bubble formation in the obstructed area due to interference with off-gassing. Blood vessel disease, heart disease, lung disease, poor cardiovascular conditioning, anxiety, hypothermia, alcohol ingestion, accidental tourniquets (from dive suit bands, straps, or posturing of joints), and medications may also affect the circulation and contribute to seemingly undeserved cases of decompression sickness.

5. Obesity: Fat tissues have five times the affinity for nitrogen that other body tissues have. Thus these tissues on-gas much more nitrogen than corresponding (in terms of location, duration of exposure, and blood flow) tissues. For these reasons the risks of decompression sickness are increased in the diver who is obese.

6. Patent foramen ovale: Divers with this condition in their hearts appear to have increased susceptibility to type 2 decompression sickness. The explanation is that venous gas emboli, a ubiquitous finding during decompression, pass from the right to the left side of the heart. Ordinarily they are filtered out in the lungs, but the hole in the heart allows the filtering effects of the lungs to be bypassed, and the result is that the bubbles enter the arterial circulation. Symptoms for this presentation of

decompression sickness from this cause are identical to those for arterial gas embolism (see discussion earlier in the chapter).

7. Respiratory symptoms: The chokes, a catastrophic form of decompression sickness that interferes with ventilation, occurs more frequently in aviators than divers, perhaps because of the hypoxic conditions associated with flying.

8. Silent bubbles: Ultrasound monitoring equipment frequently detects the presence of small bubbles in the bloodstream during ascent and immediately after a dive is completed. Ordinarily, these bubbles generate no symptoms and are termed silent bubbles. However, if the ultrasound reveals large amounts of bubbles, there is a positive correlation with symptomatic decompression sickness.

9. Symptom localization: Divers are more often affected by spinal cord lesions and aviators by brain involvement. In tunnel workers, the majority of the "pain-only" symptoms occur in the knees, while in divers these symptoms occur in the shoulders. The fact that divers tend to be more horizontal in the water, while tunnel workers and aviators tend to be more vertical, may be the reason a particular target organ is hit. Also, the pressure gradient of the water forces more blood into the trunk and upper extremities, which may cause more on-gassing of nitrogen to these tissues than to the lower extremities while underwater.

Classification of Decompression Sickness

Signs and symptoms of decompression sickness, correlated with their time of onset and whether or not hyperbaric oxygen recompression therapy is needed, provide the basis for the classification of decompression sickness into five types. Table 15.2 summarizes this classification. However, the majority of the presentations of decompression system are types 1 and 2 as described earlier.

Catastrophic Decompression Sickness   When bubbles obstruct the circulation to vital organs, catastrophic symptoms occur. They are similar to those of arterial gas embolism. The symptoms of catastrophic decompression sickness usually occur during ascent or immediately after surfacing.

• Symptoms of brain involvement include unconsciousness, altered level of consciousness, dizziness, vertigo, convulsions, inability to speak, muscle paralysis or weakness, nausea, vomiting, headache, and visual disturbances.

• Spinal cord symptoms include weakness or paralysis below the neck level, numbness in these areas, and loss of bladder and bowel control. If the bubble

Table 15.2	Types of Decompression Sickness		
Type	**Symptoms**	**Areas involved**	**Comments**
0	Pruritis (itching) Rash Fatigue	Skin Liver (postulated) Muscle, gut	Usually not treated with recompression therapy; hyperbaric oxygen noted to resolve the fatigue syndrome after diving
1	Joint pain Paresthesias (pins and needles sensation) Decreased sensation	Joints Extremities	Symptoms best explained by bubbles in local pain-sensitive structures in the areas of involvement
2	Paralysis, paresis (weakness) Speech, vision disturbances Twitching, convulsions Syncope, unconsciousness Shortness of breath (the chokes) Shock Collapse	Spinal cord Brain Lungs Heart	Symptoms explained by intravascular air bubbles in the areas of involvement
3	Dizziness Vertigo Nausea Nystagmus Vomiting Incoordination Tinnitus Deafness	Ear (vestibular*) Ear (cochlear**)	Bubbles presumed to form in the inner ear structures associated with balance and hearing
4	Osteonecrosis (death of bone cells)	Bone	Bubbles thought to block the circulation to bone, then cause an inflammatory response that further damages the bone

* Vestibular = balance organ of the inner ear.
** Cochlear = hearing organ of the inner ear.

involvement occurs at the top of the spinal cord, cessation of breathing may occur.

• Symptoms of lung involvement occur less than 2 percent of the time. These symptoms, in contrast to those for the brain and spinal cord, may not appear until one to three hours after the dive is completed. The time delay represents the interval required for congestion and fluid accumulations to reach a level in the lungs great enough to interfere with ventilation. Symptoms of lung involvement include shortness of breath; coughing; and the Behnke triad of increased respiratory rate, decreased blood pressure, and decreased pulse rate.

• When decompression sickness symptoms are ascribed to inner ear involvement, the classification is type 3 decompression sickness. Any serious decompression sickness symptoms such as balance problems, dizziness, incoordination, nausea, nystagmus (involuntary movements of the eyes), vertigo (room spinning sensations), or vomiting associated with ear involvement are highly suggestive of this serious type of decompression sickness.

Musculoskeletal Decompression Sickness and Other Type 1 Presentations   This presentation of decompression sickness is commonly referred to as "the bends." Bubbles are thought to form in pain-sensitive structures (Ruffini type 2 corpuscles) in tissues adjacent to joints, the skin, along nerve sheaths, or the internal organs in the body, or some combination of these. Bubbles that form in these areas lead to symptoms that are serious but not life threatening. Symptoms may arise from multiple sites. Whenever there is a history of diving and these types of symptoms occur, decompression sickness needs to be considered as a diagnosis. Symptoms of musculoskeletal decompression sickness may have a delayed onset from a few hours to a day or two after the dive is completed.

• Joint involvement symptoms are characterized by severe pain in the vicinity of joints. Usually the pain is poorly localized and without associated tenderness, redness, swelling, or increased temperature. Likewise, moving the involved joint does not affect the pain as it would with a traumatic injury.

• Bubble formation beneath the skin leads to a red, itching rash and marbling of the skin. Welts may also occur.

• Bubble formation in the vicinity of the internal organs is associated with fatigue and flu-like symptoms.

• Although the explanation for parathesias (pins and needles) and mild numbness symptoms of decompression sickness has not been ascertained, we believe they are due to microscopic bubble formation in advential (supporting) structures of nerves.

Delayed Onset Symptoms   Marginal or inadequate decompression over prolonged periods, especially from dives that require decompression stops, is associated with death of bone cells (osteonecrosis). This is believed to be due to bubbles blocking the circulation to the bone cells, plus the inflammatory reaction of the nitrogen bubble and the blood vessel wall. If small in amount, the condition may remain asymptomatic and be noted only on X-ray or with special imaging techniques. If the bone destruction occurs adjacent to joints and the bone collapses, joint pain, arthritis, and stiffness symptoms develop. This presentation is sometimes referred to as type 4 decompression sickness.

First-Response Interventions
The first response for decompression sickness, as for arterial gas embolism, is oxygen breathing. Supplemental interventions include improving hydration (diving leads to dehydration) and ingestion of aspirin to prevent sludging inflammation. Rest is important, since activity, especially if vigorous, will likely worsen the symptoms. In remote areas, return to the water and breathing of oxygen at a 33-foot (10-meter) depth for a few minutes and then gradually ascending have been recommended but are considered controversial by many authorities in diving medicine (see chapter 3). Even if symptoms resolve with the measures described, evaluation by an undersea and hyperbaric-medicine trained physician is recommended to ascertain whether or not a washout hyperbaric oxygen recompression treatment is needed and whether or not the decompression sickness episode was deserved, as well as for recommendations regarding return to diving.

Definitive Management
Hyperbaric oxygen recompression is the definitive treatment for decompression sickness. As with arterial gas embolism, reference is made to the algorithms and treatment tables found in the manuals listed in appendix B. As in arterial gas embolism, the sooner the hyperbaric oxygen recompression treatment is done, the better the chance for complete resolution of the symptoms.

Prevention
Decompression sickness can usually be prevented by employing safe diving practices such as dive planning; not violating diving tables or dive computer limits; maintaining good hydration, fitness, and body weight; and avoiding diving if bends-proneness factors exist. Some obvious bends-proneness factors are patent foramen ovale, disturbed circulation around joints following severe injuries, coagulopathies (abnormalities in blood clotting), **polycythemia** (increased number of red blood cells), and atherosclerotic cardiovascular disease. Dive planning can help prevent disordering events from

occurring and eliminate these contributors to decompression sickness. Age itself is not a contraindication to diving but may become an increasing risk factor due to reduced exercise capacity and cardiovascular reserve. Ingesting an aspirin before or immediately after diving may afford protection from sludging of red blood cells, a finding associated with decompression sickness (see chapter 3). Other specific means of preventing decompression sickness include the following:

- Use ascent rates of 30 FSW (9.1 MSW) or slower per minute, that is, one foot (0.3 meter) of ascent every two seconds.

- Always include a three-minute rest stop at 15 FSW (4.6 MSW) for every dive; light activity such as slow swimming movements will speed off-gassing.

- Avoid repetitive dives at the end of the day if fatigue is noted or more chilling is noted with each successive dive.

- Take a one-day break after three or four consecutive days of diving excursions involving many dives per day to allow for full off-gassing of the slow tissues.

- Do not fly for 24 hours after the last SCUBA diving activity, longer if the diving included decompression stop dives.

- Avoid alcohol before and after diving activities.

- After diving, avoid sitting or falling asleep with joints in fully flexed positions or in other circumstances in which circulation might be slowed.

Return to Diving

As in arterial gas embolism, the criteria for returning to diving are quite subjective. If the diver had type 1 decompression sickness, violated diving practices, and had full resolution of symptoms with recompression, resumption of diving is permitted after a couple of weeks. The diver should be counseled about why decompression sickness occurred and about safe diving practices before being given a medical clearance to dive. If the decompression sickness was undeserved (no diving practices were violated), then the patient should be evaluated for bends-proneness factors. If no risk factors or disordering events from the dive are identified, even if all symptoms cleared with hyperbaric oxygen recompression treatment, consultation with a physician experienced in undersea medicine is recommended before allowing the diver to return to SCUBA diving. Special tests for a patent foramen ovale and injury to the nervous system may be required. Finally, if significant residual neurological deficits exist after treatments for decompression sickness, return to SCUBA diving is contraindicated.

BRINGING IT ALL TOGETHER

CASE STUDY 1

A 25-year-old inexperienced female diver had difficulties with buoyancy control while diving at a maximum depth of 33 FSW (10 MSW). Unexpectedly, she found herself on the surface. Shortly, she noted a severe headache and inability to move her right arm and leg. Her dive buddy brought her to shore where she was expediently transferred to a recompression chamber and treated for arterial gas embolism. Initially her symptoms improved at the maximum depth of 165 FSW (50 MSW), but during ascent she began to feel weakness in both lower extremities. She could not stand or walk. These symptoms persisted and improved only slowly, but incompletely, with repetitive hyperbaric oxygen treatments over the next seven days.

Comment: Although the presenting symptoms were consistent with arterial gas embolism, the delayed onset of paralysis after the hyperbaric treatment to 165 FSW is best explained by decompression sickness of the spinal cord. Even though the dive was only to 33 FSW, the bubbles from arterial gas embolism may have sensitized the blood vessels to the nitrogen load from the dive. The nitrogen load was further increased when the patient was pressurized to 165 FSW using air to treat the arterial gas embolism symptoms. The failure of the lower limb paralysis symptoms to resolve completely with repetitive hyperbaric oxygen treatments suggests that the nitrogen bubbles interacted with the blood vessels (reperfusion injury) to interfere with blood flow to the spinal cord. Pressurizing the diver to 165 FSW with nitrox mixtures (increased oxygen and decreased nitrogen percentages) would have lessened the nitrogen load and increased the washout benefits of using higher oxygen percentages.

CASE STUDY 2

A 28-year-old female diving instructor was returning home by air flight from a vacation trip to the Caribbean. At the time she boarded the plane, she felt fine. Thirty-six hours before leaving she had finished her last SCUBA dive of a series of four. All were to 50 FSW (15 MSW) or less for 30 to 45 minutes and uneventful. After awaking from a nap on the return flight, she was unable to make a fist with her right hand. She felt paresthesia in the skin of this hand. After returning home she reported to a hospital with a recompression chamber and underwent a hyperbaric recompression treatment 48 hours after the completion of the last dive. Her symptoms cleared within a few minutes after breathing pure oxygen at 66 FSW (20 MSW). The woman remained asymptomatic through the remainder of the treatment and after being examined on the surface. A washout hyperbaric treatment was given the next day, and the diver was advised not to dive for a minimum of two weeks.

Comment: The diver experienced an undeserved case of type 1 decompression sickness. The inability to make a fist was attributed to local effects of bubbles on the nerves to the hand rather than bubbles in the spinal cord. Disordered decompression occurred from the altitude excursion (equivalent to 8,000 feet/2,450 meters) with the flight and presumably from falling asleep with her right arm in a position that restricted its circulation. The delayed onset of symptoms shows that nitrogen remains in the slow tissues for more than 24 hours after completion of a dive. Identifying the disordering events made it safe to give the diver permission to return to diving.

For Further Review

1. What are the similarities and differences between arterial gas embolism and decompression sickness?

2. Why are the body's positive responses (positive feedback, protective mechanisms) to the stresses incurred from problems of ascents essentially nonexistent?

3. Why is it important to differentiate deserved from undeserved decompression sickness?

4. How is the pathophysiology (causes that lead to symptoms) different for type 1 and type 2 decompression sickness?

5. Why do symptoms sometimes not resolve completely with hyperbaric oxygen recompression treatment for arterial gas embolism and decompression sickness?

6. What must one consider in making a decision to allow a diver to return to diving after experiencing decompression sickness or arterial gas embolism?

CHAPTER 7

EMERGENCY COMPLICATIONS FROM MEDICAL PROBLEMS OF DIVING

Although the conditions discussed in this chapter happen independently of the medical problems of diving (MPD), they can also occur as complications of these problems. This chapter approaches three emergency medical conditions—near-drowning, cardiac arrest, and shock—from the latter perspective, for several reasons. First, when near-drowning,

Chapter Preview

- Significance of near-drowning and drowning in diving
- Medical problems that can cause loss of consciousness in the water
- Body's responses (positive feedback, protective mechanisms) to loss of consciousness underwater
- Cardiac arrest and shock as complications of diving
- Measures to prevent cardiac arrest and shock during diving.

shock, and cardiac arrest occur in association with diving activities, invariably they arise secondary to an underlying MPD. If the MPD is not appreciated, optimal management, for example, the need for hyperbaric oxygen recompression treatment, may be delayed. Second, the terminal event in many MPD is one or more of these conditions, for example, drowning from blackout and shock, or cardiac arrest from a marine animal injury. Third, in following the format of the preceding chapters in part III, we approach these problems as an extension of the body's positive and negative feedback responses to the underlying MPD. Finally, it is important to know the first-response interventions for these conditions because of their association with the MPD. The appropriate emergency management of these complications can be the difference between recovery and death or loss of a limb and minor injury.

Aspiration, Near-Drowning, and Drowning

Aspiration, near-drowning, and drowning are related conditions since they all involve effects of breathing while underwater. Aspiration is the inhalation of water or other substances into the lower airways. If the airways are blocked, ventilation is impaired. If foreign material enters the lung, an inflammatory reaction, infection, or both, may occur. This can interfere with ventilation. Aspiration occurs not only during immersion. More frequently it occurs in **obtunded** (impaired level of consciousness) patients whose laryngeal reflex is depressed or absent or when a foreign object is accidentally swallowed. **Near-drowning** refers to loss of consciousness secondary to brain hypoxia (low levels of oxygen) while underwater but with the person surviving after rescue. Whether or not there are complications depends on the duration of anoxia (lack of oxygen) and whether aspiration occurred. **Drowning** is death that occurs as a result of these various events. The majority of this section deals with near-drowning since it is a treatable condition and the one that has the most ramifications for the diver.

Significance

Any loss of consciousness while in the water is significant for the diver. In some respects aspiration, near-drowning, and drowning represent a continuum of responses to forceful submersion or loss of consciousness, or both, in the water. Aspiration usually results in recovery. From near-drowning, recovery can be complete, or residuals can be so severe that the person is in left in a **vegetative** (few or no responses to stimuli) coma. Drowning and death are, of course, the endpoint of the continuum. Drowning is the fourth leading cause of accidental deaths in the United States with 4,000 to 8,000 occurring annually. The number of water-related aspirations and near-drownings is estimated to be 10-fold greater. Of the approximately 100 SCUBA diving deaths that occur each year in the United States, about half are attributed to drowning since no other MPD was listed as an antecedent problem.

Causes

The causes of aspiration, near-drowning, and drowning have already been identified. In diving they are almost always secondary to one of the MPD. Table 16.1 lists possible causes of loss of consciousness associated with diving activities. Any of these conditions can lead to aspiration, near-drowning, and drowning.

Effects on the Body (Pathophysiology)

Once a diver loses consciousness while submerged, breathing continues automatically. This is a reflex act, a positive feedback mechanism. On land

Table 16.1	Medical Conditions and Problems of Diving That Can Lead to Loss of Consciousness in the Water	
Condition	**Associated with struggling?**
Air embolism	Yes
Anoxia, hypoxia	Restlessness
Carbon dioxide toxicity	Yes
Carbon monoxide poisoning	No
Catastrophic decompression sickness	No
Drugs- and alcohol-related effects	Usually not
Entanglements	Yes
High-pressure nervous system syndrome	Yes
Hyperventilation breath-holding blackout	No
Hypothermia	Usually not
Marine animal injuries	Yes
Medical conditions	
Allergic reactions (drugs, inhalations)	Yes
Asthma	Yes
Heart rhythm abnormalities	No
Hypoglycemia (low blood sugar)	No
Myocardial infarction (heart attack)	Yes
Seizure	No
Stroke	No
Nitrogen narcosis	No
Oxygen toxicity seizure	No
Panic syndrome	Yes
Thoracic squeeze	Restlessness
Trauma (head or major bleeding)	No
Water aspiration	Possibly

it keeps the person alive and the tissues oxygenated; however, underwater the person suffocates. Because of muscle relaxation associated with the loss of consciousness, it is all but impossible that the regulator mouthpiece will be retained and used for breathing. The result is inhalation of water. Consciousness will not be regained (if ever) until an oxygen supply to the brain is restored.

Laryngeal Reflex   Usually the first breath of water causes the vocal cords to contract reflexively **(laryngeal reflex)**, which prevents water from entering the lungs. This is another positive feedback mechanism that helps to protect the drowning victim. Eventually, though, it is lost due to oxygen deprivation. A person who is still breathing unconsciously may aspirate water at this stage. However, usually breathing movements have ceased by this time. In most deaths from drowning, very little water is actually found in the lungs.

Lung Findings in Human Near-Drownings   In almost all human drownings, the amount of water aspirated is insufficient to cause any significant changes in the body's fluids and electrolytes. This contrasts sharply with what happens in dogs, which aspirate large quantities of water when submerged such that great differences in their body chemistries result from freshwater versus saltwater drownings. If fluid is found in the lungs of human drowning victims, it is usually from leakage from their own **plasma** (fluid portion of the blood). This is a consequence of the anoxic plus aspiration insults to the lung tissue. Complications from this cause portions of the lung to go unventilated; that is, the alveoli collapse. Circulation may be shunted from the ventilated portions of the lung. This results in what is termed ventilation–perfusion mismatch, a negative feedback mechanism from the injury to the lungs. When an air supply and ventilation are reestablished, the ventilation–perfusion inequalities persist. Because of this, oxygenation may be insufficient to meet the body's needs. The effects of these changes are progressive lowering of oxygen levels in tissues and progressive increases in the acidity of the blood as a consequence of anaerobic metabolism (see chapter 4). These are the findings that blood chemistries show in people who have experienced aspiration and near-drowning.

Diving Reflex As a Response to Immersion   Once the person is submerged and unconscious, a third reflex, positive feedback mechanism is manifested. This is the oxygen-conserving reflex with slowing of the heart rate, **shunting** (bypassing) of blood from noncritical to critical tissues, and anaerobic metabolism (see chapter 4). These processes improve the chances of survival and full recovery for victims of near-drowning. For example, it is not uncommon for people to be resuscitated with full recovery after 30 minutes of submersion. On land, survival of victims of cardiac arrest is substantially less. For example, only one in 10,000 witnessed arrest victims survives and recovers after 10 minutes of untreated cardiac arrest. Of course, there are substantial differences between these two groups since the heart continues to beat and the diving reflex becomes operative in the immersion group. In addition, victims of cardiac arrest typically have underlying heart conditions while victims of near-drownings tend to be active, healthy individuals engaged in water sport activities. In any case, the absence of panic and struggling, as well as immersion in water colder than 70 degrees F (21 degrees C), improves outcomes in victims of near-drowning.

Table 16.2	Clinical Findings Associated With Near-Drownings
Finding	**Comment/Cause**
Absence of breathing movements	Usually associated with prolonged (more than a couple of minutes) immersion
Absent, very rapid, or very slow (agonal rhythm) heart rate	Depends on the duration of anoxia
Bluish coloration of skin	Maximal oxygen utilization and failure of the venous blood to be returned to the heart
Coldness	Effects of the cold water and cessation of metabolic heat production
Convulsions	Lack of oxygen to the brain
Dilation of pupils; glassy stare in the eyes	Lack of oxygen to the brain
Incontinence (urine and feces)	Lack of oxygen to the brain
Unconsciousness	Lack of oxygen to the brain
Vomiting	Aspiration of water; swallowing of water

Clinical Findings in Near-Drowning   The positive and negative feedback responses to near-drowning determine what findings will be observed. Drowning is the presumptive diagnosis anytime a person is found unconscious in the water. Usually breathing movements, which are stimulated by nerve impulses from the brain, cease before the heart (which has its own pacemaker) stops beating. Findings of near-drowning are listed in table 16.2.

First-Response Interventions

First-response interventions are crucial since time is such a critical factor when oxygen supplies to the brain and heart are compromised. Unless the person is forcefully held underwater or fouled in lines or kelp, drowning is invariably associated with some other MPD. Even in the types of cases just mentioned, the people are undoubtedly affected with panic. The ABCs (airway, breathing, and circulation) of basic life support need to be started immediately upon recovery of the person from the water. If residual, correctable problems from the underlying MPD are present, they should be addressed simultaneously. Emergency treatment includes the procedures described in the following paragraphs.

• Retrieve the person from the water; only in the most extreme situations should basic life-support measures be initiated in the water. If the person is unconscious on the bottom, do not use the regulator to artificially ventilate.

This could inflate the lungs and lead to arterial gas embolism during ascent. While ascending, maintain the head in the extended position so that any expanding gas in the lungs (Boyle's Law) will be able to leave the lungs passively in response to the decreasing ambient pressure. An effective way to ascend with the person while controlling the head and neck position is to use the Red Cross head-carry position. The rescuer grasps the head with one hand over each side of the face and ears and the little fingers hooked over the jawbone. Then the head is cradled against the lower chest and upper abdomen. The rescuer should then initiate a gradual swimming ascent with a slightly tilted backward angle. It is controversial whether or not the rescuer should place the regulator into the person's mouth on the chance that the expanding gas will initiate breathing responses during ascent. It is not likely that the unconscious person will be able to use the regulator effectively, and consciousness will not be regained until an oxygen supply to the brain is reestablished. If the person and rescuer were not using SCUBA diving equipment, the rescuer must not put him- or herself in jeopardy of blackout during the ascent (see chapter 11).

- The next step is to dial 911 to alert the Emergency Medical Service (EMS) network. However, this may not be immediately feasible if one is away from the shoreline or the diving platform. The recommendation is to get the person to a platform where cardiopulmonary resuscitation (CPR) can be done effectively, and the EMS system can be alerted immediately. An emergency flare and diver sausage may be useful in signaling others that help is needed. While transiting to the shoreline or platform, maintain head and neck control. Cardiopulmonary resuscitation is not recommended while the person is in the water. It is difficult to do effectively and will delay getting to a place where CPR can be done efficiently. Also, in the water, the diving reflex and hypothermia may continue to offer some protection from anoxic (lack of oxygen) injury to the brain.

- Initiate the ABCs of CPR. These include the following:
  - Check the airway for proper position and obstructions; use the head tilt maneuver. If vomiting or regurgitation occurs, turn the head to the side and sweep away the material with fingers or a cloth.
  - Check for breathing by looking for chest movement, listening for the movement of air (place your ear near the person's mouth), and feeling for chest or air movement. If the person is not breathing, then do two mouth-to-mouth inflations of the lungs.
  - Check circulation by feeling for a carotid artery (neck) pulse; if one is present and the person is not breathing, then artificially ventilate at a

rate of about 15 times per minute. If no pulse is present, then initiate full CPR with 100 chest compressions per minute interspersed with two lung insufflations for every 15 chest compressions, whether one or two persons perform the CPR. For children and infants, the rates are now the same according to the new American Heart Association recommendations.

• Administration of oxygen through the rescuer's breathing of oxygen is controversial at this stage. The rescuer would have to inhale the oxygen and then immediately expire into the person's lungs. This could delay and interfere with the effectiveness of mouth-to-mouth breathing. However, if the diver resumes breathing spontaneously, then 100 percent oxygen should be administered.

• Keep the person cold if in a full state of arrest, that is, if there is no heartbeat or breathing effort, while continuing CPR. This sounds paradoxical, but the reason is that rewarming may initiate spontaneous heart beating. Typically, the heart rhythm after a period of arrest is one of **ventricular fibrillation** (very rapid, irregular, nonfunctional heart activity) or **ventricular tachycardia** (very rapid beating of the heart). This will rapidly and irreparably damage the heart and calls for immediate management with advanced life-support measures, including electrical shock and intravenous medications. If the EMS network has responded by this time and has this equipment available, then rewarming is appropriate.

• Treat for shock by elevating the lower extremities. About two units (two pints; one quart) of blood are stored in each lower extremity. Do not administer clear fluids unless the person has recovered and is alert enough to swallow without aspiration. If there is bleeding, for example, from a traumatic injury (boat propeller) or marine animal bite, it should be controlled with a pressure dressing or a tourniquet if necessary. If the person resumes spontaneous heartbeats and breathing, then rewarming is appropriate at this time.

• Transport the person to the nearest medical center for definitive treatment. Hopefully at this point the paramedics are available and emergency medical care can be transferred from the rescuer(s) to the paramedics for transport and initiation of advanced life-support measures.

Definitive Management

Once the diver is at a medical center, advanced life-support measures are continued with intubation, artificial ventilation, and intravenous fluids. If no spontaneous heartbeat or breathing is present on arrival at the emergency department, the prognosis for recovery is very bleak. A decision to pronounce the person dead may be made by a physician at this time. However, if the person is markedly hypothermic, he or she is rewarmed while advanced life-support interventions are performed until core temperatures are normalized. Then a decision to continue life-support measures is made. Medications are administered as indicated, for example, anti-arrhythmic medications for irregular heartbeat, possibly steroids if aspiration is noted on chest X-ray, antibiotics if lung infection is a concern, and sedatives–paralyzing agents if the person is resisting the ventilator. Blood tests and X-rays will help in decision making about management at this stage.

Once advanced life-support measures are instituted, it is necessary to decide whether or not hyperbaric oxygen recompression is needed. If decompression was omitted or arterial gas embolism occurred, then recompression should be initiated as soon as possible. Another consideration, which is controversial, is whether to use hyperbaric oxygen for brain resuscitation for the anoxic brain insult. In this latter situation the decision to use hyperbaric oxygen must be made conjointly by the family, the attending primary care physician, and the hyperbaric medicine specialist.

Once the person has stabilized, a process that may take days to weeks, decisions for subsequent management are made. If the person is recovering well, rehabilitation measures are instituted. If the person is in a persistent vegetative coma, transfer to a long-term care facility may be the only option. The prognosis for recovery depends primarily on the severity of the brain injury from lack of oxygen. An electroencephalogram (brain wave study) may be helpful in determining long-term prognosis. Usually, critical care management can resolve the lung injury problems.

Prevention

Aspiration, near-drowning, and drowning are prevented by knowledge of water safety.

Dive planning and properly maintained equipment can help to avoid situations that can lead to these events. The buddy system with first-response interventions is often the key consideration in whether or not the recovery of a near-drowning victim is successful. The location of the emergency medical resources available at or near the dive site should be known so that emergency help can be obtained immediately.

Return to Diving

If the period of unconsciousness associated with near-drowning is brief, rescue is immediate, and recovery is complete, return to water sport activities is permissible after a couple of days' rest. If residuals occur in the form of lung scarring or brain injury, return to diving is not advised. However, surface-type water activities such as swimming and snorkeling are highly recommended as rehabilitation techniques if the person is functional enough to do these.

BRINGING IT ALL TOGETHER

A 23-year-old well-trained, well-conditioned diver was asked by his buddies to retrieve a dropped weight belt in 30 FSW (9.1 MSW). Rather than using the buddy system, the diver used a line from the surface tied to his wrist. Each 30 seconds he was to respond to two tugs from tenders on the surface with two reply tugs. After a couple of minutes on the bottom he no longer responded to the line tugs. A standby diver, already suited up, immediately entered the water. On the bottom the standby diver found the person unconscious with the regulator out of his mouth. The person was brought to the surface with appropriate head control and was retrieved from the water. Immediate cardiopulmonary resuscitation measures were instituted. Spontaneous heartbeat and breathing movements appeared a few moments later, but the diver remained confused, lethargic, and restless. The diver was transported to a recompression chamber for suspected arterial gas embolism, and over the next four and one-half hours he was treated with hyperbaric oxygen recompression. He was momentarily compressed to 165 FSW (50 MSW) for maximum bubble compression. Throughout the treatment he remained restless and confused.

Immediately upon completion of the treatment the diver was transferred to a medical center. A chest X-ray showed whiting out of his lungs consistent with pulmonary edema secondary to aspiration of water. Blood gas studies revealed that blood oxygen was insufficient due to the lung condition. The diver was intubated and advanced life measures were instituted. Subsequently, his lungs stiffened and pneumothoraces (lung collapse) resulted from the positive pressure of the ventilator required to maintain blood oxygenation. Over several weeks' time these resolved, and the diver rehabilitated with almost full recovery. Subsequent chest X-rays and pulmonary function studies showed that scarring had occurred in his lungs. Resumption of diving was not recommended.

Comment: The reason for the loss of consciousness underwater was never determined despite a thorough investigation of the equipment and gas supply. Undoubtedly the reason was one of the no-panic syndromes (see chapter 11) with a heart arrhythmia as one of the prime considerations. It was obvious that the person had aspirated water and experienced near-drowning. Whether or not arterial gas embolism actually occurred is questionable. The symptoms the diver had after spontaneous resumption of breathing and heart activity were consistent with both hypoxia from near-drowning and brain involvement from aspiration. Since the diagnosis of arterial gas embolism was a possible consideration, hyperbaric oxygen was appropriate. Whenever there is doubt and a history of breathing compressed air under pressure, a trial of recompression is indicated. The stiffening of the lungs was consistent with a lung injury from aspiration and oxygen deprivation. Whether or not the high-pressure oxygen exposures during the hyperbaric treatment contributed to this via pulmonary oxygen toxicity mechanisms (see chapter 14) remains unanswerable.

Cardiac Arrest

Cardiac arrest is the complete cessation (stoppage) of the heart's activity. If it is recognized immediately, resuscitation efforts may be effective. Naturally, the terminal event in all diving-related deaths is cardiac arrest. As in near-drowning, MPD invariably precede the arrest. Diving activities, if done appropriately, usually are not stressful. However, certain portions of the dive are more stressful than others (see chapter 2). Emergency problems associated with diving can generate maximal exertional stresses as the person struggles to extricate him- or herself from the situation.

Significance

The effects of cardiac arrest are catastrophic, since the brain (as well as the other body tissues) cannot survive without adequately supplied and oxygenated blood. Within seconds after the heart stops beating, a person loses consciousness from lack of blood supply to the brain. The pumping action of the heart is usually one of the last bodily functions to cease when a person dies. Conversely, blockage of blood flow to the heart or irregular heart rhythms can abruptly halt cardiac activity. Cold water, panic, and breath-holding stresses of diving contribute to these problems.

Causes

The causes of cardiac arrest are not always easy to identify. Conditions in which heart muscles are deprived of oxygen, exposed to poison, or shocked by electricity are obvious causes. However, many factors may interact in generating a cardiac arrest. During a strenuous activity, factors ordinarily thought to be insignificant can contribute. Table 16.3 presents frequently occurring contributing causes of cardiac arrest. Virtually every medical and emotional disorder has some effect on the heart's blood supply, rate, and rhythm. The magnitude and duration of the insult, as well as the patient's physical condition, determine whether the challenge will be well tolerated (positive feedback mechanism) or whether it will lead to injury to the heart, cardiac arrest, or both.

Effects on the Body (Pathophysiology)

Ineffective cardiac action occurs when the heart beats too slowly, beats too rapidly, is too weak to pump the blood within it, or ceases to beat altogether. Tissues deprived of blood and oxygen stop functioning and die. The symptoms and signs of cardiac arrest, which reflect these effects, include the following:

- Loss of consciousness
- Collapse and loss of muscle tone
- Inability to feel pulses or to hear heartbeats in the chest
- Coldness—especially over arms and legs
- **Cyanosis** (deep blue coloration)—especially of lips, fingertips, and toes

Table 16.3	Cardiac Arrest: Contributing Causes
Cause	**Effect/Comment**
Air embolism and catastrophic decompression sickness	Bubbles block blood flow to heart
Anoxia	Reduces heart's O_2 supply
Blood vessel disease (hardening of the arteries)	Reduces blood supply to the heart (both heredity and environmental factors are contributors)
Cholesterol, high lipids	Contribute to blood vessel disease with hardening and narrowing of the arteries; ruptured cholesterol plaques may be the terminal event in blockage of the blood vessel
Cigarette smoking	Contributes to heart, blood vessel, and lung disease; indirectly reduces oxygen supply to the heart; in some people, nicotine actually causes narrowing of the cardiac blood vessels
Drowning	Deprives heart muscles of their oxygen supply
Electrical shock	Stops heart activity
Hypothermia	Slows heart rate; reduces blood supply to the heart
Nitrogen narcosis	Depresses heart activity; indirectly reduces cardiac blood supply
Overexertion	Oxygen demands of the exertion may exceed the heart's ability to meet the demands
Panic	Speeds heart rate; heart works less efficiently; end result is reduction in the relative blood supply in relation to the amount of pumping work; may cause arrhythmias
Shock	Inadequate blood circulation to the heart

- Dilation (enlargement) of pupils (in the eye) and failure of pupils to constrict (narrowing) with bright light—pupil responses can be altered by drugs like morphine, epinephrine, and atropine
- Glassy stare in the eyes

First-Response Interventions

Emergency treatment of cardiac arrest must be instituted immediately. Basic life support (BLS) and **advanced cardiac life support (ACLS;** interventions that use special equipment and medications to resuscitate, maintain life, or both) should be initiated as soon as possible. The ABCs of BLS were described in the previous section of this chapter. These should be continued until care of the person is assumed by a more qualified medical provider, the person is transported by paramedics to a medical center, or the rescuer is too fatigued to continue effective cardiopulmonary resuscitation.

Definitive Management

Definite treatment for cardiac arrest or insufficiency is twofold: first, sustaining adequate cardiac function to meet tissue oxygen demands, and second, correcting the causes that have led to the problem. All the interventions used to manage near-drowning may be required. In addition, electrical pacing of the heart, medications to dissolve blood clots, insertion of stents to open the blood vessels of the heart, and coronary bypass surgery may be done. If other MPD need to be addressed such as decompression sickness, hyperbaric oxygen recompression can be performed as long as the patient does not struggle during the treatment. Hyperbaric oxygen has been used to treat heart attacks and is thus not a contraindication for treating the diver with this problem and concomitant decompression sickness or arterial gas embolism symptoms.

Prevention

Prevention of cardiac arrest includes medical screening for those at risk for cardiac arrest, as well as dive planning to reduce the stresses of diving. Cardiac risk factors such as high blood pressure, obesity, diabetes, smoking, elevated cholesterol levels, and a positive family history of heart problems need to be paired with the diver's level of condition, age, and previous diving experiences. Today much can be done to determine whether diving would be reasonably safe for those with risk factors. Studies that can help provide this information include stress electrocardiograms, angiography (dye studies of blood flow to the heart), ultrasound studies of heart muscle contractility, and monitoring of heart activity over 24 hours. The use of heart medications is not an absolute contraindication to diving (see chapter 10). However, if cardiac function is impaired even with medications, diving should not be done.

Return to Diving

Return to diving after a cardiac arrest depends on if the cause was corrected, heart damage occurred, the fitness of the individual, and the motivation to return to diving. Generally, clearance by a cardiologist and a physician with knowledge of diving medicine is needed before resumption of diving is allowed. The diagnostic techniques just described provide a basis for the decision. Finally the patient should be counseled regarding ways to minimize the stresses of diving, such as diving in warm waters so that thick wet suits and heavy weight belts are not needed, shortening dive times, diving from boats in order to minimize surface swims, and limiting the number of dives each day.

Shock

Shock is a clinical condition characterized by failure of the circulatory system to maintain adequate perfusion (blood flow) to tissues. It occurs when the body's positive feedback mechanisms for dealing with the causes of shock are overwhelmed. Like the other complications of the MPD, shock invariably has antecedent causes, and some of them can occur from diving.

Significance

Medical problems of diving can lead to multiple types or forms of shock. Hypovolemic shock may result from massive bite injuries. Envenomations from marine animal toxin injuries may cause cardiogenic shock. Anoxic injuries may also cause this form of shock. Massive intravascular bubbling from explosive decompression or arterial gas embolism, or a combination of the two, is another diving-related cause of shock. Any type of shock represents a very serious, life-threatening situation. Immediate action must be initiated in order to save the diver's life.

Causes

Shock is manifested whenever the body's effective blood circulation falls below a certain critical level. The effective blood circulation is the amount of blood that is in circulation to supply the body tissues' oxygen and nutrition requirements.

It is easy to appreciate how bleeding can lower the effective blood circulation to a critical point. However, there are other disorders that also cause the effective blood circulation to fall below the critical level.

- Blood loss or hypovolemic ("hypo" = lowered, "volemic" = blood volume) shock: Caused by external bleeding or internal bleeding such as ulcers or rupture of aneurysms (expansions of blood vessels).

- Cardiogenic ("cardio" = heart, "genic" = origin) shock: From heart attack, heart failure, or arrhythmias; once the heart ceases to circulate the blood effectively, the result is similar to that with the other types of shock.

- Neurogenic ("neuro" = nerve) shock: From loss of nerve control of the blood vessels; the capacity of the vascular system exceeds the blood volume by a factor of 20 or more (see chapter 3). If blood is not highly regulated by the nervous system, it may be diverted from the critical tissues like the brain or remain in reservoirs. Fainting from the sight of a needle, pain, or a frightening experience is a form of neurogenic shock. *Distributive* is now the preferred term for this type of shock and also refers to shock from anaphylaxis (allergic reactions).

- Septic (sick from an infectious process) shock: Toxins produced by certain types of bacteria have an effect on the body similar to that of neurogenic shock. In neurogenic, cardiogenic, and septic shock, blood loss is not a factor. That is why the phrase "effective circulation" is used in association with shock.

Effects on the Body (Pathophysiology)

Although the exact mechanism of shock is not fully understood (hence the frequently used term *shock syndrome*), it is thought to arise when certain critical body tissues are deprived of an adequate blood supply. In the compensated phase, positive feedback mechanisms make adjustments to maintain oxygenation of critical tissues. Increased pulse and respiratory rates are manifestations of these positive feedback mechanisms. As long as the insult or injury is not too severe, the body can make appropriate adjustments, and the person's life is not threatened. For example, a shark attack may cause massive body tissue losses and bleeding. The uncontrollable bleeding leads to shock and lowering of the blood pressure. The lowered blood pressure slows the blood loss. Even though lowering the blood pressure is an effect of shock, it keeps the person from bleeding to death as rapidly as would be the case otherwise.

In the decompensated phase of shock, the feedback mechanisms are no longer able to maintain an effective blood circulation, and progressive deterioration occurs. Unless the body's compensating mechanisms are bolstered with oxygen, medical treatments, blood transfusions, and medications, the person's life is in jeopardy. The problems that lead to the decompensated phase of shock, such as a heart attack or bleeding from a wound, must also be managed simultaneously. The effects of shock can contribute to its progression, as illustrated in figure 16.1. An example is seen in cardiogenic shock; here the heart requires more oxygenated blood, but its pumping action is so compromised that it cannot effectively circulate the oxygenated blood. This becomes a vicious circle.

Whether the body can institute positive feedback mechanisms, coupled with appropriate management, and reverse the process depends on the duration, severity, and extent of injury. If treatment or correction of the underlying injury or insult can intersect and mediate the vicious circle, the shock syndrome is said to be reversible. At a certain point shock becomes irreversible: The tissues have been so deprived of oxygen that they are no longer able to recover. When this happens, death occurs regardless of the treatment. Duration of shock is a critical factor in whether or not the patient will survive; after an hour or so of decompensated shock, it invariably becomes irreversible.

Symptoms of shock are manifestations of the effects from the effective circulation's falling below a critical level. They include rapid heart rate, lowered blood pressure, cyanosis, sweating, paleness, altered level of consciousness to the point of fainting, and coldness.

First-Response Interventions

Treatment of shock is designed to eliminate the cause of the initial injury and to improve the effectiveness of circulation. Emergency treatment of shock includes the following steps:

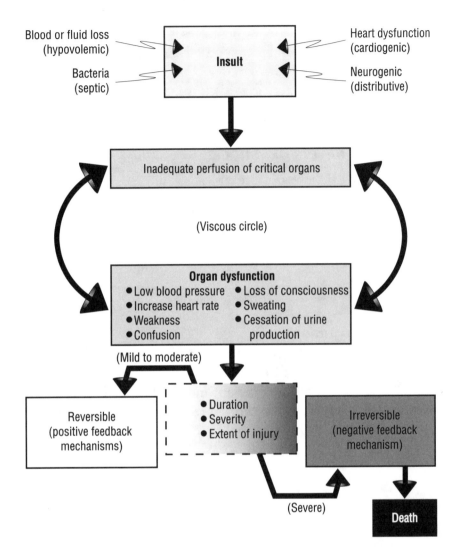

FIGURE 16.1 Self-perpetuation of the shock syndrome. Inadequate blood flow (perfusion) to critical organs leads to their dysfunction.

- Eliminate or correct the cause. For example, in blood loss, stop the bleeding; in cardiac arrest or drowning, administer 100 percent oxygen and resuscitation measures.

- Elevate the legs: Two-fifths of the body's total blood volume may be stored in the lower extremities. Elevating the legs can act like a blood transfusion and restore this stored blood to the effective circulation.

- Keep the patient warm.

- Administer clear fluids if the patient is alert; water, juices, and clear soups can be rapidly absorbed and can thereby contribute to the effective circulation. Ingestion of alcoholic beverages is harmful since these tend to relax the musculature around the blood vessels, lower the blood pressure, and diminish the effective circulation.

- Administer 100 percent oxygen; this helps to compensate for the lack of effective blood circulation by making the blood more efficient in carrying oxygen. Hyperbaric oxygen is 10 times more efficient in this regard than breathing room air and is used in critical shock situations such as those associated with blood loss in Jehovah's Witness patients and crises in patients with sickle cell anemia.

Diving Physics: Reversible Shock

When laboratory animals have been bled to the point at which they go into shock, they survive if blood is returned to them within an hour. Shock in this situation is said to be reversible. If the animals are bled to the same level but are not retransfused until three or four hours later, they die from irreversible shock.

Definitive Management

Definitive management is aimed toward elimination or correction of the cause of shock. For divers in shock from a massive decompression illness event, hyperbaric oxygen recompression therapy may be the only intervention that can save their lives. Advanced life-support techniques, as mentioned earlier, may be required in the management of shock.

BRINGING IT ALL TOGETHER

A 46-year-old male with several cardiac risk factors including smoking, overweight, poor level of conditioning, and elevated cholesterol levels decides to begin SCUBA diving with the goal of improving his conditioning. He completes the pool training sessions without problems. During his first open water dive he suits up and then descends a 50-foot (15-meter) pathway to the beach. He feels uncomfortable in the equipment and notes that he is sweating profusely as he reaches the beach. He disregards these symptoms since it is a warm day and he is wearing a thick wet suit. Upon entering the water, which is about 25 degrees C cooler than the air temperature, he collapses. The dive instructor immediately rescues him, initiates the emergency response system, and begins basic life-support measures. A faint pulse is detected, but by the time the paramedics arrive the person is pulseless. He does not respond to resuscitation efforts.

Comment: The diagnosis of cardiogenic shock best explains the events described. Whether it was due to a fatal arrhythmia or a massive heart attack (it takes time for changes from lack of blood supply to the heart muscles to occur) could not be determined by the coroner. A thorough pre-dive medical screening might have been able to detect that the person was at risk for a cardiac event. From this information, it would have been possible to institute corrective measures or recommend against diving.

Prevention

The way to prevent shock is to avoid accidents and other factors that lead to the various presentations of shock. For example, treating an infection early prevents septic shock. Dive planning can help reduce the likelihood of a diving accident that could lead to shock. The pre-dive medical evaluation can reveal risk factors for diving and provide the basis for initiating corrective actions or making the recommendation against diving (see chapter 10).

Return to Diving

The guidelines regarding return to diving after cardiac arrest are apropos for shock also. Resumption of diving is appropriate when the cause of shock was an extrinsic factor such as blood loss or infection and when recovery, conditioning, and fitness are restored to the pre-injury state.

For Further Review

1. How do the complications of MPD differ from the actual medical problems themselves?

2. What are the predispositions to cardiac events that have relevance to divers? Which ones can be modified to make diving more safe?

3. How do aspiration, near-drowning, and drowning differ?

4. Why is fluid aspiration rarely great enough to cause changes in blood chemistries when drownings occur in humans? How does this differ for dogs?

5. What secondary complications can occur from near-drowning?

6. What must one consider before allowing a person who has had a complication from one of the MPD to resume diving?

DIVING MEDICINE FROM A TO Z

This reference is an easy way to quickly review subjects mentioned in this text. It is not meant to be all-inclusive or to summarize all the information on a subject. The items under each alphabet letter are limited to six or less. One or more chapters that include further information on the subject are listed in parentheses. The chapter listed first is the one that contains the primary or most complete information on a given subject. In general, the more important items relating to each topic are near the top of the list.

A = Arterial Gas Embolism (Chapters 15, 1)

- The most serious of the medical problems of diving
- Irreversible brain damage may occur if hyperbaric recompression therapy is not started immediately
- Often associated with panic or equipment problems, or both, leading to too rapid ascents
- The proposed mechanism is breath-holding during ascent with resultant gas expansion (Boyle's Law) in the lungs and explosive rupture of alveoli and adjacent blood vessels
- Accounts for about 20 percent of the approximately 100 yearly SCUBA diving deaths

B = Blackout, Causes of (Chapters 11, 14, 16)

- Hyperventilation and breath-holding with alteration of normal signaling mechanisms to breathe
- Reverse diffusion of oxygen from the blood into the lungs after deep breath-hold dives
- Dilution of oxygen associated with using closed-circuit diving systems
- Cardiac causes such as cardiac arrest, irregular heart rhythms, and heart attack
- Nitrogen narcosis
- Carbon monoxide poisoning

C = Cardiopulmonary Resuscitation (Chapter 16)

- Activate the Emergency Medical Services system (i.e., dial 911 to call for help)

- *Airway:* check position, look, listen, feel for breathing
- *Breathing:* two mouth-to-mouth insufflations
- *Cardiac activity:* feel for carotid (neck artery) pulse
- Rates: for an adult, 100 chest compressions and 15 artificial ventilations per minute

D = Decompression Sickness (Chapters 15, 3, 5)

- The "price" divers may "pay" for breathing compressed gases underwater
- Occurs infrequently; two to three occurrences for every 10,000 SCUBA dives
- The reason dive tables and dive computers are essential for planning dives
- Occurrences about equally divided between deserved (violations of diving practices) and undeserved (disordered decompression, bends-proneness factors, or both)
- Treated with hyperbaric oxygen recompression
- If no residual problems after treatment and no bends-proneness factors identified, return to diving usually permitted after a couple of weeks

E = Environmental Problems (Chapters 12, 1)

- Probably the most important cause of diver morbidity (i.e., interruption of or temporary loss of diving time) from the medical problems of diving
- Swimmer's ear
- Sunburn
- Hypothermia
- Hyperthermia

F = Fast Tissues (Chapters 3, 15)

- On- and off-gas (the inert gas) very rapidly, within seconds or minutes
- Lungs almost instantaneously equilibrate with the new ambient (outside) pressure of the inert gas
- Blood, heart, and brain tissue also believed to be very fast tissues
- Diving tables and many diving computers do not consider on- and off-gassing of the very fast tissues
- Slow ascent rates and the three-minute 15-FSW (4.6-MSW) rest stop are usually sufficient to prevent decompression sickness in the fast tissues

G = Gas Laws (Chapters 1, 5, 11, 13-15)

- Boyle's: the volume of a gas in a flexible enclosed structure is inversely related to the pressure exerted on the structure

- Charles': the volume of a gas increases directly with the temperature and vice versa (Kelvin temperatures must be used in the computations)
- Dalton's: the total pressure of gases in a system is equal to the sum of the partial pressures of the individual gases
- Henry's: in a closed liquid–gas system, the amount of gas forced into the liquid phase is proportional to the pressure of the gas
- Universal gas law: the combination of Boyle's and Charles' Laws, that is, $PV = nRT$ or $P_1V_1/T_1 = P_2V_2/T_2$ where P = pressure, V = volume, T = temperature (degrees Kelvin), n = number of gas molecules, and R = the universal gas constant

H = Hyperbaric Oxygen Indications (Chapters 6, 14, 15)

- Decompression sickness
- Arterial gas embolism
- Carbon monoxide poisoning
- Near-drowning and other causes of hypoxic encephalopathy (brain dysfunction from lack of oxygen) are investigational uses
- Adjunct to healing of problem wounds (diabetic, radiation induced, gas gangrene, flesh-eating bacteria, etc.); about 90 percent of the clinical uses of hyperbaric oxygen are discussed
- Crush injuries

I = Immersion Effects (Chapters 4, 5, 7)

- Initiation of the diving reflex: (a) bradycardia (slowing of the heart), (b) peripheral vasoconstriction (decreased blood flow to the extremities), and (c) anaerobic metabolism
- Shifting of fluids from the core to the central circulation
- Decreased lung capacity in humans
- Increased urine production in humans
- Hypothermia in cold water

J = Joint Pains (Chapters 15, 3)

- Found in about 50 percent of the cases of decompression sickness (DCS)
- Actual causes in DCS yet to be identified; likely due to microscopic bubble formation in joint capsules (Ruffini type 2 corpuscles) and stretching of these pain-sensitive structures from bubble enlargement
- Musculoskeletal injuries associated with climbing aboard boats or lifting of equipment are a common cause of joint pains in divers

- With a history of compressed air diving and joint pains, a trial treatment of hyperbaric oxygen recompression should always take place
- The basis for the common term for DCS, the bends, is the bent-over posture that bridge caisson workers had when walking after experiencing DCS

K = Kinesiology (Chapter 8)

- The science of movements based on muscles, joints, and lever systems
- Diving mammals have adaptations for movement through the water, including (a) body shape, (b) improved mechanical advantages of muscle–joint systems, (c) subcutaneous fatty tissues, and (d) heat exchange systems
- Sport divers move through the water less than 1/12 as fast as diving mammals
- Many choices are available for swim fins, each with advantages and disadvantages

L = Limiting Factors for Depth of Sport Diving (Chapters 2, 3, 5, 13-15)

- Pure oxygen: 33 FSW (10 MSW) for about 30 minutes
- Nitrox-36: 110 FSW (33 MSW) for 30 minutes
- Sport SCUBA diving with air: 130 FSW (40 MSW) for 10 minutes
- Nitrox-32: 130 FSW for 20 minutes
- Predicted thoracic squeeze depth threshold for a breath-hold dive in an average-sized male: 132 FSW (40 MSW)
- Helium–oxygen and trimix (oxygen, helium, and nitrogen): 380 FSW (116 MSW) with deep sea diving rig, or 1,000 FSW (305 MSW) or greater using saturation diving techniques

M = Metabolism (Chapters 4, 10, 7)

- Provides energy for body functions, including movement through the water
- Increases in human divers with high-protein diet and conditioning (acclimatizations) to cold water
- Metabolism with oxygen is about 20 times more efficient (in generating energy) than anaerobic (without oxygen) metabolism
- About 3,600 kilocalories of energy production is needed to lose one pound (0.5 kilogram) of weight
- Exercising at a moderate level of activity requires about 600 kilocalories of energy utilization an hour; that is, it takes about six hours of exercise to lose one pound

N = Nystagmus (Dizziness, Light-Headedness, Vertigo–Room Spinning Sensations, Confusion) (Chapters 13, 14-16)

- Nystagmus refers to involuntary rapid movements of the eyeball; this and the other conditions all indicate potentially serious problems with brain or inner ear function when they are associated with diving

- Many medical problems of diving can lead to these problems, including (a) lack of oxygen to the brain from arterial gas embolism and decompression sickness, (b) decompression sickness of the inner ear, (c) eardrum perforation and entry of cold water into the middle ear space, (d) most of the medical problems associated with the bottom phase of a dive, (e) head injury, (f) strokes, and (g) shock and marine animal envenomations

- Whenever any of these symptoms are experienced, diving activities must be stopped immediately

- Immediate medical evaluation is required for any of these symptoms

O = Oxygen Toxicity (Chapters 14, 1)

- A complication of breathing oxygen under increased partial pressures

- High exposures lead to seizures, and lower exposures for longer durations lead to pulmonary edema (fluid in the lungs); precursor symptoms may include anxiety, ringing in the ears, tremors, and tunnel vision

- Seizure thresholds are variable depending on oxygen partial pressure, duration of exposure, activity, anxiety, thermal comfort, and previous seizure history

- Nitrox and closed-circuit SCUBA diving with pure oxygen alter oxygen partial pressures and increase the risks of oxygen toxicity during diving

- A guideline for oxygen exposure limits (the U.S. Navy has modified this somewhat) is two atmospheres absolute oxygen exposure for 30 minutes

- This guideline is equivalent to a 33-FSW (10-MSW) dive using 100 percent oxygen for 30 minutes or an open-circuit air dive to about 300 FSW (91 MSW) for the same period of time

P = Panic (Chapters 11, 1, 15)

- Probably the most important (seriousness plus frequency) medical problem of diving for the sport diver

- Estimated to contribute to over 50 percent of the drowning deaths in sport SCUBA divers

- Incidence inversely related to experience

- Characterized by a loss of control and a failure to take corrective actions that would otherwise be obvious when not in a state of panic

- Self-perpetuation (vicious circle) mechanisms sustain the panic attack even if the inciting cause is no longer present
- Outcomes of panic in the water are threefold: (a) resolution, (b) drowning from exhaustion, or (c) cardiac arrest

Q = Quick References (Appendix B)

- Divers Alert Network: (919) 684-8111
- Undersea and Hyperbaric Medical Society: (301) 942-2980
- Edmonds' *Diving and Subaquatic Medicine*
- *Bennett and Elliott's Physiology and Medicine of Diving*
- *NOAA Diving Manual*
- Strauss and Borer's "Diving Medicine: Contemporary Topics and Their Controversies."

R = Reflex, Diving (Chapters 4, 11, 13, 16)

- A universal adaptation with components present in most vertebrate animals, associated with hypoxic (low oxygen) stresses
- Components: see Immersion Effects
- Initiated by immersion of the face in water
- The reflex is initiated by water stimulating the fifth (trigeminal) cranial nerve
- It is modified in humans by activity, experience, water temperature, and age

S = Stresses in Diving (Chapters 1, 3, 11, 16)

- The consequences of interacting with the underwater environment
- Most resolved without conscious effort, for example, by the need to breathe as a result of carbon dioxide elevations in the blood
- Unresolved stresses lead to an alarm reaction; in the water this can be manifested as panic
- Stress reduction and panic prevention should be an integral part of diving training
- Unresolved stresses lead to medical problems of diving, especially panic

T = Thermal Properties of Water (Chapters 1, 7, 12)

- Specific heat of water is 1,000 times greater than that of air
- Heat conduction of water is 25 times as rapid as that of air
- Survival times in water can be measured in minutes as compared to survival time in hours in air of the same temperature
- Thermal discomfort frequently is the factor that limits the duration of a dive

- Minimizing movements in cold water is more effective for conserving heat than trying to generate metabolic heat by muscle activity

U = Units for Measuring Pressure (Chapter 1)

- Selected for convenience and common usage
- Absolute pressures take into consideration the weight of the earth's atmosphere
- Conversion of one pressure unit to another is easily accomplished (table 1.1)
- The relative change in pressure during descent from an 18,000-foot (5,500-meter) altitude to sea level is equivalent to descending from sea level to 16 FSW (5 MSW)

V = Visual Challenges of Water (Chapters 1, 9)

- Vision distortion occurs unless an air interface is interposed between the water and the eyes
- Objects are magnified by about one-third when visualized underwater
- The physical properties of water limit distance vision to 100 yards (meters) or less even if the water is clear; in turbid waters visibility may be reduced to inches
- Yellow and red colors are filtered out by water; at a depth of 60 FSW (18 MSW), all brightly colored objects become a monotonous blue-gray color
- At night, underwater vision is limited to the cone of light produced by the diver's underwater lamp

W = Water Density (Chapter 1)

- Water is 775 times more dense than air
- Objects float if they weigh less than the water they displace; objects sink if they weigh more than the water they displace
- The density of water accounts for its flow properties such as currents, tides, waves, and swells
- Water density, while allowing the diver to be almost neutrally buoyant, restricts movement
- Resistance to movement through water is termed drag; diving gear, such as tanks and buoyancy compensators, markedly increases drag and slows movement through the water

X = X-Ray, A Reminder About the Importance of Fitness for Diving (Chapter 10)

- Chest X-rays generally are not required for the entry level of sport SCUBA diving

- Safe diving requires fitness; however, diving itself, if done properly, is not a good activity for aerobic conditioning
- Different types of diving require different types of medical assessments
- There are absolute, relative, and temporary contraindications for diving
- Divers over 40 years of age should have special medical exams, including X-rays, lab tests, and assessment of heart function before beginning to dive

Y = Why to Dive (Introduction, Chapters 2, 10)

- Enjoyment and pleasure
- Excitement and challenges
- An escape from the terrestrial gravity-restricted environment to a gravity-free environment
- Exploration and scientific studies
- Motivation to maintain fitness (in preparation for diving)
- Economic reasons, including dive instruction work, food harvesting, underwater construction, equipment inspection work, and treasure hunting

Z = Zero Tolerance for Unsafe Diving (Chapter 10)

- Alcohol intoxication, impaired mental function from drugs
- Medical conditions that are absolute contraindications for diving
- Residual serious medical problems originating from diving, such as paralysis
- Diving without proper training, an appropriate dive buddy, and adequate equipment
- Weather conditions that endanger the diver
- Diving without adequate knowledge, pre-dive briefing of the dive site, or both

WHERE TO GET HELP

This section has two components. First, it lists sources that a diver can consult to get information regarding a medical problem or other questions about diving. Second, it lists some well-known reference books and manuals on diving medicine and physiology. For the most part, the information in the reference texts is designed for the physician, researcher, or professional diver. A comment about each of these references accompanies the citation.

Diving Organizations

Divers Alert Network (DAN)

Web site: http://www.diversalertnetwork.org/

Diving emergency hotline: (919) 684-8111

Diving emergency hotline (collect calls): (919) 684-4326

Consultative services (weekdays 9 a.m. to 5 p.m. eastern time): (919) 684-2948

DAN is a nonprofit organization directed and staffed by experts in diving medicine. It is staffed 24 hours a day. Other activities of DAN include annual compilation of diving accident statistics, education, and research.

Diving Medicine Online

Web site: http://www.scuba-doc.com

This is a large Web site containing comprehensive updated information about diving and undersea medicine for the nonmedical diver and the non-diving medical professional; it is also an excellent reference source for the diving medical specialist.

Emergency Medical Services System

Dialing 911 almost anywhere in the United States initiates contact with the EMS system. Recovery, rescue, emergency treatment, and transportation to a medical facility can be arranged through the EMS system. If at sea, this may be through the U.S. Coast Guard; if on a shore-based dive, paramedics will likely handle the emergency.

Handicapped Scuba Association International
Web site: http://www.hsascuba.com

Phone: (949) 498-4540

Fax: (949) 498-6128

1104 El Prado, San Clemente, CA 92672-4637

The HSAI provides information about access to training and diving for individuals with physical disabilities.

International Society of Aquatic Medicine (ISAM)
Web site: www.divingdocs.org

Phone: (910) 452-1452

Fax: (910) 799-5209

E-mail: divingdocs@aol.com

6240 Turtle Hall Drive, Wilmington, NC 28409

ISAM is a society of physician divers who coordinate diving education with scuba diving activities.

National Association of Underwater Instructors (NAUI) Worldwide
Web site: http://www.nauiww.org/index-side.html

This is a worldwide diver training and certification agency. The association's training manuals detail how to use diving equipment and describe the training required for special certifications.

Occupational Safety Health Administration (OSHA)
Commercial and Scientific Diving Operations, 1999 (Washington, DC: U.S. Government Printing Office). This is a government agency that sets the standards for commercial diving activities in the United States.

Professional Association of Diving Instructors (PADI)
Web site: http://www.padi.com/

P.O. Box 7006, 30151 Tomas St., Rancho Santa Margarita, CA 92688-2128

This is another international diver training and certification agency. See NAUI for more information.

Undersea and Hyperbaric Medical Society (UHMS)
Web site: http://www.uhms.org

Phone (weekdays, eastern time): (301) 942-2980

Fax: (301) 942-7804

E-mail: uhms@uhms.org

10531 Metropolitan Ave., Kensington, MD 20895

The Undersea and Hyperbaric Medical Society is an international, nonprofit professional organization for diving and undersea medicine. It maintains a comprehensive up-to-date library and reference system, collaborates with governmental agencies for funding of diving and hyperbaric research, and provides the standards for hyperbaric oxygen therapy use in the United States. The UHMS also maintains a list of the locations of clinical hyperbaric oxygen chamber facilities in the United States.

World Recreational Scuba Training Council, Inc.

Web site: http://www.wrstc.com

E-mail: info@wrstc.com

P.O. Box 11083, Jacksonville, FL 32239-1083

This organization has representatives from the diving certifying agencies. It establishes uniform medical requirements and training standards for recreational divers.

Medical Texts, Manuals, and Reviews for Diving

Bove, A.A., and J.C. Davis, eds. 1997. *Bove and Davis' diving medicine,* 3rd ed. Philadelphia: Saunders. A good summary of the serious medical problems of diving with a comprehensive discussion of fitness for diving.

Burbakk, A.O., and T.S. Neuman, eds. 2003. *Bennett and Elliott's physiology and medicine of diving,* 5th ed. Philadelphia: Saunders. An erudite, highly referenced, multi-authored text; the most comprehensive source of physiological information on diving.

Edmonds, C., C. Lowry, J. Pennefeather, and R. Walker. 2002. *Diving and subaquatic medicine.* Boston: Butterworth. Another good source of information about medical problems of diving for physicians written in an interesting and understandable style.

Joiner, J.T., ed. 2001. *NOAA diving manual: Diving for science and technology,* 4th ed. Washington, DC: U.S. Dept. of Commerce, National Oceanic and Atmospheric Administration. A multi-authored, very well-illustrated manual that is an excellent source of information on diving equipment and diving techniques. A primary audience is the mission-oriented scientific diver.

Rahn, H., and T. Yokoyama, eds. 1965. *Physiology of breath-hold diving and the AMA of Japan, publication 1341.* Washington, D.C.: National Academy of Sciences, National Research Council. The classical and definitive source of information from field observations of breath-hold divers.

Strauss, M.B., and R.C.J.R. Borer. 2001. Diving Medicine: Contemporary Topics and Their Controversies, *American Journal of Emergency Medicine* 19:232. A streamlined article in question and answer format that discusses situations that physicians may need to answer regarding their patients who dive.

U.S. Navy diving manual (section on air diving). 1993. NAVSEA 0994-LP-001-9110. Flagstaff, AZ: Best. Like the *NOAA Diving Manual,* this resource provides diving tables for a variety of diving types and treatment tables for decompression illness, as well as other technical and medical information.

ITEMS FOR THE DIVING MEDICAL KIT

Most divers do not give much attention to having medical supplies available for their dives. When a medical problem of diving arises, it is desirable to initiate care at the dive scene. Therefore emergency medical supplies should be a component of the diver's equipment. There is overlap between equipment carried for safety reasons, prevention of injury, and treatment of injury. For example, a diving knife could be used for all three purposes. There are three levels of sophistication regarding equipment for diving medical kits: (1) the personal kit, (2) equipment for a several-day boat trip, and (3) supplies that should be carried for a dive excursion or scientific mission. Since loss of consciousness requires immediate initiation of basic life support, the most important medical "piece" of equipment a diver can have is knowledge of cardiopulmonary resuscitation. The following are suggestions for medical equipment recommended for each of the three levels of sophistication of diving activities.

Personal First Aid Supplies for the Diver

Personal first aid supplies are items the diver may carry in the pockets of a buoyancy compensator or bring to the dive site in the diving bag. Items to prevent medical problems of diving, like much of the safety equipment a diver carries, should be considered no less valuable than items used to actually treat a problem. According to the philosophy of preventive medicine, prevention is more important as compared to the less desirable choice of treating a problem that could have been prevented. Although the list seems long, about half the items are considered standard equipment for the diver, and another third are probably routinely carried by the well-prepared diver. The items in this list encompass almost everything needed to treat the medical problems of diving that occur frequently but are not serious—those for which medical help is not usually sought.

Item	Role
Afrin or pseudoephedrine-type nose drops	Prevention of an ear squeeze before a dive; treatment of one after a dive
Aspirin	A first-line ancillary measure for managing decompression sickness; treatment of minor aches, pains, and headaches not related to diving problems
Band-Aids (several sizes)	To cover minor cuts and scratches; often help with pain control from these injuries
Benedryl	A multiple-use over-the-counter medication for allergic reactions, sedation, nausea, seasickness
Candy bar, high-protein bar, non-diet soda pop	For management of hypoglycemia (low blood sugar); especially important for persons with diabetes who dive
Cell phone	To call 911 or other agencies for emergency help
Cortisone cream	Management of skin irritations, allergic reactions from marine animal injuries
Dive knife	A safety item that can free a diver of entanglements; useful for scraping off tentacles (with talcum powder)
Dive light, strobe, waterproof signal flares, and/or cylume	Another group of safety items that have relevance to diving accidents; used to signal for help, pickup, or rescue, especially during nighttime diving activities
Dive sausage	Another safety item; raising and lowering it in series of three is a universal sign of need for help (see Whistle)
Dive skins (Lycra dive suit)	Protection (preventive medicine) equipment for sunburn, marine animal injuries, and hypothermia
Ear drops (alcohol + acetic acid or proprietary)	Ear canal hygiene; prevention of swimmer's ear
Ibuprofen (Advil, Motrin, Nuprin, Aleve)	For muscle soreness that is attributed to a minor injury or overuse; not to be used to mask decompression sickness symptoms
Seasickness pills (Bonine, Antivert, meclizine)	Prevention of seasickness; seasickness can mimic many other serious problems associated with diving
Sudafed tablets	Prevention of ear and sinus squeezes; treatment if they occur
Sunglasses	Eye protection between dives; select lenses that have both UV (ultraviolet) A and B protection
Sunscreen	Prevention of sunburn; select a product that has an SFA (sun protection factor) over 25 and is waterproof
Talcum powder	To coalesce tentacles of jellyfish so they can be scraped off the skin; also helpful for "slipping into" neoprene exposure suits
Tourniquet (a piece of small-sized rope or rubber tubing)	Useful as a "be prepared" item for tying on loose objects, but in the rare situation of uncontrolled bleeding (shark bite, propeller injury) can be lifesaving

Item	Role
Water	To manage dehydration associated with a dive; another first-line ancillary management for the conscious, alert diver with suspected decompression sickness
Whistle	Another safety item; whistle blasts in series of three signal that immediate help is needed

Equipment for Daily or Several-Day Dive Boat Trips

With the increasing sophistication of sport diving boat operations, most of the items included in the following table are routinely carried in the dive boat medical locker. These items, by virtue of their expense, size, or training requirements for proper use, are better suited to a dive boat than for inclusion as personal medical items.

Item	Role
Alcohol, ammonia, and/or baking soda	For inactivating the poisons from marine animal sting injuries
Antidiarrhea agents	Pepto Bismol, Maalox, and Immodium are over-the-counter agents, useful for stomach "upset"; also, Lomotil, which requires a prescription
Automatic electrical defibrillator (AED)	For defibrillating (correcting irregular heart rhythms) and monitoring heart rhythms in the unconscious diver
Cervical collar and spine board	For the suspected traumatic spinal cord injury (from diving into shallow water, head and neck trauma from falls on the boat, etc.)
Cough syrup	Many over-the-counter choices available
Disinfectants	Betadine, for example
Dressing supplies	For wound coverage; control of bleeding
Elastic (Ace) wraps	For applying splints, holding dressings in place, protecting sprained joints, or controlling bleeding
Hot water source	For managing puncture wounds from marine animals; for rewarming for severe hypothermia
Oral airway	Helps to keep the tongue from blocking the throat
Otoscope	For examining the eardrum; if it is perforated, the diver should not return to the water; inexpensive otoscopes are available from pharmacies and from the Divers Alert Network (DAN)
Oxygen	Making portable oxygen kits available to dive operators, as well as the associated training, is one of DAN's missions; oxygen is the first intervention for decompression illness and near-drowning

(continued)

(continued)

Item	Role
Splints and slings	For immobilization of traumatic extremity injuries; often the elastic wrap is used to hold the splint or sling in place
Thermometer	For measuring temperature, for example, with hypothermia and for determining whether a diver has a fever and should not enter the water
Tylenol with codeine (Tylenol #3)	Although this pill requires a prescription, it is another multiple-use medication; for pain relief, control of coughing, and control of diarrhea
Upset stomach medications	Antacids and GERD (gastroesophageal reflux disease) medications

Supplies for a Dive Excursion or Scientific Mission

Often dive excursions or scientific activities are carried out in remote areas. Frequently a physician is in attendance. All the equipment listed in the preceding tables should be the starting point for the medical equipment for a dive excursion or scientific mission. It is important for the dive supervisor, the physician, or the medic in charge of the health of the participants to be aware of the medical conditions of the divers and the medical supplies they have brought with them. Often the preparedness of the divers and their past experiences constitute a wealth of available medical resources that could be used for other divers in case of injuries or diseases. The following additional items should be included in the dive excursion or dive mission medical kit.

Item	Role
Antibiotics	A selection of two or three agents will cover a spectrum of bacteria
Antiemetics (for control of nausea and vomiting)	Compazine, Droperidol, Tigan (available in suppository form), and others
Antimalaria pills	For diving in areas where malaria is endemic; the Communicable Disease Center in Atlanta, GA, will give current recommendations for malaria prophylaxsis
Blood pressure cuff	For monitoring blood pressure
Cardiac medications	Atropine, epinephrine, digitalis preparations, idocaine, diuretics, other anti-arrhythmic medications
Claggett needle and Heimlich valve	For pneumothorax management
Dental kit	For temporary tooth filling repairs

Item	Role
Flashlight	For checking papillary responses, for examining wounds
Foley catheter	For urinary retention, associated paraplegia (spine bends)
Intravenous solutions such as normal saline, glucose, and electrolytes; also including needles and connecting lines	For emergency hydration, treatment of shock and hypoglycemia
Laryngoscope endotracheal tubes and Ambu bag	For airway management and artificial ventilation
Metered dose inhalers	For wheezing, allergic, and asthmatic reactions; bronchodilators (albuterol), steroids, or combinations
Narcotic analgesics (painkillers)	For managing severe traumatic pain, heart attacks, pulmonary edema, puncture wounds from marine animal injuries, diarrhea, and cough
Sedative medications (Valium, Haldol)	For anxiety management; control of acute psychotic reactions, alcohol withdrawal
Special mission-oriented considerations	For example, sea snake and stone fish anti-venoms if the mission is directed at doing research on these animals
Steroids	For severe allergic reactions, asthma, and spinal cord injury
Stethoscope	For monitoring heart and lung function and measuring blood pressure
Surgical kit	For repair of minor lacerations, debridement of wounds, removal of foreign objects
Topical agents for burns, other wounds	Silvadene, antibacterial ointments, lidocaine ointment for pain relief
Vaseline gauze	For sucking chest wounds (trauma); wound coverage

LUMINARIES IN DIVING MEDICINE

Countless numbers of scientists, divers, and physicians have made substantial contributions to diving medicine. This appendix is not intended to list every person who has contributed to diving medicine, nor does it include the scientists who have contributed to the understanding of the (nonhuman) mammalian divers. With few exceptions, the luminaries included in this section are known personally to the authors or have spoken at underwater science meetings attended by the authors.

Name	Location (where work done)	Contribution
Bachrach, A.	Washington, DC (Navy)	Panic and psychological stresses of diving
Bassett, A.	San Antonio, TX	Development of the dive computer; diving and medical seminars for physicians
Behnke, A.	Washington, DC (Navy)	The father of diving medicine; helium–oxygen diving for submarine rescue; use of oxygen to treat decompression sickness
Bennett, P.	Durham, NC (Duke)	First chief executive officer of DAN; high-pressure nervous system syndrome; nitrogen narcosis; coauthor of *Physiology and Medicine of Diving*
Bert, P.	France	Cerebral oxygen toxicity; cause of decompression sickness
Bond, G.	San Diego, CA (Navy)	Saturation diving; nicknamed "Papa Topside"
Bove, A.	Philadelphia, PA	Dehydration and hemoconcentration associated with decompression sickness; diving fitness; coauthor of *Diving Medicine*
Cousteau, J.	France	Development of the SCUBA regulator; conservation of the diving environment; promoting the sport of SCUBA diving
Craig, A.	Buffalo, NY	Breath-hold diving
Edmonds, C.	Australia	Marine animal injuries, ear problems of divers; first author of *Diving and Subaquatic Medicine*

(continued)

(continued)

Name	Location (where work done)	Contribution
Egstrom, G.	Los Angles, CA	Diving safety, panic, and psychological stresses of diving (with A. Bachrach); diver performance
Elliott, D.	Great Britain	Decompression sickness, hypothermia, coauthor of *Physiology and Medicine of Diving;* diver fitness
Goodman, M.	Washington, DC (Navy)	Co-developer of the oxygen treatment tables for decompression sickness and arterial gas embolism
Haldane, J.	Great Britain	Decompression theory; the 2-to-1 ratio for safe ascents
Hallenbeck, J.	Washington, DC	Neurological complications of diving; the cause of spinal bends
Hamilton, R.	Tarrytown, NY	Technical diving; no-stop decompression
Hart, G.	Long Beach, CA (Navy)	No air-break oxygen treatment tables in monoplace hyperbaric chambers for decompression illness
Hayward, J.	Canada	Accidental hypothermia; survival in cold water
Hills, B.	Australia	Decompression theory
Jones, J.	San Francisco, CA	Dysbaric osteonecrosis (bone death from diving)
Keatinge, W.	Great Britain	Immersion hypothermia
Kindwall, E.	Milwaukee, WI	Caisson workers; dive safety
Lambertsen, C.	Philadelphia, PA	Oxygen toxicity; closed-circuit (100%) oxygen SCUBA gear
Lamphier, E.	Milwaukee, WI	Pulmonary (lung) effects of diving; dive profiles and decompression sickness
Leitch, D.	Washington, DC (Navy)	Low pressures (2.8 ATA) for treatment of decompression illness
Levin, H.	Washington, DC (Navy)	Inflammation of blood vessel linings from nitrogen bubbles
Lundgren, C.	Buffalo, NY	The effects of diving on lung physiology
Malamed, Y.	Israel	Diving safety
Modell, J.	Miami, FL	Near-drowning and drowning
Moon, R.	Durham, NC (Duke)	Decompression illness
Neuman, T.	San Diego, CA	Asthma and diving; multiorgan injury from arterial gas embolism; combined arterial gas embolism and decompression sickness

Name	Location (where work done)	Contribution
Philp, R.	Canada	Interactions between bubbles and blood components
Rahn, H.	Buffalo, NY	Breath-hold diving
Spencer, M.	Seattle, WA	Doppler detection of venous gas embolism
Strauss, M.	Long Beach, CA	Outcomes of decompression; disordered decompression; no-panic syndromes; pain science source of limb bends
Thalmann, E.	Panama City, FL (Navy)	Saturation diving; decompression theory; navy dive computer algorithms
Vann, R.	Durham, NC (Duke)	Flying after diving; decompression theory; exercise during decompression
Wienke, B.	Los Alamos, NM	Free gas phase of decompression; desirability of slowing ascent rates and the 3-minute 15-foot rest stop
Workman, R.	Washington, DC (Navy)	Oxygen treatment tables; surface decompression

GLOSSARY

absolute contraindication—Condition in which diving is absolutely prohibited because it is not safe to dive with the condition or diving will aggravate the condition.

actin—A muscle protein that is part of the muscle contraction mechanism.

adenoid—A mass of tissue in the upper part of the throat, behind the nose, that contains white blood cells and helps with the control of infections.

advanced cardiac life support (ACLS)—Interventions that use special equipment and medications to resuscitate and/or maintain life in situations of cardiac and pulmonary arrest or insufficiency.

aerobic metabolism—Metabolism that requires oxygen. This efficiently utilizes the energy potential of the glucose molecule.

agglutination—The clumping together of cells or cell products. Agglutination is associated with sludging and stasis of the blood.

agonist—A contracting muscle that is the primary mover for the motion desired; it is resisted or counteracted by another muscle, the antagonist.

air hunger—An extremely strong desire to breathe in order to increase exhalation of carbon dioxide; it is usually an indirect sign that tissue oxygen demands for aerobic metabolism are not being met.

alveolar spaces—The small air chambers in the pulmonary tissue where gas exchange takes place.

alveoli—The small sac-like structures at the end of the airway where all gas exchange between the lungs and the blood takes place.

ambient pressure—The pressure around the diver's body, which is essentially the same as the pressure of the gas the diver breathes.

anaerobic metabolism—Metabolism that does not require oxygen. This very inefficiently utilizes the energy potential of the glucose molecule.

anemia—A deficiency in red blood cells.

antagonist—A muscle that counteracts the action of another muscle, the agonist.

antibiotics—Medications that kill or stop the growth of microorganisms.

anticonvulsant—Medication that prevents or reduces convulsions.

antihistamine—A drug used to prevent allergic reactions.

anti-inflammatory agents—Medications that reduce inflammation.

anxiety—An unpleasant emotional state with its psychological and physiological responses to an unidentifiable danger or fear.

Archimedes' principle—An object will float if it weighs less than the weight of the water it displaces and will sink if it weighs more.

arrhythmia—Irregular heartbeat rhythm.

arterial gas embolism—A medical condition in which air bubbles introduced into arteries block the circulation of the arteries.

aspiration—The inhalation of substances such as water, food, or vomitus into the lungs.

aspirin—A medication that has many effects, including pain relief and reduction of fever and inflammation. For diving, its anti-sludging effect may offer protection from decompression sickness and the reperfusion injury.

asthma—A disease causing reversible narrowing of the bronchi (lung passageways). Its primary effect is the interference with the passive, exhalation phase of respiration.

atmosphere—The gaseous mass or envelope surrounding the Earth and retained by the Earth's gravitational field.

ATP—Adenosine triphosphate, a high-energy phosphate compound present in all living cells that serves as the primary energy source for many metabolic processes.

atropine—A medication that blocks activity of special types of nerves, for example, those that slow the heart rate.

autochthonous—Bubbles originating spontaneously in the tissues.

barotrauma—Injury that results from changes in pressure.

bends-proneness factors—Conditions that predispose the diver to decompression sickness.

bends resistance—Factors that offer resistance to decompression sickness.

bioluminescence—Light production from living sources, for example, the firefly.

blackout—Temporary loss of consciousness usually without warning, premonitions, or anxieties.

body insulation capacity—The difference between rectal (core) and skin temperatures divided by the rate of heat loss from the skin.

Bohr effect—An increased ability to off-load oxygen from hemoglobin when the blood becomes more acidic.

Boyle's law—As the pressure is increased on a volume of gas, the volume decreases and vice versa.

bradycarolia—Slowing of the heart rate.

breath-hold break point—The point at which there is an irresistible desire to breathe and it is impossible to further breath-hold.

breath-hold diving (skin diving, free diving)—Diving that relies on breath-holding ability to stay underwater.

bronchi—The two main branches of the trachea, leading directly to the lungs as they divide into smaller and smaller divisions.

buoyancy—The capacity to float in a liquid.

caisson—A watertight boxlike structure that can be pressurized with air to keep water out while building footings for bridges and other structures that are underwater.

cardiac arrest—Complete cessation of cardiac activity (heartbeat).

cardiac output—The amount of blood that the heart pumps per minute.

cardiovascular—Pertaining to the heart and blood vessels.

carotid sinus—A slight dilation in the carotid artery at its bifurcation into the external and internal carotid arteries, it contains baroreceptors (pressure sensors). When these sensors are stimulated, they cause reflex slowing of the heart, dilation of the blood vessels (vasodilation), and a fall in blood pressure.

carotid sinus syndrome—Stimulation of a carotid sinus, resulting in symptoms from stimulating the carotid sinus; consciousness may be lost.

cataract—The opacification of the lens of the eye; exposure to sunlight is a cause.

Charles' Law—The volume of a gas increases as the temperature of the gas increases and vice versa.

chilling—The feeling of discomfort in a cold environment; at this stage, core temperature is maintained.

chokes—A type of decompression sickness where bubbles in the lungs cause breathing difficulties.

chromosomes—Structures within cells that contain genetic material and have the ability to replicate themselves.

cilia—Microscopic hairlike projections in the respiratory tract (as well as other locations in the body) that beat in a rhythmic fashion to move mucus through the tract.

citric acid cycle—The aerobic phase of metabolism of glucose.

claustrophobia—Morbid fear of confined or closed-in places.

closed-circuit SCUBA—A diving technique where air is exhaled into breathing bags and rebreathed as oxygen is added and carbon dioxide is removed.

commercial diving—Diving for pay.

computerized tomography—A special type of X-ray that makes cross-section images of tissues and with the help of a computer is able to re-format them to aid in interpretations.

conduction—Heat transfer through an object such as a frying pan, which conducts heat from the flame to the food being cooked.

congestion—Distension of blood vessels.

conjunctiva—A clear membrane that coats the inner aspect of the eyelids and the outer surface of the eye.

contraceptive agents—Medications that prevent pregnancy.

convection—Heat transfer of bodies of gas or fluid such as a hair dryer moving heated air.

convulsion—Involuntary contraction or series of contractions of muscles initiated by abnormal nerve activity in the brain; also called a seizure.

core—The central portion of the body. This refers to the structures contained within the thorax, abdomen, head, and neck.

core temperature—Temperature in the central portion of the body, which contains the vital organs such as the heart, brain, lungs, liver, and kidneys.

cornea—The transparent structure forming the front portion of the eye.

coronary occlusion—Blockage of a blood vessel to the heart; this leads to a heart attack and possibly death of heart muscle (myocardial infarction).

critical tissue—The tissue (actually the theoretical tissue compartment, for example, five-minute tissue, ten-minute tissue, etc.) that has the highest nitrogen saturation during the off-gassing portion of the dive and determines whether or not further ascent can be done safely.

current—The movement of one mass of water through another.

cyanosis—A bluish discoloration of skin and mucous membranes due to excessive concentration of reduced (unoxygenated) hemoglobin in the blood.

Dalton's Law—The total pressure exerted by a mixture of gases is equal to the sum of the pressures that would be exerted by each of the gases if it alone were present and occupied the total volume.

dead space—The portion (volume) of airways that is not involved in gas exchange, that is, all structures of the bronchial tree except the alveoli.

decompression sickness—A wide spectrum of conditions, from skin itches; to joint pains; to breathing problems; to paralysis, following reductions in ambient pressure.

deep vein thrombosis—The clotting of blood in the veins usually associated with injury, slow blood flow, or changes in the clotting characteristics of blood.

dehydration—The condition that results from fluid depletion in the body.

density—Mass per unit volume.

deoxyribonucleic acid (DNA)—The molecule that encodes genetic information in the chromosome; it determines the structure, function, and behavior of the cell.

deserved decompression sickness—Decompression sickness due to the violation of dive computers or dive tables.

diaphragm—The thin muscle below the lungs and the heart that separates the chest from the abdomen and is the main muscle used for inspiration of air into the lungs.

diastole—The time between ventricular contractions (systole); the heart fills with blood during this phase of the cardiac cycle.

diastolic blood pressure—The blood pressure at the end of the diastolic period of the cardiac cycle.

dilation—Widening, increase in circumference as can be observed in a blood vessel.

disordered decompression—Factors, that are usually one-time occurrences, that interfere with the orderly off-gassing of nitrogen from the body.

dive computer—A computer for diving that pairs depths with durations at each depth and then computes safe dive times, ascent rates, and need for decompression stops. Also, the computer may give information about when it is safe to fly after diving.

dive profile—Refers to the shape of a curve that occurs when the depth of the dive is plotted against the time progression of the dive.

diving reflex—A reflex initiated by immersion (especially of the face) in water causing bradycardia, peripheral vasoconstriction, and anaerobic metabolism.

downers—A slang expression for drugs that depress the nervous system.

drowning—Death due to immersion in the water; suffocation in the water.

dry suit—A garment worn by divers for thermal protection. Usually a body suit constructed of various watertight materials. It functions by preventing water from coming into contact with a diver's body. Thermal undergarments are worn under the dry suit.

echo location—An auditory orientation mechanism involving the emission of low-frequency sounds that are then reflected from an object back to the emitter; the biological equivalent of SONAR.

ectomorphic somatotype—Tall, thin, lean type of body build; largest possible surface area-to-body mass ratio of the three body builds.

electrocardiogram—The recording of the electrical activity of the heart on a moving strip of paper.

emphysema—The disease condition (commonly referred to as chronic obstructive pulmonary disease [COPD]) where the alveoli lose their elasticity and no longer passively move the air in them to the bronchial tubes for exhalation.

emphysematous blebs—Out-pouchings or pockets in the lungs that have weak walls and may be easily ruptured.

endomorphic somatotype—Short, squatty type of body builds; smallest possible surface area-to-body mass ratio of the three body builds.

endothelial cell—A thin, flattened cell that lines the inside surfaces of blood vessels, lymph vessels, and internal body cavities.

enzyme—Proteins that break down food into its component parts that then can be absorbed into the blood through the gut.

epithelium—A special tissue or covering that lines the sinuses.

euphoria—A feeling of great happiness or well-being.

fast tissue—A tissue that on-gasses and off-gasses nitrogen rapidly, meaning it has a short tissue half-time.

fast-twitch fibers—Muscle fibers that utilize anaerobic metabolism for their actions and thereby are capable of brief, maximal outputs of energy such as seen in sprinters and weightlifters.

foramen ovale—An opening in the septum between the right and left atria of the heart, present in the fetus but usually closed soon after birth; it remains patent in about 15 percent of the population.

free radical—An atom or molecule that contains a chemical charge and readily combines with other chemicals.

gastroesophageal reflux—A backflow of the contents of the stomach into the esophagus, caused by relaxation of a properly functioning lower esophageal sphincter (valve) or an incompetent valve; this is frequently referred to as GERD (gastroesophageal reflux disease).

gauge pressure—The reading on a diving or chamber pressure gauge. This eliminates having to subtract the pressure of the atmosphere.

generalized alarm reaction—A three-stage response—alarm, resistance, and exhaustion—to stress; the panic syndrome incorporates these features.

glycolysis—A complex series of cellular biochemical reactions, not requiring oxygen, that split glucose, glycogen, or other carbohydrates into pyruvic, or lactic, acid while storing energy in ATP molecules.

gradient pressure—The difference in pressure between two different portions of a structure such as the middle ear.

habituation—Unresponsiveness after continued exposures to a stimulus; this is a form of acclimatization.

Haldane 2-to-1 ratio—The amount the ambient pressure can be reduced (according to JBS Haldane), expressed as a ratio, without bubble formation when the tissue is fully saturated.

Heimlich valve—A valve device that connects to a chest tube or needle; it allows air to be expelled from the collapsed lung cavity during exhalation, re-expansion of the lung, and maintenance of the negative intrathoracic pressure.

hematocrit—The percentage of red blood cells in the blood.

hemodynamic—Pertaining to the flow of blood.

hemoglobin—The oxygen-carrying protein of the red blood cell expressed as grams of hemoglobin per 100 cubic centimeters of blood. The hemoglobin measurement is approximately 1/3 the hematocrit value.

hemolyzed blood—Blood in which there is destruction of the red blood cells.

Henry's Law—The amount of a gas that will dissolve in a liquid relates directly to the pressure of the gas.

hilum—Central portion of the lung where the bronchi begin to branch off.

hormone—A naturally occurring substance secreted by specialized cells that affects the metabolism or function of other cells.

hot water suit—A garment worn by divers for thermal protection. Hot water is pumped through a hose to the diver's suit to continuously bathe the diver in warm water.

hydrodynamics—The principles of movement through water and other fluids.

hyperbaric oxygen therapy—The breathing of pure oxygen at greater than 1 ATA in a pressurized chamber.

hyperthermia—Abnormally high body temperature.

hyperventilation—Increase in rate and depth of respirations, either vouluntary or involuntary; at rest this reduces carbon dioxide levels in tissues but does not add to oxygen stores.

hypesthesia—A diminution in sensation.

hypoglycemia—Low blood sugar levels that lead to weakness, confusion, sweating, and loss of consciousness.

hypothalamus—A portion of the brain that lies beneath the thalamus and secretes substances that regulate metabolism.

hypothermia—Abnormally low body temperature.

hypoxia—Reduction of oxygen supply to tissue below levels needed to maintain consciousness and/or keep other body tissues functioning.

impairment—A physical or mental condition that reduces the level of function of the involved body part.

inert gas—A gas that forms no chemical combinations with other substances; a gas that does not participate in metabolic processes in the body.

inhibition—Slowing or restraint of a process.

involuntary diuresis—The excretion of urine without voluntary control.

iris—The colored, contractile mechanism in the front portion of the eye with a perforation, the pupil.

isometric—Muscle contraction without change in length.

labyrinthitis—Inflammation of the inner ear, often accompanied by an impaired sense of balance.

lactic acid—The end product of anaerobic metabolism.

laryngeal reflex—The closing of the vocal cords in response to aspiration; this is a very strong reflex, one of the last reflexes to be lost before death.

larynx—The part of the respiratory tract that lies between the pharynx (back of the throat) and the trachea. It contains the vocal cords, which are needed for speaking. A trapdoor valve above the larynx, the epiglottis, prevents food and water in the throat from entering the larynx when swallowing.

lung function testing—Diagnostic procedure that measures lung volumes and speed at which air goes in and out of the lung.

malabsorption—Inability or insufficiency of the absorption of food products by the gut for utilization by the body for metabolism, growth, and repair.

mammals—Warm-blooded animals that possess hair, have bony vertebral columns, breathe air, and breast-feed their young.

martini law—An adage for appreciating the effects of nitrogen narcosis; each 50 FSW (15 MSW) of descent is equivalent to the effect of drinking one martini.

mediastinum—A potential space between the breastbone and the heart.

medical standards for diving—Level of physical and mental health that is necessary for diving.

Menière's disease—A malfunctioning of the semicircular canal of the inner ear, characterized by dizziness, nausea, vomiting, or a buzzing in the ear.

meningitis—Inflammation of the meninges as the result of infection by bacteria or viruses.

mesomorphic somatotype—Strong, muscular type of body build in between the endomorphic and ectomorphic builds.

metabolism—The sum of all the chemical processes taking place in the organism to produce energy; to tear down and recycle (catabolism) and to buildup and reform (anabolism) body tissues.

morbidity—Illness.

M-value—The maximum (i.e., "M") permitted level of supersaturation of each tissue half time based on Workman's calculations (US Navy) before autochthonous bubbles form. The M-values are greater than Haldane's 2:1 ratio for fast tissue and less than his 2:1 ratio for slow tissues.

myocardial infarction—The death of muscle tissue in the heart from interruption of the blood supply to the heart; a heart attack.

myoglobin—A protein found in skeletal muscle. It has a higher affinity for oxygen than hemoglobin has. It stores oxygen in muscle tissues for use under anaerobic conditions.

myoglobinuria—The passage of red-brown urine secondary to the release of myoglobin from muscles; this occurs when muscles are deprived of oxygen and from the venom of sea snakes.

myosin—A muscle protein that interacts with actin as part of the contraction mechanism.

narced—A slang expression for the effects of nitrogen narcosis.

narcosis—A condition of deep stupor or unconsciousness produced by a drug or other chemical substance.

near-drowning—Loss of consciousness due to immersion in the water with subsequent survival.

nitrox (enriched air) mixture—Gas mixtures used in SCUBA diving that have increased concentrations of oxygen and decreased concentrations of nitrogen; this extends bottom times and reduces the risks of decompression sickness.

no-panic syndromes—A diverse group of medical problems of diving characterized by blackout in the water.

nutrition—The science of food values and diet recommendations.

obtunded—Impaired level of consciousness.

open-circuit SCUBA—A diving technique in which each breath that is inhaled is exhaled into the water.

osteoma—A tumor composed of bony tissue.

osteonecrosis—Death of bone; "osteo" means bone, "necrosis" refers to death.

oxidation—The reaction and combination of a substance with oxygen.

oxygen deficit (debt)—The amount of oxygen required to metabolize the waste products of anaerobic metabolism.

panic—An uncontrolled psychological stress.

paralysis—Loss of motor function (movement); in diving this is usually due to injury to the spinal cord.

paraplegia—Complete paralysis of the lower half of the body, including both legs, the bladder, and the bowel, usually caused by damage to the spinal cord.

paresthesia—An abnormal pins-and-needles-like sensation.

partial pressure—The proportion of the total pressure contributed by a single gas in the mixture.

Pascal's principle—A fluid or gas in a closed container transmits a change in pressure equally and undiminished to all portions of the container.

perfusion—The amount of blood flow to a body part.

periphery—The portion of the body outside the core. Typically, this refers to the appendages (arms and legs) and the skin and subcutaneous (below the skin) tissues of the core.

phrenic nerve—The nerve that transmits impulses from the brain to the diaphragm. Normally impulses are initiated automatically from the brain but can be overridden by conscious effort such as hyperventilating or breath-holding.

plasma—The fluid portion of the blood; the remaining portion of blood after the red and white blood cells are removed.

platelet—A type of blood cell that aids in the clotting process.

pleural cavity—The potential space that lies between the pleura (the lining) that covers the lungs and the pleura that lines the inside of the thoracic cavity.

pneumothorax—Collapse of the lung.

poison—A substance that injures or kills tissues when introduced into the body.

polycythemia—A pathological condition characterized by an abnormal increase in the number of red blood cells in the blood.

premenstrual syndrome—A combination of emotional, physical, psychological, and mood disturbances that occurs after ovulation and normally ends with the onset of the menstrual flow.

pressure—Force per unit area.

pressure gradient—A difference between the ambient pressure and the pressure within an object.

propulsion—The mechanics of moving an object.

pulmonary embolism—The dislodging of clots from deep venous thromboses and transport in the bloodstream to the lungs where they can cause a life-threatening condition.

pupil—The aperture (hole) in the iris of the eye.

radiation—Heat transfer through a medium to a remote object; the sun radiates heat to the earth without warming the intervening space itself.

rapture of the deep—A picturesque expression for nitrogen narcosis.

Raynaud's phenomenon—A disease condition in which minimal cooling challenges lead to constriction of blood flow to the hands and feet.

recompression—The method of treating decompression sickness and air embolism by placing the diver in a chamber and then pressurizing it to reduce the size of bubbles.

recompression chamber—A vessel that can safely withstand pressurization. It is used to treat diving problems and other medical conditions.

red blood cell (erythrocyte)—A cell specialized for oxygen transport that contains hemoglobin.

refraction—The deviation of a light ray from a straight line in passing from one transparent medium to another of a different density.

refractive index—The refractive power of any substance as compared to air.

regulator—A device that reduces high-pressure gas in SCUBA tanks to levels that will not injure the diver, compensates for the ambient pressure of the water, and allows the diver to inhale and exhale on demand.

relative contraindication—Condition in which diving is generally not recommended but under special circumstances may be permitted.

reperfusion injury—The cessation of blood flow due to white blood cells adhering to the lining of blood vessels and the release of their toxic radicals (the chemicals that kill bacteria). The toxic radicals cause cessation of blood flow. Nitrogen bubbles may initiate the white blood cell adherence reaction.

residual lung volume—Volume of the air in the lungs after full expiration.

residual nitrogen time—The amount of nitrogen remaining in the tissues after a dive.

respiratory gases—The gases involved with ventilation, namely oxygen and carbon dioxide.

resuscitation—The restoration to life or consciousness of one apparently dead.

retina—The light-receiving layer at the back of the eyeball that converts visual images into nerve impulses for transmission to the brain for interpretation.

rods and cones—The two photoreceptor cell types in the retina. The rods are more sensitive to lightness and darkness than the cones. The cones detect color.

Ruffini type 2 corpuscle—A fluid-filled sensory organelle (microscopic organ) embedded in joint capsules that detects stretch sensations.

saturated tissue—A tissue that has equilibrated with nitrogen at a given ambient pressure.

serous otitis media—Fluid collection in the middle ear; possibly a manifestation of breathing increased partial pressures of oxygen.

shock—Failure of the circulatory system to maintain adequate perfusion to organs and tissues.

shunt—To bypass.

silent bubbles—Venous gas bubbles that are believed to be a normal occurrence during decompression and ordinarily do not cause symptoms.

skip breathing—Technique, now frowned upon, where breathing with SCUBA gear is delayed to nearly the breath-hold break point.

slow tissue—A tissue that on-gasses and off-gasses nitrogen slowly, meaning it has a long tissue half-time.

slow-twitch fibers—Muscle fibers that utilize aerobic metabolism for their actions and thereby are capable of sustained action as observed in marathon runners.

sludging—Aggregation of red blood cells forming a mass that can impede circulation.

snorkel diving—A variant of breath-hold (free) diving where a snorkel, a short breathing tube, is used to improve efficiency.

SONAR—A system that uses underwater sound transmission and its reflection off of objects for the detection and location of the objects; the engineering equivalent of echolocation.

sport diving—Diving for enjoyment without consideration for remuneration.

stress—A challenge, stimulus, or other signal that initiates a response in the organism.

surge—The back-and-forth movement of water between waves.

swell—Upward and downward movement of water generated and propelled by wind.

swimmer's ear—Inflammation of the external ear canal commonly associated with people who swim regularly, as competitive swimmers do.

systole—The time when the ventricles of the heart contract.

systolic blood pressure—The highest point of the blood pressure, which coincides with the end of systole.

temperature afterdrop—The decline in core temperature after exiting cold water. It is due to obliteration of the shunting reflex and the return of cold blood from the periphery to the core.

temporary contraindication—Condition in which diving is temporarily contraindicated, but once the condition is resolved, diving is OK to resume.

tendon—A strong cord-like fibrous structure that connects muscle to bone.

teratogenic—Causing malformations of a fetus.

thermocline—The junction between warmer and colder masses of water.

thoracic squeeze—A rare MPD that is the lung counterpart of an ear squeeze.

tinnitus—Ringing in the ear.

tissue half-time—The time it takes for a tissue to become 50 percent saturated with nitrogen at the new ambient pressure.

toxicity—The disease or injury condition resulting from substances that are normally present in the body but cause harm only when their concentrations increase.

trachea—The windpipe, a tube lined with mucous membrane passing from the larynx to the bronchi.

trigeminal nerve—The nerve that is responsible for transmitting sensation from over the face to the brain. The stimulus of water coming in contact with sensors at the ends of this nerve initiates the diving reflex.

turbulence—A localized current effect that occurs when a current is deflected off another object.

undeserved decompression sickness—The occurrence of decompression sickness without the apparent violation of dive computers or dive tables.

vagus nerve—The nerve that innervates (transmits messages from the brain to) the gut, heart and larynx. Stimulation of the vagus nerve via the diving reflex slows the heart rate.

Valsalva maneuver—Forced expiratory effort against a closed airway, which decreases cardiac filling and the amount of blood ejected from the heart.

vasoconstrictors—Medications that increase blood pressure by stimulating contraction of the muscular layer of arteries and arterioles.

vascularity—The amount of blood vessels to a particular tissue.

vegetative—Few or no responses to stimuli, as in a coma.

ventilation—The process of breathing in oxygen and the exhalation of carbon dioxide.

ventricular fibrillation—Disordered, chaotic nonfunctional heart activity; if not immediately corrected with electrical shock and medications, the heart will become irreparably damaged.

ventricular tachycardia—Very rapid beating of the heart.

vertigo—A sensation of the room spinning.

vicious circle—A condition in which one problem gives rise to another which, in turn, affects the first so that the condition becomes self-perpetuating.

viscosity—The thickness or resistance to flow of a liquid or gas.

vitreous humor—The gelatinous substance that fills the eyeball between the lens and the retina.

wave—The resultant contour of the water surface as a swell that approaches the shallow water of the shoreline.

wet suit—A garment worn by divers for thermal protection constructed of neoprene. A thin layer of water warmed by the diver's body heat remains trapped in the neoprene.

REFERENCES

Adrian, M.J., S. Mohan, and P.V. Karpovich. 1966. Energy cost of leg kick, arm and stroke, and whole crawl stroke. *J Appl Physiol* 21:1763.

Andersen, H.T. 1964. Stresses imposed on diving vertebrates during prolonged underwater exposure. *Symp Soc Exper Biol* 18:109.

Andersen, H.T. 1966. Physiological adaptation in diving vertebrates. *Physiol Rev* 46:212.

Andersen, L.K. 1960. Energy cost of swimming. *Acta Chirug Scand Suppl* 235:169.

Beckman, E.L. 1963. Thermal protection during immersion in cold water. *Proceedings second symposium on underwater physiology.* Washington, DC: National Academy of Sciences-National Research Council, 247.

Behnke, A.R., and C.P. Yaglou. 1951. Physiological responses of men to chilling in ice water and to slow and fast rewarming. *J Appl Physiol* 3:591.

Bond, G.F. 1966. Effects of new and artificial environments on human physiology. *Arch Environ Health* 12 (1, January):85-90.

Carley, L.D., E. Karl, K.E. Schaefer, and J.A. Harry. 1955. Effect of skin diving on lung volume. *J Appl Physiol* 8:519.

Carlson, L.D., A.C.L. Hsieh, F. Fullington, and R. Elsner. 1958. Immersion in cold water and body tissue insulation. *J Aviat Med* 29:145.

Chryssanthou, C., F. Teichner, and W. Antopol. 1971. Studies on dysbarism. IV. Production and prevention of decompression sickness in "non-susceptible" animals. *Aerosp Med* 42 (8, August):864-867.

Cross, E.R. 1965. Taravana: Diving syndrome in the Tuamotu diver. In *Physiology of breath-hold diving and the Ama of Japan,* ed. H. Rahn. Washington, DC: National Academy of Sciences. National Research Council Publication 1341, 207-220.

Donald, K.W., and W.M. Davidson. 1954. Oxygen uptake of "bottled" and "fin swimming" divers. *J Appl Physiol* 7:31.

Elsner, R.R. 1969. Cardiovascular adjustments to diving. In *The biology of marine mammals,* ed. H.T. Andersen. New York: Academic Press, 117-145.

Elsner, R.R., and P.F. Scholander. 1965. Circulatory adaptations to diving in animals and man. *Physiology of breath-hold diving and the AMA of Japan* 281.

Elsner, R.W., and P.F. Sholander. 1963. Selective ischemia in diving man. *Am Heart J* 65:571.

Elsner, R.W., P.F. Scholander, A.R. Craig, E.G. Dimond, L. Irving, M. Pilson, K. Johansen, and E. Bradstreet. 1964. A venous oxygen reservoir in diving elephant seal. *Physiologist* 7:124.

Glaser, E.M., F.R. Berridge, and K.M. Prior. 1950. Effects of heat and cold on the distribution of blood within the human body. *Clin Science* 9:181.

Guyton, A.C., and J.E. Hall. 2000. *Textbook of medical physiology,* 10th ed. Philadelphia: Saunders.

Hong, S.K., J. Henderson, A. Olszowka, W.E. Hurford, K.J. Falke, J. Qvist, P. Radermacher, K. Shiraki, M. Mohri, H. Takeuchi et al. 1991. Daily diving pattern of Korean and Japanese breath-hold divers (Ama). *Undersea Biomed Res* 18 (5-6, September-November):433-443.

Hong, S.K., H. Rahk, D.H. Kang, S.H. Song, and B.S. Kang. 1963. Diving pattern, lung volumes and alveolar gas of Korean diving women (Ama). *J Appl Physiol* 18:457.

Hong, S.K., D.W. Rennie, and Y.S. Park. 1986. Cold acclimatization and deacclimatization of Korean women divers. *Exerc Sport Sci Rev* 14:231-268.

Irving, L. 1938. The insensitivity of diving animals to CO_2. *Am J Physiol* 124:729.

Irving, L., D.M. Solandt, D.Y. Solandt, and K.C. Fisher. 1935. Respiratory characteristics of the blood of the seal. *J Cell Comp Physiol* 7:393.

Kang, B.S., S.H. Song, C.S. Suh, and S.K. Kong. 1963. Changes in the body temperatures and basal metabolic rate of Ama. *J Appl Physiol* 18:483.

Kang, D.H., P.K. Kim, B.S. Kange, S.H. Song, and S.K. Hong. 1965. Energy metabolism and body temperature of the Ama. *J Appl Physiol* 20:46.

Kang, D.H., Y.S. Park, Y.D. Park, I.S. Lee, D.S. Yeon, S.H. Lee, S.Y. Hong, D.W. Rennie, and S.K. Hong. 1983. Energetics of wet-suit diving in Korean women breath-hold divers. *J Appl Physiol* 54 (6, June):1702-1707.

Keatinge, W.R. 1961. The effect of work and clothing on the maintenance of the body temperature in water. *Quart J Exper Physiol and Cognate Med Sci* 46:69.

Keatinge, W.R., and J.S. Nadel. 1965. Immediate respiratory response to sudden cooling of the skin. *J Appl Physiol* 20:65.

Lanphier, E. 1954. Oxygen consumption in underwater swimming. *Fed Proc* 13:84.

Lanphier, E.H., and H. Rahn. 1961. Gas exchange during simulated breath-hold dive. *Fed Prog* 20:424.

Lilly, J.C. 1961. *Man and dolphin.* Garden City, NY: Doubleday.

Moon, R.E., E.M. Camporesi, and J.A. Kisslo. 1989. Patent foramen ovale and decompression sickness in divers. *Lancet* 1 (8637, March 11):513-514.

Murdaugh, H.V., E.D. Robin, J.E. Millen, and W.F. Drewry. 1965. Cardiac output determinations by the dye-dilution method in Squalus acanthias. *Am J Physiol* 209 (4, October):723-726.

NAVMED. 1956. *Submarine medical practice.* Washington, DC: U.S. Government Printing Office, P-5054, pp. 259.

Odend'hal, S., and T.C. Poulter. 1966. Pressure regulation in the middle ear cavity of sea lions: A possible mechanism. *Science* 153 (737, August 12):768-769.

Olsen, R.C., D.D. Fanestil, and P.F. Scholander. 1962. Some effects of breath and apneic diving on cardiac rhythm in man. *J Appl Physiol* 17:461.

Paulev, P.E. 1965. Decompression sickness following repeated breath-hold dives. *J Appl Physiol* 20:1028-1031.

Paulev, P.E. 1967. Nitrogen tissue tensions following repeated breath-hold dives. *J Appl Physiol* 22 (4):714-718.

Rahn, H. 1965. The physiological stresses of the Ama. In *Physiology of breath-hold diving and the Ama of Japan,* ed. H. Rahn. Washington, DC: National Academy of Sciences. National Research Council Publication 1341, 113.

Rennie, D.W. 1965. Thermal insulation of Korean diving women and non-divers in water. In *Physiology of breath-hold diving and the Ama of Japan,* ed. H. Rahn. Washington, DC: National Academy of Sciences. National Research Council Publication 1341, 315.

Schaefer, K.E. 1954. Group differences in carbon dioxide in the physiology of human diving. *Fed Proc* 13:128.

Schaefer, K.E. 1963. Effect of prolonged diving training. *Proceedings second symposium on underwater physiology.* Washington, DC: National Academy of Sciences-National Research Council, 271.

Schaefer, K.E., R.D. Allinson, J.H. Dougherty, C.R. Carey, R. Walker, F. Jost, and D. Parker. 1968. Pulmonary and circulatory adjustment determining the limits of depths in breath-hold diving. *Submarine Medical Research Laboratory,* Report No. 531, June.

Scholander, P.F., L. Irving, and S.W. Grinnell. 1942a. Aerobic and anaerobic changes in seal muscles during diving. *J Biol Chem* 142:431.

Scholander, P.F., L. Irving, and S.W. Grinnell. 1942b. On the temperature and metabolism of the seal during diving. *J Cell and Comp Physiol* 19:67.

Skreslet, S., and F. Aarefjord. 1968. Acclimatization to cold in man induced by frequent scuba diving in cold water. *J Appl Physiol* 24 (2, February): 177-181.

Specht, H.L., L.G. Goff, H.F. Brubach, and R.G. Bartett. 1957. Work efficiency and respiratory response of trained underwater swimmers using a modified self-contained underwater breathing apparatus. *J Appl Physiol* 10:377.

Teague, J. 1968. Navyman's best friend: The porpoise—or is it a dolphin? *All Hands* 613:8.

Van Citters, R.L., D.L. Franklin, O.A. Smith, N.W. Watson, and R.W. Elsner. 1965. Cardiovascular adaptation to diving in the northern elephant seal *(mirounga ongustirostis)*. *Comp Biochem and Physiol* 16:267.

SUGGESTED READINGS

Chapter 1

Adolfoson, J., and T. Berghage. 1974. *Perception and performance underwater.* New York: Wiley.

Bachrach, A.J., and G.H. Egstrom. 1999. *Stress and performance in diving.* Flagstaff, AZ: Best Publishing Company.

Bookspan, J. 1998. *Diving physiology in plain English.* Kensington, MD: Undersea and Hyperbaric Medical Society.

Graver, D.K. 1999. *Scuba diving.* Champaign, IL: Human Kinetics.

Lin, Y.C. 1988. Applied physiology of diving. *Sports Med* 5 (1, January) 41-56.

Martin, L. 1998. *Scuba diving explained—questions and answers on physiology and medical aspects.* Flagstaff, AZ: Best Publishing Company.

Morgan, W.P. 1995. Anxiety and panic in recreational scuba divers. *Sports Med* 20 (6, December):398-421.

Nevo, B., and S. Breitstein. 2000. *Psychological and behavioral aspects of diving.* Flagstaff, AZ: Best.

Chapter 2

Barsky, S. 1999. *The simple guide to snorkeling fun.* Flagstaff, AZ: Best.

Barsky, S., M. Ward, and M. Thurlow. 1998. *Simple guide to rebreather diving.* Flagstaff, AZ: Best Publishing Company.

Berger, K., R. Hildebrand, and F. Hildebrand. 2000. *Scuba diving.* New York: Norton.

Bozanic, J.E. 2002. *Mastering rebreathers.* Flagstaff, AZ: Best Publishing Company.

Clinchy, R.A., and G. Egstrom. 1993. *Advanced sport diver: Workbook.* St. Louis: Moseby.

Gilliam, B., R. Von Maier, and J. Crea. 1995. *Deep diving, an advanced guide to physiology, procedures and systems.* San Diego: Watersport.

Lettnin, H.K. 2000. *International textbook of mixed gas diving.* Flagstaff, AZ: Best Publishing Company.

Lippmann, J. 1997. *The essentials of deeper sport diving.* Locust Valley, NY: Aqua Quest.

Rossier, R.N. 2000. *Recreational nitrox diving.* Flagstaff, AZ: Best Publishing Company.

Chapter 3

Butler, F.K., and D. Southerland. 2001. The U.S. Navy decompression computer. *Undersea Hyperb Med* 28 (4):213-228.

Doolette, D.J., and S.J. Mitchell. 2001. The physiological kinetics of nitrogen and the prevention of decompression sickness. *Clin Pharmacokinet* 40 (1, January):1-14.

Egi, S.M., and N.M. Gurmen. 2000. Computation of decompression tables using continuous compartment half-lives. *Undersea Hyperb Med* 27 (3, fall):143-153.

Gerth, W.A., and R.D. Vann. 1997. Probabilistic gas and bubble dynamics models of decompression sickness occurrence in air and nitrogen-oxygen diving. *Undersea Hyperb Med* 24 (4, winter):275-292.

Homer, L.D., and P.K. Weathersby. 1985. Statistical aspects of the design and testing of decompression tables. *Undersea Biomed Res* 12 (3, September): 239-249.

Lewis, J.E., and K.W. Shreeves. 1990. *The recreational diver's guide to decompression theory, dive tables, and dive computers.* Santa Ana, CA: Professional Association of Diving Instructors.

Weathersby, P.K., and L.D. Homer. 1980. Solubility of inert gases in biological fluids and tissues: A review. *Undersea Biomed Res* 7 (4, December): 277-296.

Weathersby, P.K., S.S. Survanshi, L.D. Homer, E. Parker, and E.D. Thalmann. 1992. Predicting the time of occurrence of decompression sickness. *J Appl Physiol* 72 (4, April):1541-1548.

Wienke, B.R. 1989. Tissue gas exchange models and decompression computations: A review. *Undersea Biomed Res* 16 (1, January):53-89.

Chapter 4

Andersen, H.T. 1967. Cardiovascular adaptations in diving mammals. *Am Heart J* 74 (3, September):295-298.

Butler, P.J., and D.R. Jones. 1997. Physiology of diving of birds and mammals. *Physiol Rev* 77 (3, July):837-899.

Doubt, T.J. 1996. Cardiovascular and thermal responses to SCUBA diving. *Med Sci Sports Exerc* 28 (5, May):581-586.

Elsner, R.W., and P.F. Scholander. 1963. Selective ischemia in diving man. *Am Heart J* 65:571.

Gooden, B.A. 1994. Mechanism of the human diving response. *Integr Physiol Behav Sci* 29 (1, January-March):6-16.

Hayashi, N., M. Ishihara, A. Tanaka, T. Osumi, and T. Yoshida. 1997. Face immersion increases vagal activity as assessed by heart rate variability. *Eur J Appl Physiol Occup Physiol* 76 (5):394-399.

Moon, R.E., E.M. Camporesi, and J.A. Kisslo. 1989. Patent foramen ovale and decompression sickness in divers. *Lancet* 11 (8637, March 11):513-514.

Paulev, P.E., M. Pokorski, Y. Honda, B. Ahn, A. Masuda, T. Kobayashi, Y. Nishibayashi, Y. Sakakibara, M. Tanaka, and W. Nakamura. 1990. Facial cold receptors and the survival reflex "diving bradycardia" in man. *Jpn J Physiol* 40 (5):701-712.

Russell, C.J., A. McNeill, and E. Evonuk. 1972. Some cardiorespiratory and metabolic responses of scuba divers to increased pressure and cold. *Aerosp Med* 43 (9, September):998-1001.

Strauss, M.B. 1970. Physiological aspects of mammalian breath-hold diving: A review. *Aerosp Med* 41 (12, December):1362-1381.

Chapter 5

Falke, K.J., R.D. Hill, J. Qvist, R.C. Schneider, M. Guppy, G.C. Liggins, P.W. Hochachka, R.E. Elliot, and W.M. Zapol. 1985. Seal lungs collapse during free diving: Evidence from arterial nitrogen tensions. *Science* 229: 556-558.

Ferretti, G. 2001. Extreme human breath-hold diving. *Eur J Appl Physiol* 84 (4, April):254-271.

Irving, L. 1938. The insensitivity of diving animals to CO_2. *Am J Physiol* 124:729.

Kooyman, G.L., and G.L. Kooyman. 1973. Respiratory adaptations in marine mammals. *Am Zoologist* 13:457-468.

Laurence, I. 1939. Respiration in diving mammals. *Physiol Rev* 19:112.

Liner, M.H., and D. Linnarsson. 1994. Tissue oxygen and carbon dioxide stores and breath-hold diving in humans. *J Appl Physiol* 77 (2, August): 542-547.

Schaefer, K.E. 1963. Effect of prolonged diving training. *Proceedings second symposium on underwater physiology*. Washington, DC: National Academy of Sciences-National Research Council, 271.

Snyder, G.K. 1983. Respiratory adaptations in diving mammals. *Respir Physiol* 54 (3, December):269-294.

Williams, T.M., R.W. Davis, L.A. Fuiman, J. Francis, B.J. Le Boeuf, M. Horning, J. Calambokidis, and D.A. Croll. 2000. Sink or swim: Strategies for cost-efficient diving by marine mammals. *Science* 288 (5463, April 7):133-136.

Chapter 6

Castellini, M.A., J.M. Castellini, and P.M. Rivera. 2001. Adaptations to pressure in the RBC metabolism of diving mammals. *Comp Biochem Physiol A Mol Integr Physiol* 129 (4, July):751-757.

Diercks, K.J., and P.T. Eisman. 1977. Hematologic changes after daily asymptomatic dives. *Undersea Biomed Res* 4 (4, December):325-331.

Eckenhoff, R.G., and J.S. Hughes. 1984. Hematologic and hemostatic changes with repetitive air diving. *Aviat Space Environ Med* 55 (7, July):592-597.

Espersen, K., H. Frandsen, T. Lorentzen, I.L. Kanstrup, and N.J. Christensen. 2002. The human spleen as an erythrocyte reservoir in diving-related interventions. *J Appl Physiol* 92 (5, May):2071-2079.

Marabotti, C., F. Chiesa, A. Scalzini, F. Antonelli, R. Lari, C. Franchini, and P.G. Data. 1999. Cardiac and humoral changes induced by recreational scuba diving. *Undersea Hyperb Med* 26 (3, fall):151-158.

Noren, S.R., and T.M. Williams. 2000. Body size and skeletal muscle myoglobin of cetaceans: Adaptations for maximizing dive duration. *Comp Biochem Physiol A Mol Integr Physiol* 126 (2, June):181-191.

Philp, R.B., P.B. Bennett, J.C. Andersen, G.N. Fields, B.A. McIntyre, I. Francey, and W. Briner. 1979. Effects of aspirin and dipyridamole on platelet function, hematology, and blood chemistry of saturation divers. *Undersea Biomed Res* 6 (2, June):127-146.

Taylor, W.F., S. Chen, G. Barshtein, D.E. Hyde, and S. Yedgar. 1998. Enhanced aggregability of human red blood cells by diving. *Undersea Hyperb Med* 25 (3, fall):167-170.

Wickham, L.L., R. Elsner, F.C. White, and L.H. Cornell. 1989. Blood viscosity in phocid seals: Possible adaptations to diving. *J Comp Physiol* [B] 159 (2):153-158.

Chapter 7

Bridgman, S.A. 1991. Peripheral cold acclimatization in Antarctic scuba divers. *Aviat Space Environ Med* 62 (8, August):733-738.

Nunneley, S.A., E.H. Wissler, and J.R. Allan. 1985. Immersion cooling: Effect of clothing and skinfold thickness. *Aviat Space Environ Med* 56 (12, December):1177-1182.

Park, Y.S., and S.K. Hong. 1991. Physiology of cold-water diving as exemplified by Korean women divers. *Undersea Biomed Res* 18 (3, May):229-241.

Skreslet, S., and F. Aarefjord. 1968. Acclimatization to cold in man induced by frequent scuba diving in cold water. *J Appl Physiol* 24 (2, February): 177-181.

Chapter 8

Capelli, C., D.R. Pendergast, and B. Termin. 1998. Energetics of swimming at maximal speeds in humans. *Eur J Appl Physiol Occup Physiol* 78 (5, October):385-393.

Feldkamp, S.D. 1987. Swimming in the California sea lion: Morphometrics, drag and energetics. *J Exp Biol* 131 (September):117-135.

Pendergast, D.R., M. Tedesco, D.M. Nawrocki, and N.M. Fisher. 1996. Energetics of underwater swimming with SCUBA. *Med Sci Sports Exerc* 28 (5, May):573-580.

Starling, R.D., D.L. Costill, T.A. Trappe, A.C. Jozsi, S.W. Trappe, and B.H. Goodpaster. 1995. Effect of swimming suit design on the energy demands of swimming. *Med Sci Sports Exerc* 27 (7, July):1086-1089.

Sumich, J.L. 1983. Swimming velocities, breathing patterns, and estimated costs of locomotion in migrating gray whales, *Eschrictius robustus*. *Can Jr Zool* 61:647-652.

Yamaguchi, H., F. Shidara, N. Naraki, and M. Mohri. 1995. Maximum sustained fin-kick thrust in underwater swimming. *Undersea Hyperb Med* 22 (3, September):241-248.

Zamparo, P., D.R. Pendergast, B. Termin, and A.E. Minetti. 2002. How fins affect the economy and efficiency of human swimming. *J Exp Biol* 205 (Pt 17, September):2665-2676.

Chapter 9

Jarchow, T., and F.W. Mast. 1999. The effect of water immersion on postural and visual orientation. *Aviat Space Environ Med* 70 (9, September):879-886.

Luria, S.M., and J.A. Kinney. 1975. Vision in the water without a facemask. *Aviat Space Environ Med* 46 (9, September):1128-1131.

Lythgoe, J.N. 1976. Underwater vision. *Proc R Soc Med* 69 (1, January): 67-68.

Norman, D.A., R. Phelps, and F. Wightman. 1971. Some observations on underwater hearing. *J Acoust Soc Am* 50 (2, August):544-548.

Pack, A.A., and L.M. Herman. 1995. Sensory integration in the bottlenosed dolphin: Immediate recognition of complex shapes across the senses of echolocation and vision. *J Acoust Soc Am* 98 (2 Pt 1, August):722-733.

Wells, M.J., and H.E. Ross. 1980. Distortion and adaptation in underwater sound localization. *Aviat Space Environ Med* 51 (8, August):767-774.

Chapter 10

Fitness

Cresswell, J.E., and M. St Leger-Dowse. 1991. Women and scuba diving. *BMJ* 302 (6792, June 29):1590-1591.

Edge, C.J., A.P. Grieve, N. Gibbons, F. O'Sullivan, and P. Bryson. 1997. Control of blood glucose in a group of diabetic scuba divers. *Undersea Hyperb Med* 24 (3, September):201-207.

Harrison, L.J. 1992. Drugs and diving. *J Fla Med Assoc* 79 (3, March):165-167.

Rump, A.F., U. Siekmann, and G. Kalff. 1999. Effects of hyperbaric and hyperoxic conditions on the disposition of drugs: Theoretical considerations and a review of the literature. *Gen Pharmacol* 32 (1):127-133.

St Leger-Dowse, M., P. Bryson, A. Gunby, and W. Fife. 2002. Comparative data from 2250 male and female sport divers: Diving patterns and decompression sickness. *Aviat Space Environ Med* 73 (8, August):743-749.

Taylor, D.M., K.S. O'Toole, and C.M. Ryan. 2002. Experienced, recreational scuba divers in Australia continue to dive despite medical contraindications. *Wilderness Environ Med* 13 (3, fall):187-193.

Tetzlaff, K., C.M. Muth, and L.K. Waldhauser. 2002. A review of asthma and scuba diving. *J Asthma* 39 (7, October):557-566.

Walsh, J.M. 1974. Amphetamine effects on timing behavior in rats under hyperbaric conditions. *Aerosp Med* 45 (7, July):721-726.

Nutrition

DeBolt, J.E., A. Singh, B.A. Day, and P.A. Deuster. 1988. Nutritional survey of the US Navy SEAL trainees. *Am J Clin Nutr* 48 (5, November):1316-1323.

Dwyer, J. Nutritional requirements and dietary assessment. In *Harrison's principles of internal medicine, online version*. New York: McGraw-Hill, chapter 73.

Hayden, J.D., J.B. Davies, and I.G. Martin. 1998. Diaphragmatic rupture resulting from gastrointestinal barotrauma in a scuba diver. *Br J Sports Med* 32 (1, March):75-76.

Singh, A., P.A. Deuster, B.A. Day, D.J. Smith, J.E. DeBolt, and T.J. Doubt. 1988. Nutritional status of land-based U.S. Navy divers. *Undersea Biomed Res* 15 (2, March):135-145.

Chapter 11

Panic

Baddeley, A., and C. Idzikowski. 1985. Anxiety, manual dexterity and diver performance. *Ergonomics* 28 (10, October):1475-1482.

De Moja, C.A., M. Reitano, and P. De Marco. 1987. Anxiety, perceptual and motor skills in an underwater environment. *Percept Mot Skills* 65 (2, October):359-365.

Mears, J.D., and P.J. Cleary. 1980. Anxiety as a factor in underwater performance. *Ergonomics* 23 (6, June):549-557.

Morgan, W.P. 1995. Anxiety and panic in recreational scuba divers. *Sports Med* 20 (6, December):398-421.

Strauss, M.B. 1973. The panic syndrome. *Phys and Sport Med* June; 1:39-42.

Blackout

Bove, A.A., A.L. Pierce, F. Barrera, G.A. Amsbaugh, and P.R. Lynch. 1973. Diving bradycardia as a factor in underwater blackout. *Aerosp Med* 44 (3, March):245-248.

Craig, A.B., Jr. 1976. Summary of 58 cases of loss of consciousness during underwater swimming and diving. *Med Sci Sports* 8 (3, fall):171-175.

Diehl, R.R., D. Linden, B. Bunger, M. Schafer, and P. Berlit. 2000. Valsalva-induced syncope during apnea diving. *Clin Auton Res* 10 (6, December): 343-345.

Hill, P.M. 1973. Hyperventilation, breath holding and alveolar oxygen tensions at the breaking point. *Respir Physiol* 19 (2, November):201-209.

Strauss, M.B, and S.L. Shane. 1988. The no-panic syndromes in underwater diving. *SPUMS J* 18 (1, March):16-22.

Temple, J.D., R.T. Bosshardt, and J.H. Davis. 1975. SCUBA tank corrosion as a cause of death. *J Forensic Sci* 20 (3, July):571-575.

Chapter 12

Environmental Problems

Gentile, D.A., and P.S. Auerbach. 1987. The sun and water sports. *Clin Sports Med* 6 (3, July):669-684.

Lippitt, M.W., and M.L. Nuckols. 1983. Active diver thermal protection requirements for cold water diving. *Aviat Space Environ Med* 54 (7, July): 644-648.

Lloyd, E.L. 1979. Diving and hypothermia. *BMJ* 2 (6191, September 15):668.

Strauss, M.B., and R.L. Dierker. 1987. Otitis externa associated with aquatic activities (swimmer's ear). *Clin Dermatol* 5 (3, July-September):103-111.

Wells, J.M. 1991. Hyperthermia in divers and diver support personnel. *Undersea Biomed Res* 18 (3, May):225-227.

Injuries From Marine Animals

Auerbach, P.S. 1984. Hazardous marine animals. *Emerg Med Clin North Am* 2 (3, August):531-544.

Brown, C.K., and S.M. Shepherd. 1992. Marine trauma, envenomations, and intoxications. *Emerg Med Clin North Am* 10 (2, May):385-408.

Evans, R.J., and R.S. Davies. 1996. Stingray injury. *J Accid Emerg Med* 13 (3, May):224-225.

Kizer, K.W. 1983-1984. Marine envenomations. *J Toxicol Clin Toxicol* 21 (4-5):527-555.

Pearn, J. 1995. The sea, stingers, and surgeons: The surgeon's role in prevention, first aid, and management of marine envenomations. *J Pediatr Surg* 30 (1, January):105-110.

Soppe, G.G. 1989. Marine envenomations and aquatic dermatology. *Am Fam Physician* 40 (2, August):97-106.

Strauss, M.B., and R.I. MacDonald. 1976. Hand injuries from sea urchin spines. *Clin Orthop* January-February; 114:216-218.

Strauss, M.B., and W.L. Orris. 1974. Injuries to divers by marine animals: A simplified approach to recognition and management. *Mil Med* 139 (2, February):129-130.

Chapter 13

Ear and Sinus Squeezes

Becker, G.D., and G.J. Parell. 2001. Barotrauma of the ears and sinuses after scuba diving. *Eur Arch Otorhinolaryngol* 258 (4, May):159-163.

Edmonds, C., and F.A. Blackwood. 1975. Disorientation with middle ear barotrauma of descent. *Undersea Biomed Res* 2 (4, December):311-314.

Kieser, J., and D. Holborow. 1997. The prevention and management of oral barotrauma. *NZ Dent J* 93 (414, December):114-116.

Molvaer, O.I., and G. Albrektsen. 1988. Alternobaric vertigo in professional divers. *Undersea Biomed Res* 15 (4, July):271-282.

Money, K.E., I.P. Buckingham, I.M. Calder, W.H. Johnson, J.D. King, J.P. Landolt, J. Laufer, and H. Ludman. 1985. Damage to the middle ear and the inner ear in underwater divers. *Undersea Biomed Res* 12 (1, March): 77-84.

Mutzbauer, T.S., P.H. Mueller, O. Sigg, K. Tetzlaff, and B. Neubauer. 2000. Underwater application of nasal decongestants: Method for special operations. *Mil Med* 165 (11, November):849-851.

Sheridan, M.F., H.H. Hetherington, and J.J. Hull. 1999. Inner ear barotrauma from scuba diving. *Ear Nose Throat J* 78 (3, March):181, 184, 186-187 passim.

Shupak, A., I. Doweck, E. Greenberg, C.R. Gordon, O. Spitzer, Y. Melamed, and W.S. Meyer. 1991. Diving-related inner ear injuries. *Laryngoscope* 101 (2, February):173-179.

Thoracic Squeeze

Craig, A.B., Jr. 1968. Depth limits of breath hold diving (an example of Fennology). *Respir Physiol* 5 (1, June):14-22.

Kiyan, E., S. Aktas, and A.S. Toklu. 2001. Hemoptysis provoked by voluntary diaphragmatic contractions in breath-hold divers. *Chest* 120 (6, December):2098-2100.

Leith, D.E. 1989. Adaptations to deep breath-hold diving: Respiratory and circulatory mechanics. *Undersea Biomed Res* 16 (5, September): 345-354.

Liner, M.H. 1994. Cardiovascular and pulmonary responses to breath-hold diving in humans. *Acta Physiol Scand Suppl* 620:1-32.

Raper, A.J., D.W. Richardson, H.A. Kontos, and J.L. Patterson, Jr. 1967. Circulatory responses to breath holding in man. *J Appl Physiol* 22 (2, February):201-206.

Schaefer, K.E., R.D. Allison, J.H. Dougherty, Jr., C.R. Carey, R. Walker, F. Yost, and D. Parker. 1968. Pulmonary and circulatory adjustments determining the limits of depths in breathhold diving. *Science* 162 (857, November 29):1020-1023.

Strauss, M.B., and P.W. Wright. 1971. Thoracic squeeze diving casualty. *Aerosp Med* 42 (6, June):673-675.

Chapter 14

Nitrogen Narcosis

Biersner, R.J. 1987. Emotional and physiological effects of nitrous oxide and hyperbaric air narcosis. *Aviat Space Environ Med* 58 (1, January):34-38.

Fowler, B., K.N. Ackles, and G. Porlier. 1985. Effects of inert gas narcosis on behavior—a critical review. *Undersea Biomed Res* 12 (4, December): 369-402.

Fowler, B., and J. Adams. 1993. Dissociation of the effects of alcohol and amphetamine on inert gas narcosis using reaction time and P300 latency. *Aviat Space Environ Med* 64 (6, June):493-499.

Hamilton, K., M.F. Laliberte, and B. Fowler. 1995. Dissociation of the behavioral and subjective components of nitrogen narcosis and diver adaptation. *Undersea Hyperb Med* 22 (1, March):41-49.

Monteiro, M.G., W. Hernandez, N.B. Figlie, E. Takahashi, and M. Korukian. 1996. Comparison between subjective feelings to alcohol and nitrogen narcosis: A pilot study. *Alcohol* 13 (1, January-February):75-78.

Turle, N., A. Saget, B. Zouani, and J.J. Risso. 1998. Neurochemical studies of narcosis: A comparison between the effects of nitrous oxide and hyperbaric nitrogen on the dopaminergic nigro-striatal pathway. *Neurochem Res* 23 (7, July):997-1003.

Oxygen Toxicity

Ahmad, S., C.W. White, L.Y. Chang, B.K. Schneider, and C.B. Allen. 2001. Glutamine protects mitochondrial structure and function in oxygen toxicity. *Am J Physiol Lung Cell Mol Physiol* 280 (4, April):L779-791.

Arieli, R., A. Yalov, and A. Goldenshluger. 2002. Modeling pulmonary and CNS O(2) toxicity and estimation of parameters for humans. *J Appl Physiol* 92 (1, January):248-256.

Butler, F.K., Jr., and E.D. Thalmann. 1986. Central nervous system oxygen toxicity in closed circuit scuba divers II. *Undersea Biomed Res* 13 (2, June): 193-223.

Clark, J.M., C.J. Lambertsen, R. Gelfand, N.D. Flores, J.B. Pisarello, M.D. Rossman, and J.A. Elias. 1999. Effects of prolonged oxygen exposure at 1.5, 2.0, or 2.5 ATA on pulmonary function in men (predictive studies V). *J Appl Physiol* 86 (1, January):243-259.

Lemaitre, F., N. Meunier, and M. Bedu. 2002. Effect of air diving exposure generally encountered by recreational divers: Oxidative stress? *Undersea Hyperb Med* 29 (1, spring):39-49.

Nuckols, M.L., J. Clarke, and C. Grupe. 1998. Maintaining safe oxygen levels in semiclosed underwater breathing apparatus. *Life Support Biosph Sci* 5 (1):87-95.

Strauss, M.B., L. Sherrod, and R.W. Cantrell. 1974. Serous otitis media in divers breathing 100% oxygen. *Aero Space Med* 45 (April):4034-4037.

Carbon Dioxide Toxicity

Fothergill, D.M., W.F. Taylor, and D.E. Hyde. 1998. Physiologic and perceptual responses to hypercarbia during warm- and cold-water immersion. *Undersea Hyperb Med* 25 (1, spring):1-12.

Henning, R.A., S.L. Sauter, E.H. Lanphier, and W.G. Reddan. 1990. Behavioral effects of increased CO2 load in divers. *Undersea Biomed Res* 17 (2, March):109-120.

Morrison, J.B., J.T. Florio, and W.S. Butt. 1981. Effects of CO2 insensitivity and respiratory pattern on respiration in divers. *Undersea Biomed Res* 8 (4, December):209-217.

Anoxia

Craig, A.B., Jr. 1961. Causes of loss of consciousness during underwater swimming. *Appl Physiol* 16:583-586.

Edmonds, C.W., and D.G. Walker. 1999. Snorkelling deaths in Australia, 1987-1996. *Med J Aust* 171 (11-12, December 6-20):591-594.

Melamed, Y., and D. Kerem. 1988. Ventilatory response to transient hypoxia in O2 divers. *Undersea Biomed Res* 15 (3, May):193-201.

Nuckols, M.L., J. Clarke, and C. Grupe. 1998. Maintaining safe oxygen levels in semiclosed underwater breathing apparatus. *Life Support Biosph Sci* 5 (1):87-95.

Sausen, K.P., M.T. Wallick, B. Slobodnik, J.M. Chimiak, E.A. Bower, M.E. Stiney, and J.B. Clark. 2001. The reduced oxygen breathing paradigm for hypoxia training: Physiological, cognitive, and subjective effects. *Aviat Space Environ Med* 72 (6, June):539-545.

Sekar, S., K.F. MacDonnell, P. Namsirikul, et al. 1980. Survival after prolonged submersion in cold water without neurological squele. *Arch Intern Med* 140(6):775-779.

Carbon Monoxide Poisoning

Allen, H. 1992. Carbon monoxide poisoning in a diver. *Arch Emerg Med* 9 (1, March):65-66.

Bloom, J.D. 1972. Some considerations in establishing divers' breathing gas purity standards for carbon monoxide. *Aerosp Med* 43 (6, June):633-666.

Furgang, F.A. 1972. Carbon monoxide intoxication presenting as air embolism in a diver: A case report. *Aerosp Med* 43 (7, July):785-786.

Weaver, L.K., R.O. Hopkins, K.J. Chan, S. Churchill, C.G. Elliott, T.P. Clemmer, J.F. Orme, Jr., F.O. Thomas, and A.H. Morris. 2002. Hyperbaric oxygen for acute carbon monoxide poisoning. *N Engl J Med* 347 (14, October 3):1057-1067.

High-Pressure Nervous System Syndrome

Bennett, P.B., R. Coggin, and J. Roby. 1981. Control of HPNS in humans during rapid compression with trimix to 650 m (2131 ft). *Undersea Biomed Res* 8 (2, June):85-100.

Rostain, J.C., C. Lemaire, M.C. Gardette-Chauffour, J. Doucet, and R. Naquet. 1983. Estimation of human susceptibility to the high-pressure nervous syndrome. *J Appl Physiol* 54 (4, April):1063-1070.

Simon, S., Y. Katz, and P.B. Bennett. 1975. Calculation of the percentage of a narcotic gas to permit abolition of the high pressure nervous syndrome. *Undersea Biomed Res* 2 (4, December):299-303.

Chapter 15

Extra-Alveolar Air Syndromes (Including Arterial Gas Embolism)

Curley, M.D., H.J. Schwartz, and K.M. Zwingelberg. 1988. Neuropsychologic assessment of cerebral decompression sickness and gas embolism. *Undersea Biomed Res* 15 (3, May):223-236.

Gorman, D.F. 1989. Decompression sickness and arterial gas embolism in sports scuba divers. *Sports Med* 8 (1, July):32-42.

Hart, G.B. 1974. Treatment of decompression illness and air embolism with hyperbaric oxygen. *Aerosp Med* 45 (10, October):1190-1203.

Leitch, D.R., and R.D. Green. 1986. Pulmonary barotrauma in divers and the treatment of cerebral arterial gas embolism. *Aviat Space Environ Med* 57 (10 Pt 1, October):931-938.

Neuman, T.S., and A.A. Bove. 1990. Combined arterial gas embolism and decompression sickness following no-stop dives. *Undersea Biomed Res* 17 (5, September):429-436.

Newton, H.B. 2001. Neurologic complications of scuba diving. *Am Fam Physician* 63 (11, June 1):2211-2218.

Pearson, R.R., and R.F. Goad. 1982. Delayed cerebral edema complicating cerebral arterial gas embolism: Case histories. *Undersea Biomed Res* 9 (4, December):283-296.

Ries, S., M. Knauth, R. Kern, C. Klingmann, M. Daffertshofer, K. Sartor, and M. Hennerici. 1999. Arterial gas embolism after decompression: Correlation with right-to-left shunting. *Neurology* 52 (2, January 15):401-404.

Strauss, M.B., and R.C. Borer, Jr. 2001. Diving medicine: Contemporary topics and their controversies. *Am J Emerg Med* 19 (3, May):232-238.

Tetzlaff, K., M. Reuter, B. Leplow, M. Heller, and E. Bettinghausen. 1997. Risk factors for pulmonary barotrauma in divers. *Chest* 112 (3, September):654-659.

Weiss, L.D., and K.W. Van Meter. 1995. Cerebral air embolism in asthmatic scuba divers in a swimming pool. *Chest* 107 (6, June):1653-1654.

Decompression Sickness

Bove, A.A., J.M. Hallenbeck, and D.H. Elliott. 1974. Changes in blood and plasma volumes in dogs during decompression sickness. *Aerosp Med* 45 (1, January):49-55.

Carturan, D., A. Boussuges, P. Vanuxem, A. Bar-Hen, H. Burnet, and B. Gardette. 2002. Ascent rate, age, maximal oxygen uptake, adiposity, and circulating venous bubbles after diving. *J Appl Physiol* 93 (4, October): 1349-1356.

Dick, A.P., and E.W. Massey. 1985. Neurologic presentation of decompression sickness and air embolism in sport divers. *Neurology* 35 (5, May): 667-671.

Elliott, D.H., J.M. Hallenbeck, and A.A. Bove. 1974. Acute decompression sickness. *Lancet* 2 (7890, November 16):1193-1199.

Germonpre, P., P. Dendale, P. Unger, and C. Balestra. 1998. Patent foramen ovale and decompression sickness in sports divers. *J Appl Physiol* 84 (5, May):1622-1626.

Hallenbeck, J.M., A.A. Bove, and D.H. Elliott. 1975. Mechanisms underlying spinal cord damage in decompression sickness. *Neurology* 25 (4, April):308-316.

Hart, G.B., M.B. Strauss, and P.A. Lennon. 1986. The treatment of decompression sickness and air embolism in a monoplace chamber. *J Hyperb Med* 1 (1):1-7.

Hills, B.A. 1979. Mechanical vs. ischemic mechanisms for decompression sickness. *Aviat Space Environ Med* 50 (4, April):363-367.

Moon, R.E., and P.J. Sheffield. 1997. Guidelines for treatment of decompression illness. *Aviat Space Environ Med* 68 (3, March):234-243.

Neuman, T.S., R.G. Spragg, P.D. Wagner, and K.M. Moser. 1980. Cardiopulmonary consequences of decompression stress. *Respir Physiol* 41 (2, August):143-153.

Strauss, M.B., and R.L. Samson. 1986. Decompression sickness: An update. *Phys and Sport Med* 3 (14, March):196-205.

Toklu, A.S., and M. Cimsit. 2001. Dysbaric osteonecrosis in Turkish sponge divers. *Undersea Hyperb Med* 28 (2, summer):83-88.

Chapter 16

Aspiration and Near-Drowning

Conn, A.W., J.E. Montes, G.A. Barker, and J.F. Edmonds. 1980. Cerebral salvage in near-drowning following neurological classification by triage. *Can Anaesth Soc J* 27 (3, May):201-210.

Golden, F.S., M.J. Tipton, and R.C. Scott. 1997. Immersion, near-drowning and drowning. *Br J Anaesth* 79 (2, August):214-225.

Gonzalez-Rothi, R.J. 1987. Near drowning: Consensus and controversies in pulmonary and cerebral resuscitation. *Heart Lung* 16 (5, September):474-482.

Gooden, B.A. 1992. Why some people do not drown. Hypothermia versus the diving response. *Med J Aust* 157 (9, November 2):629-632.

Keatinge, W.R. 1977. Accidental immersion hypothermia and drowning. *Practitioner* 219 (1310, August):183-187.

Martin, T.G. 1984. Neardrowning and cold water immersion. *Ann Emerg Med* 13 (4, April):263-273.

Modell, J.H. 1993. Drowning. *N Engl J Med* 328 (4, January 28):253-256.

Oakes, D.D., J.P. Sherck, J.R. Maloney, and A.C. Charters 3rd. 1982. Prognosis and management of victims of near-drowning. *J Trauma* 22 (7, July):544-549.

Orlowski, J.P., M.M. Abulleil, and J.M. Phillips. 1989. The hemodynamic and cardiovascular effects of near-drowning in hypotonic, isotonic, or hypertonic solutions. *Ann Emerg Med* 18 (10, October):1044-1049.

Quan, L. 1993. Drowning issues in resuscitation. *Ann Emerg Med* 22 (2 Pt 2, February):366-369.

Cardiac Arrest and Shock

American Heart Association. 1997-1999. *Basic life support for healthcare providers.* Dallas: American Heart Association.

Slade, J.B., Jr., T. Hattori, C.S. Ray, A.A. Bove, and P. Cianci. 2001. Pulmonary edema associated with scuba diving: Case reports and review. *Chest* 120 (5, November):1686-1694.

Tabib, A., A. Miras, P. Taniere, and R. Loire. 1999. Undetected cardiac lesions cause unexpected sudden cardiac death during occasional sport activity. A report of 80 cases. *Eur Heart J* 20 (12, June):900-903.

INDEX

Note: The italicized *f, t,* and *ph.* refer to figures, tables, and photographs, respectively

ABOUT THE AUTHORS

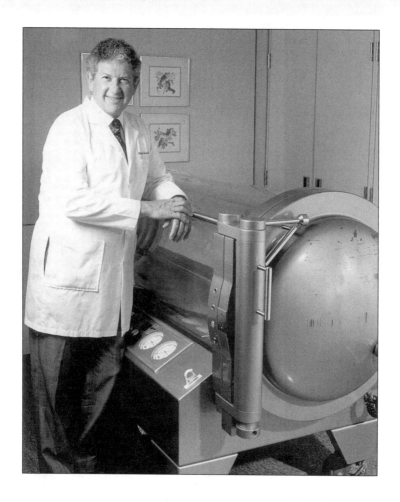

Michael B. Strauss, MD, is medical director of the department of hyperbaric medicine at Long Beach Memorial Medical Center in Long Beach, California. An experienced diver, he is familiar with almost all types of equipment, from snorkel to closed-circuit SCUBA to tethered diving out of a personal transfer capsule.

In more than 30 articles on diving medicine, Dr. Strauss has formulated an explanation for pain-only bends, delineated the outcomes of decompression, and detailed the causes of blackout (no-panic syndromes). In addition, he has about 100 other publications on wound care, orthopaedics, and hyperbaric oxygen.

Dr. Strauss is a member of the Undersea and Hyperbaric Medical Society and is a tertiary provider for referrals of medical problems of diving for the Divers Alert Network. He is a U.S. navy undersea medical officer and was a doctor for U.S. Navy SEAL teams. He is board certified in undersea and hyperbaric medicine.

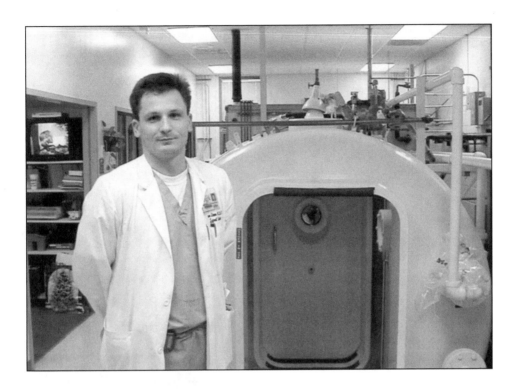

Igor V. Aksenov, MD, PhD, works in the department of medicine at the University of Florida at Gainesville. Dr. Aksenov has a diverse background in medicine, including internal, critical care, clinical toxicology and pharmacology, and hyberbaric and diving.

Dr. Aksenov worked as associate dean, professor, and director of the hyberbaric medicine program at Saba University School of Medicine in Saba, Netherlands Antilles (Dutch Caribbean). He was also the medical director of the Saba Marine Park. While in these positions, Dr. Aksenov dealt with various diving accidents and conducted research on decompression sickness in recreational divers. He was trained as a navy physician at the Military Medical Academy in St. Petersburg, Russia, and worked as head physician of the intensive care unit and director of the hyperbaric medicine unit at one of the Military Medical Academy clinics.

Dr. Aksenov is a prolific writer. He has more than 60 published scientific papers in several areas of medicine. He is a member of the Undersea and Hyperbaric Medical Society.

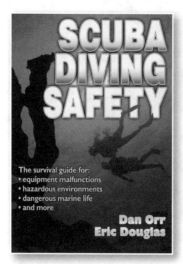
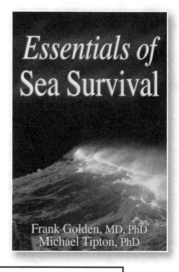